Study Guide for
FAMILY NURSE PRACTITIONER CERTIFICATION EXAMINATION AND PRACTICE PREPARATION

Margaret A. Fitzgerald

MS, APRN, BC, NP-C, FAANP
President, Fitzgerald Health Education Associates
North Andover, Massachusetts
Family Nurse Practitioner
Greater Lawrence Family Health Center
Lawrence, MA

Study Guide for
FAMILY
NURSE
PRACTITIONER
CERTIFICATION
EXAMINATION
AND PRACTICE
PREPARATION

 FA DAVIS COMPANY • PHILADELPHIA

F. A. Davis Company
1915 Arch Street
Philadelphia, PA 19103
www.fadavis.com

Printed in the United States of America

Last digit indicates print number: 10   9   8   7   6   5   4   3   2

Acquisitions Editor: Joanne P. DaCunha, RN, MSN
Production Editors: Michael Schnee, Janet Domingo
Cover Designer: Louis J. Forgione

As new scientific information becomes available through basic and clinical research, recommended treatments and drug therapies undergo changes. The author and publisher have done everything possible to make this book accurate, up to date, and in accord with accepted standards at the time of publication. The author, editors, and publisher are not responsible for errors or omissions or for consequences from application of the book, and make no warranty, expressed or implied, with regard to the contents of the book. Any practice described in this book should be applied by the reader in accordance with professional standards of care used with regard to the unique circumstances that may apply in each situation. The reader is advised always to check product information (package inserts) for changes and new information regarding dose and contraindications before administering any drug. Caution is especially urged when using new or infrequently ordered drugs.

Library of Congress Cataloging-in-Publication Data

Authorization to photocopy items for internal or personal use, or the internal or personal use of specific clients, is granted by F.A. Davis Company for users registered with the Copyright Clearance Center (CCC) Transactional Reporting Service, provided that the fee of $.10 per copy is paid directly to CCC, 222 Rosewood Drive, Danvers, MA 01923. For those organizations that have been granted a photocopy license by CCC, a separate system of payment has been arranged. The fee code for users of the Transactional Reporting Service is: 8036-0593/01 0 + $.10.

To the newest members of our family
Mouhammed Ahmadou Thiam (DOB 7.6.98)
And
Margaret Ania Ashley (DOB 12.30.99)
With wishes for a bright future filled with hope and happiness
Love, hugs and kisses from Nana

Introduction

This book represents a perspective on learning and practice that I have developed from my experience as a family nurse practitioner, providing multigenerational primary care at the Greater Lawrence (MA) Family Health Center and as a NP faculty. In addition, my experience in the years of helping thousands of NP achieve professional success through conducting NP Certification and Practice Preparation Courses influenced the development and presentation of the information held within.

The scope of practice of the nurse practitioner is wide, encompassing the care of the young, the old, the sick and the well. This book has been developed to help the nurse practitioner develop the knowledge and skills to successfully enter NP practice as well as achieve certification, an important landmark in professional achievement.

This book is not intended to be a comprehensive primary care text, but rather a source to reinforce learning and a guide for the development of the information base needed for NP practice. The reader is encouraged to answer the questions given in each section and then to check on the accuracy of response. The discussion section is intended to enhance learning through highlighting the essentials of primary care NP practice. The numerous tables can serve as a quick-look resource not only as the NP prepares for entry to practice and certification but also in the delivery of ongoing primary care.

Margaret A. Fitzgerald, MS, APRN, BC, NP-C, FAANP
PRESIDENT, FITZGERALD HEALTH EDUCATION ASSOCIATES, INC.
NORTH ANDOVER, MA
FAMILY NURSE PRACTITIONER
GREATER LAWRENCE (MA) FAMILY HEALTH CENTER

Acknowledgments

This book represents a sum of the efforts of many people.

I thank Diane Blodgett, development editor, for her tireless and accurate work, good humor and patience.

I thank Joanne DaCunha, Nursing Acquisitions Editor, at F.A. Davis for convincing me to take on this task as well as her ongoing encouragement.

I thank my family, especially my husband and business partner Marc Comstock, for their good nature as they lived through this experience.

I thank the staff of Fitzgerald Health Education Associates for sharing me with this project for many months.

I thank the patients and staff of the Greater Lawrence (MA) Family Health Center as they continue to serve as a source of inspiration as I developed this book.

Last but not least, I thank the thousands nurse practitioners who, over the years, have attended the Fitzgerald Health Education Associates Nurse Practitioner Certification and Practice Preparation courses. Your eagerness to learn, thirst for knowledge and dedication to success continue to inspire me. It is indeed a privilege to be part of your professional development.

Contents

CHAPTER

1

Health
Promotion
and Disease
Prevention

QUESTIONS

1. An example of a primary prevention measure for a 78-year-old man with chronic obstructive pulmonary disease is:

   A. reviewing the use of prescribed medications
   B. ensuring adequate illumination in the home
   C. checking pulmonary function
   D. obtaining a serum cholesterol level

2. Which of the following is the most helpful intervention to minimize fracture risk in a 76-year-old woman with osteoporosis?

   A. alendronate (Fosamax) therapy
   B. hormone replacement therapy
   C. home survey to identify fall hazards
   D. use of a back brace

3. Secondary prevention measures for a 78-year-old man with chronic obstructive pulmonary disease include:

   A. checking stool for occult blood
   B. administering influenza vaccine
   C. obtaining a serum theophylline level
   D. advising about appropriate use of car passenger restraints

4. Tertiary prevention measures for a 69-year-old woman with congestive heart failure include:

   A. administering pneumococcal vaccine
   B. adjusting therapy to minimize dyspnea
   C. skin surveying for precancerous lesions
   D. reviewing safe handling of food

ANSWERS

1. B
2. C
3. A
4. B

DISCUSSION

Primary prevention measures include activities provided to individuals to prevent the onset of a given disease. The goal of primary prevention measures is to spare the suffering, burden, and cost associated with the clinical condition. Examples include health-protecting education and counseling such as encouraging the use of car restraints and bicycle helmets and providing information on accident prevention. Immunizations and chemoprophylaxis are also examples of primary prevention measures (Table 1–1).

Secondary prevention measures include activities provided to identify and treat asymptomatic persons who have risk factors for a given disease or in preclinical disease. Examples include screening examinations for preclinical evidence of cancer, including mammography, sigmoidoscopy, and cervical examination with Papanicolaou smear. Other examples of secondary prevention activities include screening for clinical conditions with a protracted asymptomatic period such as blood pressure measurement to detect hypertension and cholesterol measurement to detect hyperlipidemia.

Tertiary prevention measures are preventive measures that are part of the management of a person with an established disease. The goal is to minimize disease-associated complications and the negative health effects of the conditions. Examples include medications and lifestyle modification to normalize blood glucose in individuals with diabetes mellitus and treatment of hyperlipidemia in patients who also have coronary heart disease.

Discussion Source

U.S. Preventative Services Task Force (1996). *Guide to Clinical Preventive Services* (2nd ed.). Baltimore: Williams and Wilkins.

TABLE 1–1.
RECOMMENDED HEALTH PROMOTION INTERVENTIONS
FOR THE GENERAL POPULATION

Age, yr	11–24	25–64	65 and Older
Leading cause of death	Motor vehicle or other unintentional injuries Homicide Suicide Malignant neoplasms Heart diseases	Malignant neoplasms Heart diseases Motor vehicle and other unintentional injuries HIV infection Suicide and homicide	Heart diseases Malignant neoplasms (lung, colorectal, breast) Cerebrovascular disease Chronic obstructive pulmonary disease Pneumonia and influenza
Interventions for the General Population			
Screening	Height and weight Blood pressure Papanicolaou (Pap) test (women) Chlamydia screen (women age < 20 yr) Rubella serology or vaccination history (women >age 12 yr) Assess for problem drinking	Blood pressure Height and weight Total blood cholesterol (men age 35–64 yr, women age 45–64 yr) Pap test (women) Fecal occult blood test, sigmoidoscopy, or both (age > 50 yr) Mammogram, clinical breast examination (women 50–69 yr) Assess for problem drinking Rubella serology or vaccination history (women of childbearing age)	Blood pressure Height and weight Fecal occult blood test, sigmoidoscopy, or both Mammogram, clinical breast examination, or both Papanicolaou (Pap) test (women) Vision screening Assess for hearing impairment Assess for problem drinking

(continued)

TABLE 1–1. (continued)

Age, yr	11–24	25–64	65 and Older
Counseling			
Injury prevention	Lap and shoulder belts Bicycle, motorcycle, All terrain vehicle helmets Smoke detectors Safe storage or removal of firearms	Lap and shoulder belts Bicycle, motorcycle, All terrain vehicle helmets Smoke detectors Safe storage or removal of firearms	Lap and shoulder belts Motorcycle and bicycle helmets Fall prevention Safe storage or removal of firearms Smoke detectors Set hot water heater to < 120–130°F CPR training for household members
Substance abuse	Avoid tobacco use Avoid underage drinking and illicit drug use Avoid alcohol and drug use while driving, swimming, boating, and so on	Tobacco cessation Avoid alcohol and drug use while driving, swimming, boating, and so on	Tobacco cessation Avoid alcohol and drug use while driving, swimming, boating, and so on
Sexual behavior	STD prevention: abstinence; avoid high-risk behavior; condoms or female barrier with spermicide Unintended pregnancy: contraception	STD prevention: abstinence; avoid high-risk behavior; condoms or female barrier with spermicide Unintended pregnancy: contraception	STD prevention; avoid high-risk sexual behavior; use condoms

(continued)

TABLE 1–1. (continued)

Age, yr	11–24	25–64	65 and Older
Diet and exercise	Limit fat and cholesterol; maintain caloric balance; emphasize grains, fruits, vegetables Adequate calcium intake (girls and women) Regular physical activity	Limit fat and cholesterol; maintain caloric balance; emphasize grains, fruits, vegetables Adequate calcium intake (women) Regular physical activity	Limit fat and cholesterol; maintain caloric balance; emphasize grains, fruits, vegetables Adequate calcium intake (women) Regular physical activity
Dental health	Regular visits to dental care provider Floss, brush with fluoride toothpaste daily	Regular visits to dental care provider Floss, brush with fluoride toothpaste daily	Regular visits to dental care provider Floss, brush with fluoride toothpaste daily
Immunizations	Tetanus and diphtheria (Td) boosters (age 11–16 yr) Hepatitis B MMR (age 11–12 yr) Varicella (age 11–12 yr) Rubella (women age > 12 yr)	Tetanus and diphtheria (Td) boosters Rubella (women of childbearing age)	Pneumococcal vaccine Influenza Tetanus and diphtheria (Td) boosters
Chemoprophylaxis	Multivitamin with folic acid (women planning or capable of pregnancy)	Multivitamin with folic acid (women planning or capable of pregnancy) Discuss hormone prophylaxis (peri- and post-menopausal women)	Discuss hormone prophylaxis (peri- and post-menopausal women)

Reference: Adapted from U.S. Preventative Services Task Force (1996). *Guide to Clinical Preventive Services* (2nd ed.). Baltimore: Williams and Wilkins.

QUESTIONS

5. When advising a patient about influenza immunization, the NP considers the following about the vaccine:

   A. Its use is contraindicated during pregnancy.
   B. Its use is limited to children older than age 6 years.
   C. It contains live virus.
   D. It is recommended for household members of high-risk patients.

6. A middle-aged man with lung disease who is about to receive influenza vaccine should be advised that:

   A. It is more than 90% effective in preventing influenza.
   B. It is contraindicated in the presence of eczema.
   C. Localized reactions from the immunization are fairly common.
   D. Short, intense flulike syndrome typically occurs after immunization.

7. Which of the following best describes amantadine or rimantadine use in the care of patients with influenza?

   A. Initiation of therapy early in acute influenza illness may minimize the severity of disease.
   B. Its primary action is in preventing influenza A during outbreaks.
   C. Amantadine is active against influenza A and B.
   D. Its use is an acceptable alternative to influenza vaccine.

8. A 24-year-old woman with asthma presents asking for influenza vaccine. She is currently taking ciprofloxacin for treatment of a urinary tract infection, does not have a fever, and is feeling better. You advise that she:

   A. should return for the immunization after completing her antibiotic therapy.
   B. needs evidence of a negative pregnancy test before taking being immunized.
   C. can receive the immunization today.
   D. is not a candidate for influenza vaccine.

ANSWERS

5. **D**
6. **C**
7. **B**
8. **C**

DISCUSSION

Influenza is a viral illness that typically causes many days of incapacitation and suffering as well as the risk of death. The vaccine is about 70–80% effective in preventing influenza A or B or reducing the severity of the disease.

Mild illness or taking an antibiotic is not a contraindication to any immunization, including influenza immunization. Annual influenza vaccine is recommended for those age 65 years and older as well as for patients with some other disorders, including asthma. The vaccine does not contain live virus and is not shed; therefore, there is no risk of shedding an infectious agent to household contacts.

Influenza vaccine may be used during pregnancy. If possible, delaying immunization until the second or third trimester is recommended. However, women who will be in the second and third trimester of pregnancy during the flu season should receive the vaccine. This vaccine may be given to infants as young as age 6 months. Influenza vaccine is recommended for household members of high-risk patients in order to avoid transmission of infection.

If taken during the flu season, amantadine and rimantadine are approximately 70–90% effective in preventing influenza A. These medications carry a less favorable adverse reaction profile than influenzae vaccine at a significantly higher cost and have no activity against influenza B. As a result, active immunization against influenza A and B by administering the flu shot is the preferred method of disease prevention.

Discussion Source

U.S. Preventative Services Task Force (1996). *Guide to Clinical Preventive Services* (2nd ed.). Baltimore: Williams and Wilkins.

QUESTIONS

9. When considering an adult's risk for measles, mumps, and rubella (MMR), the NP considers the following:

   A. Those born before 1957 are likely immune because of natural infection.

   B. Considerable mortality and morbidity occur with all three diseases.

   C. Most cases in the United States occur in infants.

   D. The use of the vaccine is often associated with protracted arthralgia.

10. Which of the following is true about measles, mumps, and rubella (MMR) vaccine?

   A. It contains inactivated virus.
   B. Its use is contraindicated in patients with a history of egg allergy.
   C. Revaccination of an immune person is associated with risk of allergic reaction.
   D. Two doses 1 month apart is recommended for young adults who have not been previously immunized.

11. A 22-year-old woman is starting a job in a college health center and needs proof of German measles and measles immunity. She received childhood immunizations and supplies documentation of MMR at age 1.5 years. Your best response is to:

   A. Obtain rubella and rubeola titers.
   B. Give MMR immunization now.
   C. Advise her to obtain immune globulin if she has been exposed to measles or rubella.
   D. Advise her to avoid individuals with rashes.

ANSWERS

   9. **A**
   10. **D**
   11. **B**

DISCUSSION

The MMR vaccine is a live, attenuated vaccine. Two immunizations 1 month apart is recommended for adults born after 1957 because those born before then are considered immune as a result of native infection. As with all vaccines, giving additional doses to those with an unclear immunization history is safe. Active immunization through the use of vaccines provides long-term protection from disease. The use of vaccines is preferred to passive immunization through the use of immune globulin (IG). IG given after exposure provides only temporary protection.

Rubella, also known as German measles, typically causes a relatively mild, 3- to 5-day illness with little risk of complication to the person infected. However, when rubella is contracted during pregnancy, the effects to the fetus can be devastating. Immunizing the entire population against rubella protects unborn children from the risk of contracting congenital rubella syndrome. Measles can cause severe illness with serious sequelae, including encephalitis and pneumonia; sequelae of mumps includes orchitis.

In the past, a history of egg allergy was considered a contraindication to receiving MMR vaccine. However, its use now appears safe, although a 90-minute observation is recommended. The MMR vaccine is safe to use during lactation, but its use in pregnancy is discouraged because of possible risk of congenital rubella syndrome from the live virus contained in the vaccine. However, this is likely a more theoretical than actual risk. MMR vaccine is well tolerated, with rare reports of mild, transient adverse reaction such as rash and sore throat.

Discussion Source

U.S. Preventative Services Task Force (1996). *Guide to Clinical Preventive Services* (2nd ed.). Baltimore: Williams and Wilkins.

QUESTIONS

12. When advising a patient about pneumococcal immunization, the NP considers the following about the vaccine:

    A. It contains inactivated bacteria.
    B. It is contraindicated after splenectomy.
    C. It protects against pneumonia caused by atypical pathogens.
    D. It is generally well tolerated.

13. Of the following, who is at greatest risk for invasive pneumococcal infection?

    A. a 68-year-old man with chronic obstructive pulmonary disease
    B. a 34-year-old woman who underwent splenectomy after a motor vehicle accident
    C. a 50-year-old man with a 15-year history of type 2 diabetes
    D. a 75-year-old woman with decreased mobility caused by rheumatoid arthritis

ANSWERS

12. D
13. B

DISCUSSION

Pneumococcal disease causes significant mortality and morbidity. The pneumococcal vaccine contains purified polysaccharide from 23 of the most common strains *of Streptococcus pneumoniae*. These strains account for 90% of the bacteremic disease associated with this pathogen. The pneumococcal vaccine protects against pneumonia caused *by S. pneumoniae*, the leading cause of pneumonia death in the United States. However, it is ineffective against pneumonia caused by other infectious agents including *Mycoplasma pneumoniae* and *Chlamydia pneumoniae* that cause atypical pneumonia.

Pneumococcal vaccine is recommended for those aged 65 years and older as well as institutionalized individuals aged 50 years and older; persons aged 2 years or older with chronic cardiac or pulmonary condition or diabetes mellitus; and those who are asplenic. In particular, this vaccine is recommended for those with particular risk for invasive pneumococcal disease, including individuals with alcoholism, cirrhosis, chronic renal failure, nephrotic syndrome, congenital, or acquired immune deficiency, or malignancy, or who are asplenic.

It is reasonable to consider repeating the vaccine every 5 years in those who are immunocompromised. Reaction to pneumococcal vaccine is rare, but a mild local reaction may be seen, particularly with re-immunization.

Discussion Source

U.S. Preventative Services Task Force (1996). *Guide to Clinical Preventive Services* (2nd ed.). Baltimore: Williams and Wilkins.

QUESTIONS

14. Concerning hepatitis B virus (HBV) vaccine, which of the following is true?

   A. It contains live, whole HBV.

   B. Adults should have anti-HBs titers after three doses of vaccine.

   C. The vaccine should be offered during treatment for sexually transmitted diseases.

   D. Serologic testing for HBsAg should be checked before initiating hepatitis B vaccine in adults.

15. In which of the following groups is routine hepatitis B surface antigen screening recommended?

    A. hospital laboratory workers

    B. recipients of hepatitis B vaccine series

    C. pregnant women

    D. college students

16. You see a woman who has been sexually involved with a man newly diagnosed with acute hepatitis B. You advise her that she should:

    A. start a hepatitis B immunization series

    B. limit the number of sexual partners

    C. be tested for HbsAb

    D. receive hepatitis B immunoglobulin and hepatitis B immunization series

ANSWERS

14. C

15. C

16. D

DISCUSSION

Hepatitis B is caused by a small double-stranded DNA virus that contains an inner core protein of hepatitis B core antigen and an outer surface of hepatitis surface antigen. The virus is transmitted through exchange of body fluids. Hepatitis B infection can be prevented by limiting exposure to blood and body fluids as well as through immunization. Recombinant hepatitis B vaccine, which does not contain live virus, is well tolerated.

Infants who become infected perinatally with HBV have an estimated 25% lifetime chance of developing hepatocellular carcinoma or cirrhosis. As a result, all pregnant women should be screened with hepatitis B surface antigen (HBsAg) at the first prenatal visit regardless of HBV vaccine history. Because the HBV vaccine is not 100% effective, a woman may have carried hepatitis B surface antigen (HBsAg) before becoming pregnant. As a result, HBsAg screening is recommended for pregnant women regardless of hepatitis B vaccine immunization history.

About 90–95% of those who receive the vaccine develop HBsAb (anti-HBs) after three doses, implying protection from the virus. As a result, routine testing for the presence of HBsAb after immunization is not routinely recommended. However, consider HBsAb testing to confirm the development of HBV protection in those with high risk for infection (e.g., health-care workers, injection drug uses, sex workers) as well as those at risk for poor immune response (e.g., dialysis patients, immune-suppressed patients).

Administration of hepatitis B immune globulin (HBIG) after exposure with a repeat dose in 1 month is about 75% effective in protecting patients from hepatitis B after percutaneous, sexual, or mucosal exposure to HBV. HBV vaccine series should be started with post-exposure HBIG.

Discussion Sources

Friedman, L. (1999). Liver, biliary tract and pancreas. In Tierney, L., McPhee, S., & Papadakis, M. *Current Diagnosis and Treatment* (38th ed.) Norwalk, CT: Appleton & Lange. Pp. 638–677.

Margolis, H., Moyer, L. (1998). Ask the experts; Hepatitis B. Available at *http://www.medscape.com*/scp/IIM/1998v15.n06

U.S. Preventative Services Task Force (1996). *Guide to Clinical Preventive Services* (2nd ed.). Baltimore: Williams and Wilkins.

QUESTIONS

17. With the varicella vaccine, which of the following is correct?

    A. It contains killed varicella zoster virus.
    B. Its use is associated with an increase in reported cases of shingles.
    C. It should be offered to older adults who have a history of chicken pox.
    D. Although highly protective against invasive varicella disease, mild cases of chicken pox have been reported in immunized patients.

18. For which of the patients should a NP order varicella antibody titers?

    A. a 14-year-old with an unsure chicken pox history
    B. a health-care worker who reports having varicella as a child
    C. a 22-year-old woman who received two varicella immunizations 6 weeks apart
    D. a 72-year-old with shingles

19. A woman who has been advised to varicella-zoster immune globulin asks about its risks. You respond that immune globulin is a:

    A. synthetic product that is well tolerated

    B. pooled blood product that often transmits infectious disease

    C. blood product obtained from a single donor

    D. pooled blood product with an excellent safety profile

ANSWERS

17. D

18. B

19. D

DISCUSSION

The varicella-zoster virus (VZV) causes the highly contagious, systemic disease commonly known as chickenpox. Varicella infection usually confers lifetime immunity. However, reinfection may be seen in immunocompromised patients. More often, reexposure causes an increase in antibody titers without causing disease.

The VZV virus can lie dormant in sensory nerve ganglion. Later reactivation causes shingles, a painful, vesicular-form rash in a dermatomal pattern. About 15% of those who have had chickenpox develop shingles at least once during their lifetimes. Shingles rates are markedly reduced in individuals who have received varicella vaccine compared with those who have had chickenpox.

A patient-reported history of varicella is considered a valid measure of immunity, with 97–99% having serologic evidence of immunity. Among adults with an unclear or negative varicella history, the majority are also seropositive. Confirming varicella immunity through varicella titers, even in the presence of a history varicella infection, should be done in health-care workers because of their risk of exposure and potential transmission of the disease.

Although the majority of cases are seen in children younger than age 18 years, the greatest varicella mortality is found in those aged 30 to 49 years.

The varicella vaccine, which contains attenuated virus vaccine, is administered in a single dose after the first birthday. Older children (age ≥13 years) and adults with no history of varicella infection or previous immunization should receive two immunizations at 4 to 8 weeks apart.

In particular, health-care workers, family contacts of immunocompromised patients, and day care workers should be targeted for varicella vaccine, as well as adults who are in environments with high risk of varicella transmission, such as college dormitories, military barracks, and long-term care facilities. The vaccine is highly protective against severe, invasive varicella. However, mild cases of chickenpox may be reported after immunization.

Varicella immune globulin, as with all forms of IG, provides temporary, passive immunity to infection. IG is a pooled blood product with an excellent safety profile.

Discussion Sources

Isada, C., Kasten, B., Goldman, M., Gray, L., Aberg, J. (1997). *Infectious Disease Handbook* (2nd ed.). Columbus, OH: Lexicomp.
U.S. Preventative Services Task Force (1996). *Guide to Clinical Preventive Services* (2nd ed.). Baltimore: Williams and Wilkins.

QUESTIONS

20. An 18-year-old man has no primary tetanus immunization series documented. Which of the following represents the immunization needed?

    A. 3 doses of Diphtheria, Tetanus, acellular Pertussis vaccine (DTaP) 2 months apart
    B. tetanus immune globulin now and 2 doses of tetanus-diphtheria (Td) vaccine 1 month apart
    C. Td now and repeated in 1 and 6 months
    D. Td as a single dose

21. Which wound presents the greatest risk for tetanus infection?

    A. a wound obtained while gardening
    B. a laceration obtained while trimming beef
    C. a human bite
    D. an abrasion obtained by falling on a sidewalk

ANSWERS

20. C
21. A

DISCUSSION

Tetanus infection is caused by *Clostridium tetani*, an anaerobic, gram-positive, spore-forming rod. This organism is found in soil, particularly if it contains manure. The organism enters the body through a contaminated wound, causing a life-threatening systemic disease characterized by painful muscle weakness and spasm ("lockjaw"). Diphtheria, caused by *Corynebacterium diphtheriae*, a gram-negative bacillus, is typically transmitted from person to person or through contaminated liquids such as milk. This organism causes severe respiratory tract infection, including the appearance of pseudomembranous pharyngitis.

Tetanus and diphtheria are uncommon infections because of widespread immunization. Because protective titers wane over time and adults are frequently lacking in up-to-date immunization, most cases of tetanus occur in those older than age 50 years.

A primary series of three tetanus-diphtheria (Td) vaccine injections sets the stage for long-term immunity. A booster Td dose every 10 years is recommended, but protection is likely for up to 20 to 30 years after a primary series. Using Td rather than tetanus toxoid for primary series and booster doses in adulthood assists in keeping diphtheria immunity as well.

At the time of wound-producing injury, tetanus immune globulin affords temporary protection for those who have not received tetanus immunization.

Discussion Sources

Isada, C., Kasten, B., Goldman, M., Gray, L., Aberg, J. (1997). *Infectious Disease Handbook* (2nd ed.). Columbus, OH: Lexicomp.
U.S. Preventative Services Task Force (1996). *Guide to Clinical Preventive Services* (2nd ed.). Baltimore: Williams and Wilkins.

QUESTIONS

22. The most common source for hepatitis A infection is:

    A. needle sharing
    B. raw shellfish
    C. contaminated water supplies
    D. intimate person-to-person contact

23. When answering questions about hepatitis A vaccine, you consider that it:

   A. contains live virus

   B. should be offered to those who frequently travel to developing countries

   C. usually is a required immunization for health-care workers

   D. is protective after a single injection

ANSWERS

22. C

23. B

DISCUSSION

Hepatitis A infection is caused by HAV (hepatitis A virus), a small RNA virus. Transmitted primarily by fecal-contaminated drinking water and food supplies, hepatitis A is typically a self-limiting infection with a very low mortality rate. Although raw shellfish growing in contaminated water can be problematic, fecal-contaminated water supplies are the most common source of infection. In developing countries with limited pure water, the majority of the children contract this disease by age 5 years. In North America, adults aged 20 to 39 years account for nearly 50% of the reported cases.

    The hepatitis A vaccine, which contains dead virus, is given in two injections 6 months apart. Candidates include those who reside in or travel to areas where disease is endemic. Consideration should be given to offering this vaccine to food handlers, day care and long-term care workers, and military and laboratory personnel. Intravenous drug users may also benefit from the vaccine. However, hepatitis A is rarely transmitted sexually or from needle sharing; rather, intravenous drug users often live in conditions that facilitate the oral-fecal transmission of the hepatitis A virus. In addition, coinfection with hepatitis A and C may lead to a rapid deterioration in hepatic function.

Discussion Sources

Friedman, L. (1999). Liver, biliary tract and pancreas. In Tierney, L., McPhee, S., & Papadakis, M. *Current Diagnosis and Treatment* (38th ed.). Norwalk, CT: Appleton & Lange. Pp. 638–677.

U.S. Preventative Services Task Force (1996). *Guide to Clinical Preventive Services* (2nd ed.). Baltimore: Williams and Wilkins.

QUESTIONS

24. Which of the following is the most effective method of cancer screening?

   A. skin examination
   B. stool for occult blood
   C. pelvic examination
   D. chest radiograph

25. An HIV-positive, 30-year-old man has two young children living with him. Which of the following best represents advice you should give him about immunizing his children?

   A. Immunizations should take place without concern of his health status.
   B. The children should not receive influenza vaccine because of the risk of viral shedding.
   C. The children should receive a hepatitis B series.

ANSWERS

24. A
25. A

DISCUSSION

Polioviruses are highly contagious and capable of causing paralytic, life-threatening infections. Transmitted fecal-orally, rates of infection among household contacts may be as high as 96%. However, since 1994, North and South America have been declared free of indigenous poliomyelitis, largely because of the efficacy of the oral poliovirus vaccine (OPV). This live virus vaccine is given orally with a small amount of the poliovirus shed through the stool. This shedding presents household members with possible exposure to poliovirus. Virtually all cases of paralytic poliomyelitis currently found in the United States have been associated with vaccines (i.e., vaccine-associated paralytic poliomyelitis [VAPP]). Using inactivated poliovirus vaccine instead of oral poliovirus vaccine (OPV), a recommendation in the presence of patient immunosuppression or immunosuppressed household contact, should eliminate VAPP.

Discussion Source

Zimmerman, R., Spann, S. (1999). Poliovirus vaccine options. *American Family Physician* 59 (1) 113–118.

QUESTIONS

26. When working with an obese middle-aged man on weight reduction, a NP considers that one of the first actions should be to:

    A. add an exercise program while minimizing the need for dietary changes
    B. ask the patient about what he believes contributes to his weight problem
    C. refer to a nutritionist for diet counseling
    D. ask for a commitment to lose weight

27. A sedentary, obese 52-year-old woman is diagnosed with hypertension. What is the least helpful response to her statement, "It is going to be too hard to diet, exercise, and take these pills"?

    A. "Try taking your medication when you brush your teeth."
    B. "You really need to try to improve your health."
    C. "Tell me what you feel will get in your way of improving your health."
    D. "Could you start with reducing the amount of salt in your diet?"

ANSWERS

26. **B**
27. **B**

DISCUSSION

Possessing information about methods for preventing disease and maintaining health is an important part of patient education. However, knowledge alone does not ensure a change in behavior. NPs need to consider a number of factors in patient counseling and education (Box 1–1).

Discussion Source

U.S. Preventative Services Task Force (1996). *Guide to Clinical Preventive Services* (2nd ed.). Baltimore: Williams and Wilkins.

**BOX 1–1
AN ORDERLY APPROACH TO PATIENT EDUCATION AND COUNSELING**

- Assess patient knowledge base about factors contributing to the problem.
- Evaluate the contribution of the patient's belief system to the problem.
- Ask about perceived barriers to action as well as supporting factors.
- Match patient teaching to patient perception of the problem.
- Inform patients about the purpose and benefit of an intervention.
- Give an anticipated onset of effect of a therapy.
- Suggest small rather than large changes in behavior.
- Give accurate, specific information.
- Consider adding new positive behaviors rather than attempting to discontinue established behavior.
- Link desired behavior with established behavior.
- Give a strong, personalized message about the seriousness of health risk.
- Ask for a commitment from the patient.
- Use a combination of teaching strategies such as visual, oral, and written methods.
- Strive for an interdisciplinary approach to patient education and counseling with all members of the team giving the same message.
- Maintain frequent contact to monitor progress.
- Expect gains and periodic setbacks.

Adapted from U.S. Preventive Services Task Force (1996). *Guide to clinical preventive services* (2nd ed.). Baltimore: Williams and Wilkins.

2
CHAPTER

Neurological Disorders

QUESTIONS

1. Assessing vision and visual fields involves testing cranial nerve (CN):

   A. I
   B. II
   C. III
   D. IV

2. You perform an extraocular movement test on a middle-aged patient. He is unable to move his eyes upward and outward. This indicates a possibility of paralysis of CN:

   A. II
   B. III
   C. IV
   D. V

3. Loss of corneal reflex is seen in dysfunction of CN:

   A. III
   B. IV
   C. V
   D. VI

ANSWERS

   1. B
   2. B
   3. C

DISCUSSION

Knowledge of the cranial nerves is critical for performing an accurate neurological assessment. Since these are paired nerves arising largely from the brainstem, a unilateral CN dysfunction is common, often reflecting a problem in the ipsilateral cerebral hemisphere.

Discussion Source

Hektor Dunphy, L. (1999). *Management Guidelines for Adult Nurse Practitioners*. Philadelphia: FA Davis. Pp. 104–105.

QUESTIONS

4. You examine a 29-year-old woman who has a sudden onset of right-sided facial asymmetry. She is unable to tightly close her right eyelid, frown, or smile on the affected side. Her examination is otherwise unremarkable. This may represent paralysis of CN:

   A. III
   B. IV
   C. VII
   D. VIII

5. Which represents the most appropriate diagnostic test for the patient in the previous question?

   A. complete blood count with white blood cell differential
   B. Lyme disease antibody titer
   C. computed tomography (CT) scan of the head with contrast
   D. blood urea nitrogen and creatinine levels

6. In prescribing prednisone for the person with Bell's palsy, the NP considers that its use:

   A. helps in reversing facial paralysis even when given late in the course of illness
   B. should be initiated at the onset of facial paralysis
   C. will likely help minimize ocular symptoms
   D. may prolong the course of the disease

ANSWERS

4. C
5. B
6. B

DISCUSSION

Bell's palsy is an acute paralysis of CN VII (in the absence of brain dysfunction) that is seen in the absence of other signs and symptoms. Because this condition can be a complication of Lyme disease, it is important to get the appropriate antibody titer. A head CT scan with contrast would be indicated if there were a question of space-occupying lesion such as a brain tumor. Because the patient's history and examination do not suggest the presence of a tumor, a CT scan is not indicated. Prednisone may help limit the length and severity of the paralysis. It is most effective when started early in the disease and of no use if therapy begins more than 10 days after the onset of symptoms. Acyclovir use in patients with Bell's palsy is controversial.

Discussion Source

Hektor Dunphy, L. (1999). *Management Guidelines for Adult Nurse Practitioners*. Philadelphia: FA Davis. Pp. 106–107.

QUESTIONS

7. A 40-year-old patient presents with a 5-week history of recurrent headaches that awaken him during the night. The pain is severe, lasts about 1 hour, and is located behind his left eye. Additional symptoms include lacrimation and nasal discharge. His physical examination is within normal limits. The most likely diagnosis is:

    A. common migraine
    B. classic migraine
    C. cluster headache
    D. increased intracranial pressure

8. Linda is a 22-year-old woman with a 3-year history of recurrent, unilateral, pulsating headaches with vomiting and photophobia. The headaches, which generally last 3 hours, can be aborted by resting in a dark room. She can usually tell that she is going to get a headache. She explains: "I see little 'squiggles' before my eyes." Her physical examination is unremarkable. This presentation is most consistent with:

    A. tension-type headache
    B. migraine without aura
    C. migraine with aura
    D. cluster headache

9. Prophylactic treatment for migraine headaches includes:

    A. propanolol
    B. ergotamine
    C. naproxen sodium
    D. enalapril

10. You are examining a 55-year-old woman who has a history of angina and migraine headache. Which of the following represents the best choice of abortive migraine therapy for this patient?

    A. verapamil
    B. ergotamine
    C. ibuprofen
    D. sumatriptan

ANSWERS

7. **C**
8. **C**
9. **A**
10. **C**

DISCUSSION

The International Headache Society (IHS) criteria for tension-type headache includes:

- Patient report of at least 10 headaches, at less than 15 days per month, lasting 30 minutes to 7 days with at least two of the following pain characteristics: pressing, nonpulsatile pain, usually in a bilateral location that is mild to moderate in intensity.
- The person with the headache is able to "work through" if needed, although often in considerable discomfort.
- The headache is not aggravated by activity. There is no vomiting, but nausea and anorexia are often reported.
- Either photophobia or phonophobia is reported.

Migraine without aura affects about 80% of those with migraine. However, upon careful questioning many patients report a migraine warning, such as agitation, jitteriness, disturbed sleep, or unusual dreams. IHS criteria for migraine without aura includes patient report of at least five attacks, lasting 4 to 72 hours with at least two of the following characteristics: unilateral location, a pulsating quality, moderate to severe in intensity, and aggravated by normal activity. Rest may be required because of pain intensity. During headache, at least one of the following is present: nausea or vomiting, photophobia, or phonophobia.

Migraine with aura is found in about 20% of those with migrainous disorders. The aura is a recurrent neurological symptom that arises from the cerebral cortex or brainstem. Typically, the aura develops over 5 to 20 minutes and last less than 1 hour and is accompanied or followed by migraine. Patients with migraines with aura do not necessarily have more severe headaches than those without aura, but the former patients are more likely to be offered a fuller range of therapies. Patients without aura may be misdiagnosed as having tension-type headaches and therefore not offered headache therapies specifically suited for migraines, such as the triptans.

Headache treatment is aimed at identifying and reducing headache triggers. In addition, acute headache treatment, called *abortive therapy*, should be offered. Prophylactic therapy, aimed at limiting the number and severity of future headaches, may also be indicated. The National Headache Foundation (NHF) sets guidelines for the appropriate use of abortive therapies, generally advising that these medications be used no more than twice a week. Excessive use of abortive therapies can lead to rebound headache.

When choosing a migraine abortive agent, a number of considerations should be kept on mind. These medications are available in a number of forms (i.e., oral, parenteral, nasal spray, suppository). Migraine headaches are also present in a number of forms. A thoughtful match between presentation of typical migraine and the form of medication is helpful. Here are some examples.

- Oral products generally take ½ to 1 hour before there is significant relief of migraine pain. These products are best suited for patients with migraine who have a slowly developing headache with minimum gastrointestinal (GI) distress. They should be used at the onset of symptoms. In general, the oral products are the least expensive treatment choice.
- Injectable products (e.g., sumatriptan and dihydroergotamine injection) have a rapid onset of action, usually within 15 to 30 minutes. These products are best suited for patients with rapidly progressing migraines accompanied by significant GI upset. Sumatriptan is the only product available as a self-injector for patient administration. Dihydroergotamine is usually given intravenously in severe migrainosis along with parenteral hydration. Injectables are usually the most expensive treatment option. If the

patient is a suitable candidate for injection therapy, sumatriptan and dihydroergotamine are both available as a nasal spray and have a similarly rapid onset of action and are tolerable in the presence of GI upset. Suppositories have a slightly longer onset of action but may be used when nausea and vomiting are present.

- Ergotamines act as 5-HT1A and 5-HT1D receptor agonists and do not alter cerebral blood flow. Because of vasoconstrictor effect, their use should be avoided in the presence of coronary artery disease and pregnancy. Ergotamines are available in a variety of forms, including oral and sublingual tablets, suppositories, injectables, and nasal sprays.
- The triptans act as selective serotonin receptor agonists and work at the 5-HT1D site, allowing an increase uptake of serotonin. Because of vasoconstrictor effect, their use is contraindicated in patients with Prinzmetal angina or coronary artery disease, those who are pregnant, and those who have recently used ergots. The triptans should be used cautiously in patients with significant heart disease risk factors. Because of the risk of serotonin syndrome, a condition of excessive availability of this neurotransmitter, the triptans should be used with caution with monamine oxidase inhibitor inhibitors (MAOIs) or selective serotonin reuptake inhibitors (SSRIs). The triptans are available in a variety of forms, including oral tablets, injectables, and nasal spray. When prescribing injectable sumatriptan, remember that the first dose should be given under observation, asking the patient about chest pain and shortness of breath, because this rapidly acting product may precipitate coronary artery vasoconstriction.
- Nonsteroidal anti-inflammatory drugs (NSAIDs) can be highly effective in both tension-type and migraine headache. These products inhibit prostaglandin and leukotriene synthesis and are most helpful when used at the first sign of headache when GI upset is not a significant issue. The NHF Guidelines advise the use of rapid onset NSAIDS in high doses with booster doses. Examples include:
  - Ibuprofen 1200 mg stat, then 600 mg every 4 hours for up to 2 doses if needed
  - Flurbiprofen (Ansaid) 100 mg, then repeat once in 1 hour if needed
  - Diclofenac (Cataflam) 50 to 100 mg as a 1 time dose
  - Ketorolac 60 mg intramuscularly as a 1 time dose
- Fioricet is a combination of caffeine, butalbital, and acetaminophen. Whereas caffeine enhances the analgesic properties of aceta-

minophen, butalbital's barbiturate action enhances select neuro-transmitter action, helping to relieve migraine and tension-type headache pain. This product is inexpensive and generally well tolerated.

- Stadol NS (butorphanol tartrate nasal spray) acts as a kappa receptor agonist, as do opioids. These products are highly analgesic but may be sedating and potentially abused.
- Midrin is a multidrug product that includes a vasoconstrictor (isometheptene mutate), analgesic (acetaminophen), and relaxant (65 mg dichloralphenazone). It should be used in multiple doses at the beginning of a migraine headache. Caution should be used when vasoconstriction is contraindicated.
- Excedrin Migraine is an aspirin, acetaminophen, and caffeine combination product. This is the only over-the-counter product given Food and Drug Administration approval for migraine therapy. Its advantages include patient ease of access to the product, excellent side-effect profile, and low cost.
- Neuroleptics may be used as adjuncts in migraine headache therapy because they help control nausea and vomiting. Because these drugs are generally highly sedating, using them in the clinician's office may make it difficult for patients to return home. Use should be limited to 3 days a week because of the risk of extrapyramidal movements (EPMs). Examples of neuroleptics are prochlorperazine (Compazine) and promethazine (Phenergan).

Consider use of prophylactic therapy of migraine, tension-type, or cluster headache if abortive headache therapy is used frequently or if inadequate symptom relief is obtained from appropriate use of these therapies. The goal of headache prophylactic therapy is a minimum of a 50% reduction in number of headaches in about two thirds of all patients along with easier-to-control headaches. Most agents work through blockade of 5HT2 receptor and need 1 to 2 months of use before effect is seen. Before headache prophylaxis is initiated, first eliminate or limit headache-inducing medications such as estrogen, progesterone, and vasodilators (Table 2–1).

Cluster headaches, also known as migrainous neuralgia, are most common in middle-aged men, particularly those with heavy alcohol and tobacco use. Sometimes called the "suicide headache" because of the severity of the associated pain, cluster headache occurs periodically in clusters of several weeks, with associated lacrimation and rhinorrhea. Treatment includes reduction of triggers, such as tobacco and alcohol use, and initiation of prophylactic therapy (as listed above plus lithium) as well as appropriate abortive therapy (triptans, high-dose NSAIDs, and high-flow oxygen).

TABLE 2–1.
MEDICATIONS FOR HEADACHE PROPHYLAXIS

Type of Medication	Example	Comments
Beta adrenergic antagonists (beta blockers, drugs with -lol suffix)	Propanolol 60–120 mg/d, nadolol 20–120 mg/d, metoprolol 100–200 mg/d	Nonselective (mixed B1 and B2) blockers may be more helpful than cardioselective (B1 selective)
Calcium channel blockers (CCB)	Verapamil 120–480 mg/d, diltiazem 90–360 mg/d, nicardipine 20–30 mg/d	Verapamil is likely the most helpful
Tricyclic antidepressants (TCA)	Desipramine 25–150 mg/d, nortriptyline 10–150 mg/d	Helpful in both tension-type and migrainous headache Usually effective at approximately 50% of dose needed for treatment of depression
Riboflavin	Vitamin B_2 (riboflavin) 400 mg/d	Mechanism not well understood Suitable for pregnant women
Lithium	Adjust dose to achieve therapeutic lithium level	Effective prophylaxis for cluster headache
Divalproex Na (Depakote, Depakene)	Doses up to 1000 mg/d in adults	Often lower than dose needed for seizure control and depression Well studied in children but may have some effect on cognitive performance Periodic hepatic and hematologic function tests required

References: Adapted from Drew-Gastes, J., Gross, R. (1999). Neurologic disorders. In Youngkin, E., Savin, K., Kissinger, J., & Israel, D. *Pharmacotherapeutics: A Primary Care Clinical Guide.* Norwalk, CT: Appleton & Lange. Pp. 621–681.

The development of the appropriate diagnosis is critical to caring for the patients who have headaches. In addition, headaches can be the presenting symptoms of a serious illness. The key points to consider in assessing the person with headache are given in Box 2–1 and Table 2–2.

Discussion Sources

Drew-Gastes, J., Gross, R. (1999). Neurologic disorders. In Youngkin, E., Sawin, K., Kissinger, J., & Israel, D. *Pharmacotherapeutics: A Primary Care Clinical Guide*. Norwalk, CT: Appleton & Lange. Pp. 621–681.
Hektor Dunphy, L. (1999). *Management Guidelines for Adult Nurse Practitioners*. Philadelphia: FA Davis. Pp. 70–73.
Solomon, S. (1997). Diagnosis of primary headache disorders: Validity of the International Headache Society criteria in clinical practice. In Matthews, N. *Neurologic Clinic*. 15(1) 107–114.

QUESTIONS

11. You examine a 28-year-old woman with a chief complaint of recurrent, bilateral headache lasting 1 to 4 hours about 4 times a month. She describes the pain as pressing and without pulsation, usually accompanied by noise intolerance. This is most consistent with a diagnosis of:

    A. migraine with aura

    B. increased intracranial pressure

    C. tension-type headache

    D. vascular headache

**BOX 2–1
HELPFUL OBSERVATIONS IN PATIENTS WITH ACUTE HEADACHE**

- History of previous identical headaches
- Intact cognition
- Supple neck
- Normal neurological examination results
- Improvement in symptoms while under observation and treatment

---

Reference: Adapted from Aminoff, M. (1999). Nervous system. In Tierney, L., McPhee, S., & Papadakis, M. *Current Diagnosis and Treatment* (38th ed.). Stamford, CT: Appleton & Lange. Pp. 932–989.

TABLE 2–2.
WARNING SIGNS IN PATIENTS WITH HEADACHE

Patient Presentation	Comment
New onset of headache in person older than age 40 yr	Because primary headache onset usually occurs in adolescence to young adulthood, secondary headache should be considered in new-onset headache in later adulthood. However, less than 15% of brain tumors have headache as a presenting symptom. In brain tumor, a new-onset seizure or personality or cognitive changes are more common.
"Worst headache ever"	More than 85% are migraine headache. However, secondary headache from sudden onset of increased intracranial pressure (ICP) should be considered.
Onset with exertion	May indicate increased ICP.
"Thunderclap" sensation	May indicate subarachnoid hemorrhage (SAH).
Decreased alertness or cognitive ability	May indicate increased ICP.
Radiation of headache pain to between the scapula	May indicate SAH.
Nuchal rigidity associated with headache, often with fever	Meningitis, SAH.
History or physical finding consistent with infection	Meningitis, encephalitis.
Worsening while being observed	May indicate increasing ICP.

Reference: Adapted from Aminoff, M. (1999). Nervous system. In Tierney, L., McPhee, S., & Papadakis, M. *Current Diagnosis and Treatment* (38th ed.). Stamford, CT: Appleton & Lange. Pp. 932–989.

12. Treatment options for the acute relief of symptoms for the patient in Question 11 include:

    A. nortriptyline
    B. ergot derivatives
    C. sumatriptan
    D. naproxen sodium

13. Prophylactic treatment options for the prevention of tension-type headaches include:

    A. desipramine
    B. lisinopril
    C. oxycodone
    D. butalbital

ANSWERS

11. C
12. D
13. A

DISCUSSION

Although much of headache care is focused on the relief and prevention of migraine, tension-type headaches are a significant source of suffering and lost function. Abortive treatment options include the use of acetaminophen; NSAIDs; and combination products such as butalbital with acetaminophen and acetaminophen, aspirin, and caffeine. Prophylactic therapies are highly effective at limiting the number and frequency of tension-type headache.

IHS criteria for tension-type headaches include the following:

- At least 10 episodes of headache described as the following: occurring less than 15 days a month and lasting at least 30 minutes to 7 days with at least two of the following pain characteristics: usually bilateral, pressing, nonpulsatile pain that is mild to moderate in intensity.
- The person is able to "work through" the pain if needed because it is not aggravated by activity. No vomiting is reported, but nausea and anorexia are common.
- Photophobia or phonophobia is present.

Discussion Sources

Drew-Gastes, J., Gross, R. (1999). Neurologic disorders. In Youngkin, E., Sawin, K., Kissinger, J., & Israel, D. *Pharmacotherapeutics: A Primary Care Clinical Guide*. Norwalk, CT: Appleton & Lange. Pp. 621–681.
Hektor Dunphy, L. (1999). *Management Guidelines for Adult Nurse Practitioners*. Philadelphia: FA Davis. Pp. 70–73.
Solomon, S. (1997). Diagnosis of primary headache disorders: Validity of the International Headache Society criteria in clinical practice. In Matthews, N. *Neurologic Clinic*. 15(1) 107–114.

QUESTION

14. A 68-year-old man presents with new onset of headaches. He describes the pain as bilateral frontal to occipital and worst when he arises in the morning and when coughing. He feels much better by mid-afternoon. The history is most consistent with headache caused by:

    A. vascular compromise
    B. increased intracranial pressure (ICP)
    C. brain tumor
    D. tension-type with geriatric presentation

ANSWER

14. B

DISCUSSION

The headache in increased ICP is usually reported as worst upon awakening, which is when brain swelling is the worst. The pain is less intense as the day progresses as it resolves. Establishing the appropriate diagnosis is critical because treatment is guided by the reason for the increased ICP. Tension-type headaches in older patients follow the typical pattern as in younger patients, with symptoms progressing as the day goes on.

Discussion Source

Hektor Dunphy, L. (1999). *Management Guidelines for Adult Nurse Practitioners*. Philadelphia: FA Davis. P. 72.

QUESTIONS

15. An 18-year-old college freshman is brought to the student health center with a chief complaint of headache and fever. On physical examination, he has positive Kernig and Brudzinski signs. The most likely diagnosis is:

    A. encephalitis
    B. meningitis
    C. subarachnoid hemorrhage
    D. epidural hematoma

16. A 19-year-old college sophomore has meningococcal meningitis. You speak to the school health officers about the possible risk to other students. You inform them that:

    A. The patient does not have a contagious disease.
    B. All students need to receive antimicrobial prophylaxis regardless of their degree of contact with the infected person.
    C. Only intimate partners need prophylaxis.
    D. Those with household-type contact with the patient should receive antimicrobial prophylaxis.

ANSWERS

15. B
16. D

DISCUSSION

Meningococcal meningitis, caused by *Neisseria meningitidis*, is one of the most common forms of bacterial meningitis. The presence of Kernig and Brudzinki signs along with headache and fever indicate a high probability of meningitis. Encephalitis is more likely viral in origin and usually presents with fewer meningeal signs.

Because *N. meningitis* is transmitted through droplets, prophylaxis should be offered to those with household-type or intimate contact with the infected person, in particular if they have had more than 4 hours of exposure to the patient the week before the onset of illness. Antimicrobial options include any of the following:

- Rifampin 600 mg orally every 12 hours in four doses
- Ciprofloxacin 500 mg orally in one dose
- Ceftriaxone 250 mg intramuscularly in one dose

Discussion Source

Gilbert, D., Moellering, R., Sande, M. (1998). *The Sanford Guide to Antimicrobial Therapy* (28th ed.). Vienna, VA: Antimicrobial Therapy, Inc. Pp. 109.

QUESTIONS

17. A 34-year-old woman has recently been diagnosed with multiple sclerosis (MS). When providing primary care for this patient, you consider that MS:

    A. has a predictable course of progressive decline in intellectual and motor function

    B. presents with a classic pattern of myalgia, blurred vision, and ataxia

    C. often is seen with a variable pattern of exacerbation and remissions

    D. is accompanied by classic central nervous system lesions detectable on skull films

18. Which of the following is most consistent with findings in patients with Parkinson's disease?

    A. rigid posture with poor muscle tone

    B. masklike facies and continued cognitive function

    C. tremor at rest and bradykinesia

    D. excessive arm swinging with ambulation and flexed posture

19. Treatment options in Parkinson's disease include:

    A. levodopa

    B. chlorpromazine

    C. prednisone

    D. baclofen

ANSWERS

17. C
18. C
19. A

DISCUSSION

Multiple sclerosis is characterized by periods of exacerbation and remission, often with an unpredictable course. The diagnosis is difficult to make because there is no "classic" presentation, but more likely recurrent fatigue, muscle weakness, and other nonspecific signs and symptoms often attributed to other disease or simply stress and fatigue. Magnetic resonance imaging is the most sensitive test for detecting demyelinating plaques, a typical finding in MS.

The presentation of Parkinson's disease consists of a combination of six features: tremor at rest, rigidity, bradykinesia, flexed posture, loss of postural reflexes, and masklike facies. At least two of these, with one being tremor at rest or bradykinesia, must be present for the diagnosis to be made. Typically, the patients with Parkinson's disease hold their arms rigidly at the sides with little movement during ambulation. Because this disease is characterized by an alteration in the dopaminergic pathway, levodopa—a metabolic precursor of dopamine—is used to minimize symptoms. The later addition of dopamine receptor agonists such as bromocriptine may help.

Discussion Source

Hektor Dunphy, L. (1999). *Management Guidelines for Adult Nurse Practitioners*. Philadelphia: FA Davis. Pp. 116–121.

QUESTIONS

20. Which of the following best describes patient presentation during an absence (petit mal) seizure?

    A. blank staring lasting 3 to 50 seconds accompanied by impaired level of consciousness
    B. awake state with abnormal motor behavior lasting seconds
    C. rigid extension of arms and legs followed by sudden jerking movements with loss of consciousness
    D. abrupt muscle contraction with autonomic signs

21. Which of the following best describes patient presentation during a simple partial seizure?

    A. blank staring lasting 3 to 50 seconds accompanied by impaired level of consciousness
    B. awake state with abnormal motor behavior lasting seconds
    C. rigid extension of arms and legs followed by sudden jerking movements with loss of consciousness
    D. abrupt muscle contraction with autonomic signs

22. Which of the following best describes patient presentation during a tonic-clonic (grand mal) seizure?

    A. blank staring lasting 3 to 50 seconds accompanied by impaired level of consciousness
    B. awake state with abnormal motor behavior lasting seconds
    C. rigid extension of arms and legs followed by sudden jerking movements with loss of consciousness
    D. abrupt muscle contraction with autonomic signs

23. Which of the following best describes patient presentation during a myoclonic seizure?

    A. blank staring lasting 3 to 50 seconds accompanied by impaired level of consciousness
    B. awake state with abnormal motor behavior lasting seconds
    C. rigid extension of arms and legs followed by sudden jerking movements with loss of consciousness
    D. abrupt muscle contraction with autonomic signs

24. Treatment options for the adult with tonic-clonic seizures include all of the following except:

    A. carbamazepine
    B. phenytoin
    C. gabapentin
    D. trandolapril

25. A preferred treatment option for absence seizures includes:

    A. valproic acid
    B. phenytoin
    C. gabapentin
    D. felbamate

26. A patient taking phenytoin may exhibit drug toxicity when concurrently taking:

   A. theophylline
   B. famotidine
   C. acetaminophen
   D. aspirin

ANSWERS

20. A
21. B
22. C
23. D
24. D
25. A
26. A

DISCUSSION

The type of seizure directs the treatment of the seizure disorder. Thus, knowledge of the presentation of the more common forms of seizures is critical (Table 2–3).

A number of standard and newer antiepileptic drugs (AED) are now available. For the control of tonic-clonic seizures, phenytoin, carbamazepine, gabapentin, and lamotrigine are among the most commonly used drugs. In absence seizures, ethosuximide, valproic acid, and clonazepam are effective, with the latter two prescribed often for myoclonic seizures. Expert knowledge of the indications and adverse reaction profiles of these medications is needed before initiating or continuing AED therapy.

Certain AEDs, including phenytoin and carbamazepine, are members of a group known as narrow therapeutic index (NTI) drugs. A certain amount of NTI drugs is therapeutic, and just slightly more than this amount is potentially toxic. Other drugs in this category include warfarin, theophylline, and digoxin. Many of these drugs have high levels of protein binding as well as significant utilization of hepatic enzymatic pathways for drug metabolism such as cytochrome P450. Phenytoin is highly (>90%) protein bound; when taken with other highly protein bound drugs, it can be displaced from its protein-binding site, leading to increased free phenytoin and a risk of toxicity. Carbamazepine can in-

TABLE 2–3.
DESCRIPTION AND TREATMENT OF COMMON SEIZURES

Seizure Type	Description of Seizure	Antiepileptic Drug of Choice	Comments
Absence (petit mal)	Blank staring lasting 3–50 sec accompanied by impaired level of consciousness	Valproic acid, ethosuximide	Usual age of onset, 3–15 yr.
Myoclonic	Awake state or momentary loss of consciousness with abnormal motor behavior lasting seconds to minutes One or more muscle groups involved, occasionally flinging patient	Valproic acid, clonazepam, ethosuximide, primidone, gabapentin, lamotrigine	Difficult to control. At least 50% also have tonic-clonic seizures. Usual age of onset, 2–7 yr.
Tonic-clonic (grand mal)	Rigid extension of arms and legs followed by sudden jerking movements with loss of consciousness. Bowel and bladder incontinence common with postictal confusion.	Carbamazepine, valproic acid, phenytoin, primidone, gabapentin, lamotrigine	Onset at any age. In adults, new onset may be found in brain tumor or after head injury.

(continued)

TABLE 2–3. (continued)			
Seizure Type	**Description of Seizure**	**Antiepileptic Drug of Choice**	**Comments**
Simple partial or focal seizure (Jacksonian)	Movement may affect any part of body, localized or generalized	Valproic acid, ethosuximide, phenobarbital	Typical age of onset, 3–15 yr.
Complex partial	Aura characterized by unusual sense of smell or taste, visual or auditory hallucinations, image or sound, stomach upset. Followed by vague stare and facial movements as well as autonomic signs.	Carbamazepine, phenytoin, phenobarbital, primidone, gabapentin, lamotrigine	Onset at any age.

References: Adapted from Aminoff, M. (1999). Nervous system. In Tierney, L., McPhee, S., & Papadakis, M. *Current Diagnosis and Treatment* (38th ed.). Stamford, CT: Appleton & Lange. Pp. 932–989.

Hektor Dunphy, L. (1999). *Management Guidelines for Adult Nurse Practitioners.* Philadelphia: FA Davis. Pp. 120–123.

Moe, P., Seay, A. (1999). Neurologic and muscular disorders. In Hay, W., Hayward, A., Levin, M., Sondheimer, J. *Current Pediatric Diagnosis and Treatment* (14th ed.). Stamford, CT: Appleton & Lange. Pp. 622–694.

crease the metabolic capacity of hepatic enzymes, leading to more rapid metabolism of the drug and reduced levels of this and other drugs. The prescriber should be familiar with the drug interactions of all AEDs and monitor therapeutic levels as well as for adverse reactions (see Table 2–3).

Discussion Sources

Aminoff, M. (1999). Nervous system. In Tierney, L., McPhee, S., & Papadakis, M. *Current Diagnosis and Treatment* (38th ed.). Stamford, CT: Appleton & Lange. Pp. 932–989.

Hektor Dunphy, L. (1999). *Management Guidelines for Adult Nurse Practitioners*. Philadelphia: FA Davis. Pp. 120–123.

QUESTIONS

27. Risk factors for transient ischemic attack (TIA) include all of the following except:

A. atrial fibrillation

B. carotid artery disease

C. oral contraceptive use

D. pernicious anemia

28. A TIA is characterized as an episode of reversible neurological symptoms that may last up to:

A. 1 hour

B. 6 hours

C. 12 hours

D. 24 hours

29. When caring for a patient with a recent TIA, you consider that:

A. Long-term antiplatelet therapy is indicated.

B. This person has a relatively low risk of future stroke.

C. Women present with this disorder more often than men do.

D. Rehabilitation will be needed to minimize the effects of the resulting neurological insult.

ANSWERS

27. D

28. D

29. A

DISCUSSION

A TIA is a neurological event in which all signs and symptoms including numbness, weakness or flaccidity as well as visual changes, ataxia, or dysarthria, resolve usually within minutes but certainly 24 hours after onset. If changes persist beyond 24 hours, the diagnosis of stroke should be entertained. Indeed, TIA should be considered a "stroke warning." Risk factors include carotid artery atherosclerosis; structural cardiac problems, such as valvular problems that lead to increased risk of embolization; and hypercoagulable conditions, such as antiphospholipid antibody and oral contraceptive use. Intervention includes minimizing risk factors through lifestyle modification (e.g., smoking cessation, diet, and exercise) as well as long-term antiplatelet therapy.

Discussion Source

Hektor Dunphy, L. (1999). *Management Guidelines for Adult Nurse Practitioners*. Philadelphia: FA Davis. Pp. 123–126.

3
CHAPTER

Skin
Disorders

QUESTIONS

1. How many grams of a topical cream or ointment are needed for a single application to the hands?

   A. one

   B. two

   C. three

   D. four

2. How many grams of a topical cream or ointment are needed for a single application to an arm?

   A. one

   B. two

   C. three

   D. four

3. How many grams of a topical cream or ointment are needed for a single application to the entire body?

   A. 10 to 30

   B. 30 to 60

   C. 60 to 90

   D. 90 to 120

ANSWERS

   1. B

   2. C

   3. B

DISCUSSION

Knowledge of the amount of a cream or ointment needed to treat a dermatologic condition is an important part of the prescriptive practice (Table 3–1). Prescribers often write prescriptions for an inadequate amount of a topical medication with insufficient numbers of refills, possibly creating a situation in which treatment fails because of an inadequate length of therapy.

Discussion Source

Ardnt, K. (1995). *Manual of Dermatologic Therapeutics* (5th ed.). Boston: Little Brown. Pp. 120–121.

TABLE 3–1.
TOPICAL MEDICATION-DISPENSING FORMULA

Area	Amount Needed in grams for One Application	Amount of Agent Needed in Twice-a-day Application for 1 Wk, g	Amount of Agent Needed in Twice-a-day Application for 1 Mo
Hands, head, face, anogenital region	2	28	120 g (4 oz)
One arm, anterior or posterior trunk	3	42	180 (6 oz)
One leg	4	56	240 g (8 oz)
Entire body	30–60	420–840 (14–28 oz)	1.8–3.6 kg (60–120 oz or 3.75–7.5 lb)

Reference: Adapted from Ardnt, K. (1995). *Manual of Dermatologic Therapeutics* (5th ed.). Boston: Little, Brown. Pp. 120–121.

QUESTIONS

4. You write a prescription for a topical agent and anticipate the greatest rate of absorption when it is applied to the:

   A. palms of the hands
   B. soles of the feet
   C. face
   D. abdomen

5. You prescribe a topical medication and want it to have maximum absorption, so you chose the following vehicle:

   A. gel
   B. lotion
   C. cream
   D. ointment

ANSWERS

4. **C**
5. **D**

DISCUSSION

Safe prescription of a topical agent for patients with dermatologic disorders requires knowledge of the best vehicle for the medication. Certain parts of the body, notably the face, axilla, and genital area are quite permeable, allowing greater absorption of medication when compared with less permeable areas such as the extremities and trunk. In particular, the thickness of the palms of the hands and soles of the feet create a barrier so that relatively little topical medication is absorbed when applied to these sites. A general rule of cutaneous drug absorption is that it is inversely proportional to the thickness of the stratum corneum. For example, hydrocortisone absorption from the arch of the foot is 0.14 of that absorbed from the forearm; forehead absorption is six times as potent.

In general, the less viscous the vehicle containing a topical medication, the less of it is absorbed. As a result, medication contained in a gel or lotion is absorbed in smaller amounts than that held in a cream or ointment. Besides enhancing absorption of the therapeutic agent, creams and ointments provide lubrication to the region, often a desirable effect in the presence of xerosis or lichenification.

Discussion Source

Robertson, D., Maibach, H. (1998). Dermatologic pharmacology. In *Katzung's Basic and Clinical Pharmacology* (7th ed.). East Norwalk, CT: Appleton & Lange. Pp. 999–1016.

QUESTION

6. One of the mechanisms of action of a topical corticosteroid preparation is as a(n):

   A. antimitotic
   B. exfolliant
   C. vasoconstrictor
   D. humectant

ANSWER

6. C

DISCUSSION

Corticorteroids are a useful class of drugs often used for treating inflammatory and allergic dermatologic disorders. Although corticosteroids reduce inflammatory and allergic reactions through a number of mechanisms (including immunosuppressive and inflammatory properties), their relative potency is based on vasoconstrictive activity—that is, the more potent topical steroids such as betamethasone (class 1) have significantly greater vasoconstricting action than the least potent agents such as hydrocortisone (class 7) (Table 3–2).

Discussion Source

Robertson, D., Maibach, H. (1998). Dermatologic pharmacology. In *Katzung's Basic and Clinical Pharmacology* (7th ed.). East Norwalk, CT: Appleton & Lange. Pp. 999–1016.

TABLE 3–2.
EXAMPLES OF TOPICAL STEROID POTENCY

Potency	Examples
Low potency	Hydrocortisone (0.5%, 1%, 2.5%) Flucocinolone acetonide 0.01% (Synalar) Triamcinolone acetonide 0.025% (Aristocort)
Intermediate potency	Flucocinolone acetonide 0.025% (Synalar) Hydrocortisone butyrate 0.1% Hydrocortisone valerate 0.2% (Westcort) Triamcinolone acetonide 0.1%
High potency	Flucocinolone acetonide 0.2% (Synalar-HP) Desoximtasone 0.25% (Topicort) Fluocinonide 0.05% (Lidex) Betamethasone dipropionate augmented 0.05% (Diprolene AF cream)
Super high potency	Betamethasone dipropionate augmented 0.05% (Diprolene gel, ointment) Clobestasol propionate 0.05% (Temovate) Halobetasol propionate 0.05% (Ultravate 0.05%)

Reference: Adapted from Robertson, D., Maibach, H. (1998). Dermatologic pharmacology. In *Katzung's Basic and Clinical Pharmacology* (7th ed.). East Norwalk, CT: Appleton & Lange. Pp. 999–1016.

QUESTION

7. The majority of oral antihistamines exhibit therapeutic effect by:

   A. inactivating circulating histamine
   B. preventing the production of histamine
   C. blocking activity at histamine receptor sites
   D. acting as a procholenergic agent

ANSWER

7. C

DISCUSSION

Antihistamines prevent action of formed histamine, a potent inflammatory mediator, and therefore can be used to control acute symptoms of itchiness and allergy. All antihistamines work by blocking H_1 (histamine 1) receptor sites, thus preventing the action of histamine.

Discussion Source

Robertson, D., Maibach, H. (1998). Dermatologic pharmacology. In *Katzung's Basic and Clinical Pharmacology* (7th ed.). East Norwalk, CT: Appleton & Lange. Pp. 999–1016.

QUESTION

8. Muprocin's (Bactroban) spectrum of antimicrobial activity includes:

    A. primarily gram-negative organisms

    B. select *Staphylococcus* and *Streptococcus* species

    C. *Pseudomonas* species and anaerobic organisms

    D. only organisms that do not produce beta-lactamase

ANSWER

8. B

DISCUSSION

Mupirocin (Bactroban) is a topical antibacterial agent effective in eradicating select gram-positive organisms such as methicillin-resistant and methicillin-sensitive *Staphylococcus aureus* and *streptococci*. As a result, mupirocin is an effective treatment option for impetigo as well as for the temporary elimination of nasal carriage of *S. aureus*.

Discussion Source

Robertson, D., Maibach, H. (1998). Dermatologic pharmacology. In *Katzung's Basic and Clinical Pharmacology* (7th ed.). East Norwalk, CT: Appleton & Lange. Pp. 999–1016.

QUESTIONS

9. Which of the following medication contributes to the development of acne vulgaris?

    A. lithium
    B. propanolol
    C. tetracycline
    D. oral contraceptives

10. First-line therapy for acne vulgaris with closed comedones includes:

    A. oral antibiotics
    B. isotretinoin
    C. benzoyl peroxide
    D. hydrocortisone cream

11. When prescribing tretinoin (Retin-A), the NP advises the patient to:

    A. use it with benzoyl peroxide to minimize irritating effects
    B. use a sunscreen because the drug is photosensitizing
    C. add a sulfa-based cream to enhance antiacne effects
    D. expect a significant improvement in acne lesions after approximately 1 week of use

12. In the treatment of acne vulgaris, which of type of lesions responds best to topical antibiotic therapy?

    A. open comedones
    B. cysts
    C. pustules
    D. superficial lesions

13. Which of the following is indicated for the treatment of acne rosacea?

    A. metronidazole gel (MetroGel)
    B. clindamycin lotion (Cleocin)
    C. erythromycin 2% solution
    D. azelaic acid 20% (Azelex cream)

14. You have initiated therapy for an 18-year-old man with acne vulgaris. You have prescribed tetracycline 500 mg twice a day. He returns in 3 weeks, complaining that his skin is "no better." Your next action is to:

    A. Counsel him that 6 to 8 weeks of treatment is often needed before significant improvement is achieved.
    B. Discontinue the tetracycline and initiate minocyline therapy.

C. Advise him that antibiotics are likely not an effective treatment for him and should be not be continued.

D. Add a second antimicrobial agent.

15. Of the following, who is the best candidate for isotretinoin (Accutane) therapy?

A. a 17-year-old patient with pustular lesions and poor response to benzoyl peroxide

B. a 20-year-old patient with cystic lesions who had tried a variety of therapies with minimal effect

C. a 14-year-old patient with open and closed comedones and a family history of "ice pick" lesions

D. an 18-year-old patient with inflammatory lesions and improvement with tretinoin (Retin-A)

16. In a 22-year-old woman using isotretinoin (Accutane) therapy, the NP ensures follow-up to monitor for all of the following tests except:

A. aspartate aminotransferase (AST)

B. triglycerides

C. pregnancy test

D. platelet count

ANSWERS

9. A
10. C
11. B
12. C
13. A
14. A
15. B
16. D

DISCUSSION

Acne vulgaris is a common pustular disorder caused by a combination of factors. An increase in sebaceous activity causes a plugging of follicles and retention of sebum, allowing an overgrowth of *Propionibacterium acnes*. This allows an inflammatory reaction with the resulting wide variety of lesions, including open and closed comedones, cysts, and pustules.

Both topical and systemic antibiotics are used to treat acne and are particularly helpful as therapy for pustular lesions. However, the mechanism of action of antibiotics in acne therapy is probably not based solely on their antimicrobial action but may be caused in part by their anti-inflammatory activity. Additional acne vulgaris agents include topical vitamin A derivatives such as tretinoin (Retin-A), synthetic retinoid (Accutane), and comeodolytics (benzoyl peroxide) (Table 3–3).

Nearly all adolescents develop acne vulgaris. Most discover that the skin clears considerably by early adulthood. Only 15% will seek treatment for this problematic condition that affects teens at a time in their lives when body image and social acceptance are usually of greater influence than they are in any other time of life. However, a number of effective treatment options are available.

Acne-inducing drugs should be avoided, if possible. However, certain medications such as lithium and phenytoin (Dilantin) may need to be used. These medications can also cause acne in adults. In any event, drug-induced acne can be treated with conventional therapy (see Table 3–3).

Discussion Source

Hektor Dunphy, L. (1999). *Management Guidelines for Adult Nurse Practitioners*. Philadelphia: FA Davis. Pp. 128–132.

QUESTIONS

17. A common infective agent in domestic pet cat bites is:

    A. rabies virus
    B. *Pasteurella multocida*
    C. *Bacteroides* species
    D. *Hemophilus influenzae*

18. A 24-year-old man arrives at the walk-in center. He reports that he was bitten in the thigh by a raccoon while walking in the woods. The examination reveals a wound that is 1 cm deep on his right thigh. The wound is oozing bright red blood. Your next best action is to:

    A. Administer high-dose parenteral penicillin.
    B. Initiate antibacterial prophylaxis with amoxicillin with clavulanate.
    C. Give rabies immune globulin and rabies vaccine.
    D. After proper cleansing, suture the wound.

TABLE 3–3.
ACNE MEDICATIONS

Acne Medication	Mechanism of Action	Comments
Benzoyl peroxide cream, lotion, various concentrations	Antimicrobial against *Propionibacterium acnes* as well as comedolytic effects	First-line therapy for mild to moderate inflammatory acne vulgaris Start with low concentration (2.5%), may increase if well-tolerated and full therapeutic effect not achieved
Azelaic acid (Azelex) 20% cream	Likely antimicrobial against *P. acnes*, keratolytic, may alter testosterone metabolism	May be used as first-line therapy in mild to moderate inflammatory acne Initial therapy should be once daily application of cream once a week, then twice daily if tolerated Expect ~ 6 wk therapy before noting improvement Mild skin irritation with redness and dryness is common Watch for hypopigmentation when used in darker-skinned patients
Tretinoin (retinoic acid) gel, cream, various concentrations	Decreases cohesion between epidermal cells, increases epidermal cell turnover, transforms closed to open comedones.	First-line therapy for mild to moderate acne vulgaris Acid form of vitamin A Should be used in lowest concentration needed to produce initial slight erythema and peeling During first 4–6 wk, expect comedones to worsen as more lesions visible. Optimal results occur at 8–12 wk Use on dry skin only at least 20 min after face washing to minimize drying effects Photosensitizing; advise patient to use sunscreen

(continued)

TABLE 3–3. (continued)

Acne Medication	Mechanism of Action	Comments
Isotretinoin (Accutane) capsules, various strengths	Likely inhibits sebaceous gland function	Aretinoid (vitamin A analog) Indicated in severe cystic acne treatment when other methods including oral antibiotics are not effective Usual course of treatment is 4–6 mo; discontinue when nodule count reduced by 70%. Repeat course only if needed after 2 mo off drug Prescribing of drug implies that clinician is fully aware of adverse reactions profile, including cheilitis, conjunctivitis, hypertriglyceridemia, dry skin, photosensitivity, and so on Periodically monitor liver enzymes, lipids, complete blood count with differential Potent teratogen; women with reproductive potential need to use highly reliable form of contraception and have periodic evaluation for pregnancy
Oral antibiotics (clindamycin, erythromycin, tetracycline)	Antimicrobial against *P. acnes*	Indicated for the treatment of moderate papular inflammatory acne Titrate up to full prescriptive dose over 1–2 wk; expect clinical improvement in about 2 mo After the skin is clear, taper off slowly over a few months while adding topical antibiotic agents; rapid discontinuation results in return of acne Risk of development of resistant organisms Oral tetracyclines and erythromycin may decrease effectiveness of oral contraceptives and result in pregnancy; advise addition of barrier method and expect breakthrough bleeding

(continued)

TABLE 3–3. (continued)

Acne Medication	Mechanism of Action	Comments
Topical antibiotics (clindamycin, erythromycin, tetracycline)	Antimicrobial against *P. acne*	Indicated in treatment of mild to moderate inflammatory acne vulgaris Less effective than oral antibiotics Generally well tolerated with some local effects such as dryness, burning, pruritus, erythema Risk of development of resistant organisms
Oral contraceptives	Reduction in ovarian androgen production, decreased sebum production	Indicated for treatment of acne vulgaris in women older than age 15 yr who have achieved menarche, desire contraception, have no known contraindications to oral contraceptives, and unresponsive to topical antiacne medications
Metronidazole gel	Likely antimicrobial action	Indicated in treatment of acne rosacea 5–8 wk of therapy needed before clinical improvement is achieved Chronic therapy usually indicated Generally well tolerated with local effects including dryness, burning, stinging

References: Adapted from Gilbert, D., Moellering, R., Sande, M. *The Sanford Guide to Antimicrobial Therapy* (28th ed.). 1998. Vienna, VA: Antimicrobial Therapy, Inc. Pp. 36–51 and Burns, C., Covey, D. (1998). Dermatologic disorders. In Youngkin, E., Savin, K., Kissinger, J., Israel, D. *Pharmacotherapeutics: A primary care clinical guide.* Norwalk, CT: Appleton & Lange. Pp. 569–603.

ANSWERS

17. **B**
18. **C**

DISCUSSION

Bite wounds should not be considered benign or inevitable. Intervention includes education to avoid further bites; therefore, patient history must include a complete history of events leading up to the bite.

All bites should be considered to carry significant infectious risk. This may vary from the relatively low rate of dog bite infection (~5%) to the very high rate with cats (~80%). Initial therapy includes vigorous wound cleansing with antibacterial agents as appropriate and debridement if necessary. Starting short-term prophylactic therapy within 12 hours of the wound should be considered, and tetanus immunization should be updated as needed (Table 3–4).

There has been a recent increase in domestic cases of rabies, primarily from bites by usually docile, often nocturnal wild animals that attack without provocation. These include bats, foxes, woodchucks, squirrels, and skunks. Check with local authorities for information on rabies when a bite involves domestic pets because the rabies risk in this situation is usually negligible, and rabies prophylaxis is not indicated.

Discussion Sources

Hektor Dunphy, L. (1999). *Management Guidelines for Adult Nurse Practitioners*. Philadelphia: FA Davis. Pp. 128–132.
Gilbert, D., Moellering, R., Sande, M. (1998). *The Sanford Guide to Antimicrobial Therapy* (28th ed.). Vienna, VA: Antimicrobial Therapy, Inc.

QUESTIONS

19. A patient presents with a painful blistering burn involving the first, second, and third digits of his right hand. The most appropriate plan of care is to:

    A. Apply an anesthetic cream to area and open the blisters.
    B. Apply silver sulfadiazine cream (Silvadene) to the area and then apply a bulky dressing.
    C. Refer the patient to burn specialty care.
    D. Loosely wrap the burn with a nonadherent dressing and prescribe an analgesic agent.

TABLE 3–4.
INFECTIOUS AGENTS AND TREATMENT IN BITES

Type of Bite	Infective Agent	Prophylaxis or Treatment of Infection
Bat, raccoon, skunk	Uncertain, significant rabies risk	For bacterial infection Primary: Amoxicillin with clavulanate 875 mg/125 mg BID Alternative: Doxycyline 100 mg BID Animal should be considered rabid and given rabies immune globulin and vaccine
Cat	*Pasteurella multocida, Staphylococcus aureus*	Primary: Amoxicillin with clavulanate 875 mg/125 mg BID Alternative: Cefuroxime 0.5 g BID, doxycyline 100 mg orally BID Switch to PCN if *P. multocida* is cultured from wound
Dog	*Viridans* spp., *P. multocida, S. aureus, Bacteroides* spp., others	Primary: Amoxicillin with clavulanate 875 mg/125 mg BID Alternative: Clindamycin 300 mg QID
Human	*Viridans* spp, *Staphylococcus epidermidis, S. corynebacterium, S. aureus, Bacteroides* spp., others	Early, not yet infected Amoxicillin with clavulanate 875 mg/125 mg BID for 5 days Later (3–24 h, signs of infections) Parenteral therapy with amoxicillin with sulbactam, cefoxitin, others
Rat	Streptobacillus monifomis	Primary: Amoxicillin with clavulanate 875 mg/125 mg BID Alternative: Doxycyline Rabies prophylaxis not indicated
Swine	Polymicrobial gram + cocci, gram − bacilli, anaerobes, *Pasteurella* sp.	Primary: Amoxicillin with clavulanate 875 mg/125 mg BID Alternative: Parenteral third-generation cephalosporin, others
Nonhuman primate	Herpes virus simiae	Acyclovir

Reference: Adapted from Gilbert, D., Moellering, R., Sande, M. (1998). *The Sanford Guide to Antimicrobial Therapy* (28th ed.). Vienna, VA: Antimicrobial Therapy, Inc. Pp. 36–51.

20. You examine a patient with a red, tender burn that has excellent capillary refill involving the anterior right leg. The estimated body surface area is appropriately:

    A. 5%

    B. 9%

    C. 13%

    D. 18%

ANSWERS

19. C

20. B

DISCUSSION

As with bites, burn intervention includes asking for a complete history of
the events leading up to the injury to develop a plan for avoiding future
events. In addition, education for burn avoidance for high-risk individuals such as children, the elderly, and smokers should be a routine part of
primary care.

In general, smaller (<10% BSA), minor (second degree or lower) burns
not involving a function area such as the hand or foot and of minimal
cosmetic consequence can be treated in the outpatient setting. Treatment
options include prevention of infection by the use of a topical antibiotic
such as silver sulfodiozine or manfenide acetate. Any burn involving
areas of high function, such as the hands and feet, or of significant cosmetic consequence, such as the face, should be referred promptly to specialty care.

First- and second-degree burns are characterized by erythema, hyper-
emia, and pain. With first-degree burns, the skin blanches with ease;
second-degree burns have blisters and a raw, moist surface. In third-
degree burns, pain may be minimal but the burns are usually surrounded
by areas of painful first- and second-degree burns. The surface of third-
degree burns is usually white and leathery. An important to estimate the
surface area of the body affected by the burn (Fig. 3–1).

Discussion Source

Hektor Dunphy, L. (1999). *Management Guidelines for Adult Nurse Practitioners*. Philadelphia:
FA Davis. Pp. 140–142.

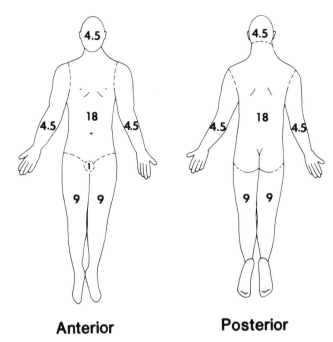

FIG. 3–1. Rule of Nines for calculating total burn surface area. (Adapted from Richard, R. and Staley, M. [1994]. *Burn Care and Rehabilitation* [p. 109]. Philadelphia: FA Davis.)

QUESTIONS

21. The most common causative organisms in cellulitis are:

    A. *Escherichia coli* and *Hemophilus influenzae*
    B. *Bacteroides* species and other anaerobes
    C. group A beta-hemolytic streptococci and *S. aureus*
    D. pathogen viruses

22. Which of the following is the best treatment option for cellulitis?

    A. cephalexin
    B. doxycyline
    C. metronidazole
    D. trimethoprim-sulfa

ANSWERS

21. C
22. A

DISCUSSION

Cellulitis is an acute infection of the subcutaneous tissue and skin. It usually spreads rapidly and is most commonly found in the extremities. The cause is usually a gram-positive organism such as group A beta-hemolytic streptococci and *S. aureus*. On occasion, particularly in immunocompromised individuals, select gram-negative organisms are the causative agent.

The antibiotic for treating cellulitis involves the choice of an agent with strong gram-positive coverage (in streptococci and staphylococci) and stability in the presence of beta-lactamase (in staphylococci). The Sanford Guide recommends the following oral agents, all demonstrating the above characteristics:

- Erythromycin
- A first-generation cephalosporin such as cephalexin (Keflex)
- Amoxicillin with clavulanate (Augmentin)
- Clarithromycin (Biaxin)
- Azithromycin (Zithromax)

Discussion Sources

Hektor Dunphy, L. (1999). *Management Guidelines for Adult Nurse Practitioners*. Philadelphia: FA Davis. Pp. 142–144.
Gilbert, D., Moellering, R., Sande, M. (1998). *The Sanford Guide to Antimicrobial Therapy* (28th ed.). Vienna, VA: Antimicrobial Therapy, Inc.

QUESTIONS

23. The most important aspect of skin care for individuals with atopic dermatitis is:

    A. frequent bathing with antibacterial soap
    B. consistent use of medium- to high-potency topical steroids
    C. application of lubricants
    D. treatment of dermatophytes

24. A common trigger agent for contact dermatitis is/are:

    A. nickel

    B. plastics

    C. soaps

    D. spicy foods

25. One of the more common sites for atopic dermatitis in the adult is:

    A. dorsum of the hand

    B. face

    C. neck

    D. flexor surfaces

ANSWERS

23. C

24. A

25. D

DISCUSSION

Atopic dermatitis, or eczema, is one manifestation of a type I hypersensitivity reaction. This type of reaction is caused when IgE antibodies occupy receptor sites on mast cells. This causes a degradation of the mast cell and subsequent release of histamine, vasodilatation, mucous gland stimulation, and tissue swelling. Within the heading of type I hypersensitivity reaction are two subgroups, atopy and anaphylaxis.

Within the atopy subgroup are a number of common clinical conditions, such as allergic rhinitis, atopic dermatitis, allergic gastroenteropathy, and allergy-based asthma. Atopic diseases have a strong familial component and tend to cause localized rather than systemic reactions. Individuals with atopic disease are often able to identify allergy-inducing agents. Treatment for atopic dermatitis includes

- Avoiding offending agents
- Minimizing skin dryness by limiting soap and water exposure
- Consistently using lubricants
- Treating the skin with care because it tends to be sensitive

When flare-ups occur, the skin eruption is largely caused by histamine release. Antihistamines and topical and systemic corticosteroids should be used to control eczema flare-ups.

Itch is a very distressing symptom; many patients say it is more distressing than pain. It is a cardinal symptom of many forms of dermatitis. Histamine contributes to the development of itching; therefore, antihistamines can provide relief. Pruritus tends to be the worst at night, often causing disturbance in sleep. In particular, providing the patient with a bedtime dose of antihistamine can yield tremendous relief of itch and improved sleep. Hydroxyzine (Atarax) appears to provide somewhat better relief of itch than other antihistamines. Certirizine (Zyrtec) is a nonsedating antihistamine that is a metabolite of hydroxyzine.

With an acute flare-up of eczema or with contact dermatitis, an intermediate- to higher-potency topical steroid is usually needed to control acute symptoms. After this is achieved, the lowest-potency topical steroid that yields the desired effect should be used (see Table 3–2).

Discussion Source

Hektor Dunphy, L. (1999). *Management Guidelines for Adult Nurse Practitioners.* Philadelphia: FA Davis. Pp. 127–149.

QUESTIONS

26. A 38-year-old woman with advanced HIV disease presents with a chief complaint of a painful, itchy rash over her trunk. Examination reveals linear vesicular lesions that do not cross the midline and are distributed over the posterior thorax. This is most consistent with:

    A. herpes zoster
    B. dermatitis herpetiformis
    C. molluscum contagiosum
    D. impetigo

27. A 17-year-old patient presents with a 48-hour history of a mildly pruritic, painful, 3-cm, round vesicular lesion on the right upper lip. The lesion exudes a small amount of serous fluid, and Tzanck smear is positive for giant multinucleated cells. This most likely represents a lesion caused by:

    A. herpes virus
    B. *S. aureus*
    C. streptococci
    D. allergic reaction

28. When caring for an adult with an outbreak of shingles, you advise that:

   A. There is no known treatment for this condition.

   B. During outbreaks, the chickenpox virus is shed.

   C. Although they are acutely painful, the lesions will heal well without scarring or lingering discomfort.

   D. This condition commonly strikes young and old alike.

ANSWERS

26. A
27. A
28. B

DISCUSSION

Herpes zoster infection, commonly known as shingles, is an acutely painful condition caused by the varicella-zoster virus, the same agent that causes chickenpox. The virus lies dormant in the dorsal root ganglia of a dermatome. When activated, the characteristic blistering lesions occur along a dermatome, not crossing the midline. Any person who has had chicken pox is at risk for shingles. However, it is usually seen in those of advanced age, those who are immunocompromised, or those with some other underlying health problem. When shingles is seen in younger adults, the possibility of HIV infection should be considered. During the acute attack, the chickenpox (varicella-zoster) virus is shed; therefore, patients may transmit this infection. Shingles, however, is not communicable person to person.

   Diagnosis of shingles is usually straightforward because of its characteristic lesions. If confirmation is needed, Tzanck smear will reveal giant multinucleated cells, a finding in all herpetic infections.

   Scarring and post-herpetic neuralgia are problematic sequelae of shingles. Initiating antiviral therapy with high-dose acyclovir (Zovirax), valacyclovir (Valtrex), or famciclovir (Famvir) preferably within the first 72 hours of herpes zoster outbreak helps limit the severity of the lesions as well as minimize the risk of postherpetic neuralgia and scarring.

   Adequate analgesia should be offered to the person with shingles. Using a combination of topical agents such as Burow's solution along with a high-potency nonsteroidal anti-inflammatory drug or opioid, or both, helps provide considerable relief. The patient should also be monitored for suprainfection of lesions. Because of the risk of complication and possible compromise of vision, expert consultation should be sought if herpes zoster involves a facial dermatome. NSAIDs should not be prescribed during varicella infection because of the risk of necrotizing fasciitis.

Discussion Source

Hektor Dunphy, L. (1999). *Management Guidelines for Adult Nurse Practitioners*. Philadelphia: FA Davis. Pp. 149–151.

QUESTIONS

29. When prescribing itraconazole (Sporanox), the NP considers that:

    A. The drug is a cytochrome P450 3A4 inhibitor.
    B. One pulse cycle is recommended for fingernail treatment, and two cycles are needed for toenail therapy.
    C. Continuous therapy is preferred in the presence of hepatic disease.
    D. Taking the drug on an empty stomach enhances the efficacy of the product.

30. When prescribing pulse dosing with itraconazole (Sporonox) for the treatment of fingernail fungus, the NP realizes that:

    A. A transient increase in AST levels may be seen.
    B. Drug-induced leukopenia is a common problem.
    C. The patient needs to be warned about excessive bleeding because of the drug's antiplatelet effect.
    D. Its use is contraindicated in the presence of iron-deficiency anemia

31. In diagnosing onychomycosis, the NP considers that:

    A. Nails often have a single midline groove.
    B. Pitting is often seen.
    C. Microscopic examination reveals hyphae.
    D. Beau's lines are present.

ANSWERS

29. A
30. A
31. C

DISCUSSION

Onychomycosis, or dermatophytosis of the nail, is a chronic disfiguring disorder. The nails are dull, thickened, and lusterless with a pithy consistency. Parts of the nail often break off. Because trauma and other conditions can cause a similar appearance, confirmation of the diagnosis with microscopic examination for hyphae of the nail scrapings mixed with potassium hydroxide (KOH) is important.

Until recently, therapeutic options were limited. Topical treatment proved to be of little value because the fungal agent is held within the nail matrix. Oral products such as griseofulvin required months of therapy because the drug was taken up by the developing nailbed and still yielded a high rate of relapse.

Antifungals such as itraconazole (Sporanox) and terbinafine (Lamsil) offer well-tolerated effective treatment for fingernail and toenail fungal infections. Both can be used in pulse cycles, with alternating times of drug use and then abstinent periods. An example of pulse dosing is itraconazole 400 mg daily for the first week of the month for 2 months to treat the fingernails and for 3 months to treat the toenails. These products are held within the nail matrix for months after therapy; this gives effective treatment at a considerably reduced cost when compared with constant therapy. In addition, all oral antifungals have hepatotoxic potential and may cause an increase in AST levels. However, pulse therapy lessens this risk considerably.

Caution is needed when prescribing itraconazole because it inhibits by cytochrome P450 3A4, a pathway also used by drugs such as diazepam, digoxin, anticoagulants, and certain HIV protease inhibitors. When these agents attempt to use this metabolic pathway, levels of both potentially increase, causing toxicity. Terbinafine has significantly fewer drug interactions.

Discussion Source

Hektor Dunphy, L. (1999). *Management Guidelines for Adult Nurse Practitioners.* Philadelphia: FA Davis. Pp. 151–152.

QUESTIONS

32. A 78-year-old woman resident of a long-term care facility complains of generalized itchiness at night that disturbs her sleep. Her examination is consistent with scabies. Which of the following do you expect to find on examination?

    A. excoriated papules on the interdigital area
    B. annular lesions over the buttocks
    C. vesicular lesions in a linear pattern
    D. honey-crusted lesions that began as vesicles

33. Which of the following represents the most accurate patient advice when using permethrin (Elimite) for treating scabies?

    A. To avoid systemic absorption, the medication should be applied over the body and rinsed off within 1 hour.
    B. The patient will notice a marked reduction in pruritus within 48 hours of using the product.
    C. Itch often persists for a few weeks after successful treatment.
    D. It is a second-line product in the treatment of scabies.

34. When advising the patient about scabies contagion, you inform her that:

    A. Mites can live for a number of weeks away from the host.
    B. Close personal contact with an infected person is usually needed to contract this disease.
    C. Casual contact with an infected person is likely to result in infestation.
    D. Bedding used by an infected person must be destroyed.

ANSWERS

32. A
33. C
34. B

DISCUSSION

Scabies is a communicable skin disease generally requiring close person contact, such as sexual relations, to achieve contagion. However, contact with used, unwashed bedding and clothing from an infected person can result in infection. As a result, bedclothes and other items used by a person with scabies must be either washed in hot water or placed in a clothes dryer for a normal cycle. As an alternative, items can be placed in plastic storage bags for at least 1 week because mites do not survive for more than 3 to 4 days without contact with the host. Mites tend to burrow in areas of warmth, such as the finger webs, axillary folds, belt line, areola, scrotum, and penis, with lesions developing in these areas. They may start with the characteristic burrows but usually progress to a vesicular or papular form, often with excoriation caused by scratching.

Permethrin (Elimite) lotion is the preferred method of treatment for scabies. The lotion must be left on for 8 to 14 hours to be effective. Despite effective therapy, individuals with scabies often have a significant problem with pruritus after permethrin treatment because of the presence of dead mites and their waste trapped in the skin, which causes an inflammatory reaction. This debris is eliminated from the body over a few weeks; therefore, the distress of itchiness passes at that time. Oral antihistamines, particularly for nighttime use, and medium-potency topical steroids should be offered to help with this problem (Table 3–5). In the past, lidane (Kwell) was used, but this product presents potential problems with neurotoxicity and a resulting seizure risk as well as lower efficacy. In particular, lidane should not be used by pregnant women, children, and the elderly.

Discussion Source

Hektor Dunphy, L. (1999). *Management Guidelines for Adult Nurse Practitioners*. Philadelphia: FA Davis. Pp. 156–157.

QUESTIONS

35. You examine a patient with psoriasis and expect to find the following lesions:

    A. lichenified areas in flexor areas
    B. red, well-demarcated plaques on the knees
    C. greasy lesions throughout the scalp
    D. vesicular lesions over the upper thorax

TABLE 3–5.
MEDICATIONS USED IN THE TREATMENT
OF IgE-MEDIATED HYPERSENSITIVITY REACTION

Medications	Mechanism of Action	Comments
Antihistamines	Antagonize H$_1$ receptor sites	First-generation products (diphenhydramine [Benadryl], chlorpheniramine [ChlorTrimeton]) Second-generation products (Loratadine [Claritin], certirizine [Zyrtec], fexofenadine [Allergra])
Cromolyn sodium (Nasalcrom, Intal)	Halts degradation of mast cells and release of histamine and other inflammatory mediators (mast cell stabilizer)	Prevents rather than treats allergic reactions; need consistent use to be helpful
Topical corticosteroids (nasal sprays, inhaled via MDI)	Inhibit eosinophilic action and other inflammatory mediators, potentiate effects of beta$_2$ agonists	Prevents rather than treats allergic reactions; need consistent use to be helpful
Epinephrine	Alpha, beta$_1$, beta$_2$, agonists; potent vasoconstrictor, cardiac stimulant, bronchodilator	Initial therapy for anaphylaxis because of its multiple modes of reversing airway and circulatory dysfunction Anaphylaxis usually responds quickly to 0.3–0.5 mL SC of 1:1000 solution Use with caution in the presence of cardiac disease
Oral corticosteroids	Inhibit eosinophilic action and other inflammatory mediators	In higher dose and with longer therapy (> 2 wk), adrenal suppression may occur No taper needed if use is short-term (< 10 days) and at lower dose (prednisone 40–60 mg/d) Potential for causing gastropathy

36. Psoriatic lesions are caused by:

A. decreased exfoliation

B. rapid cell turnover leading to decreased maturation and keratinization

C. inflammatory changes

D. lichenification

37. Anthralin (Dithrocreme) is helpful in treating psoriasis because it has what kind of activity?

A. antimitotic

B. exfoliative

C. vasoconstrictor

D. humectant

ANSWERS

35. B

36. B

37. A

DISCUSSION

Psoriasis is a chronic skin disorder caused by accelerated mitosis and rapid cell turnover leading to decreased maturation and keratinization. This process prevents the dermal cells from "sticking" together, allowing for a shedding of cells as the characteristic silvery scales and leaving an underlying red plaque. Psoriasis is typically found in extensor surfaces; therefore, it is most often found in plaquelike lesions over the elbows and knees. The scalp and other surfaces are occasionally involved.

Topical corticosteroids have some antimitotic activity, which allows for regression of psoriatic plaques. It is often effective to use a medium- to high-potency drug for short periods of time until the plaques resolve and then to use a lower-potency product three to four times a week to maintain remission. As with all dermatoses, consistent use of high-potency topical steroids is discouraged. Tar preparations can be very helpful, but they have a low level of patient acceptance because of their messiness and odor.

Additional treatment options include use of antralin (Dithrocreme), an antimitotic, and calciprotriene, a vitamin D_3 derivative. Although they do offer effective psoriasis therapy, these products are significantly more expensive than topical steroids and tars. Use should be reserved for steroid-resistant cases.

If psoriasis is generalized, covering more than 30% of body surface area, treatment with topical products is difficult and expensive. Ultraviolet B light exposure three times weekly is highly effective. Access to this care involves referral to a dermatologist. In addition, PUVA (psoralen plus ultraviolet light A) is effective in long-term management of widespread psoriasis, but it is associated with an increase in skin cancer risk.

For severe, recalcitrant psoriasis, cyclosporine, methotrexate, and systemic retinoid are also used. Referral to a dermatologist with expertise in prescribing these agents is indicated for these patients.

Discussion Source

Hektor Dunphy, L. (1999). *Management Guidelines for Adult Nurse Practitioners*. Philadelphia: FA Davis. Pp. 154–156.

QUESTIONS

38. Which of the following best describes seborrheic dermatitis lesions?

   A. flaking lesions in the antecubital and popliteal spaces
   B. greasy, scaling lesions within the scalp
   C. intensely itchy lesions in the groin folds
   D. silvery lesions on the elbows and knees

39. In counseling a patient with seborrheic dermatitis on efforts to clear lesions, you advise her to:

   A. Use antifungal preparations.
   B. Apply petroleum jelly nightly to affected area.
   C. Coat the area with high-potency steroid cream three times a week.
   D. Periodically expose the lesions to sunlight.

ANSWERS

38. B
39. A

DISCUSSION

Seborrheic dermatitis is a chronic, recurrent skin condition found in areas with a high concentration of sebaceous glands, such as the scalp, eyelid margins, nasolabial folds, ears, and upper trunk. A number of theories are proposed for its cause. Because of the lesions' response to antifungal agents, the backbone of therapy, seborrheic dermatitis is most likely caused by an inflammatory reaction to *Pityrosporium ovale*, a yeast present in the scalp of all humans. Further supporting this hypothesis is the fact that seborrhea is often found in immunocompromised patients and in those who are chronically ill (e.g., the elderly population and those with Parkinson's disease).

The use of lubricants such as petroleum jelly may help remove stubborn lesions so the lesions can be exposed to antifungal therapy (e.g., selenium sulfide or ketaconazole shampoo), but this does not constitute first-line therapy. As with any skin condition, high-potency topical corticosteroid use is discouraged because of the risk of subcutaneous atrophy, telegiectatic vessels, and other problems. Although seborrhea usually worsens in the winter and improves in the summer, exposing lesions to sunlight is not recommended because of the potential increase in skin cancer risk.

Discussion Source

Hektor Dunphy, L. (1999). *Management Guidelines for Adult Nurse Practitioners*. Philadelphia: FA Davis. Pp. 157–159.

QUESTIONS

40. A 49-year-old man presents with a lesion suspicious for malignant melanoma. You describe it as having:

    A. deep black-brown coloring throughout
    B. sharp borders
    C. a diameter of 3 mm or less
    D. variable pigmentation

41. A 72-year-old woman presents with a newly formed, painless, pearly, ulcerated nodule with an overlying telangiectasis on the upper lip. This most likely represents a (an):

    A. actinic keratosis
    B. basal cell carcinoma
    C. squamous cell carcinoma
    D. molluscum contagiosum

42. Which of the following represents the most effective method of cancer screening?

   A. skin examination
   B. stool for occult blood
   C. pelvic examination
   D. chest radiography

43. Risk factors for malignant melanoma include:

   A. Asian ancestry
   B. history of blistering sunburn
   C. use of sunscreen in childhood
   D. presence of atopic dermatitis

44. Actinic keratoses can be described as a(n):

   A. slightly rough pink or flesh-colored lesion in a sun-exposed area
   B. well-defined, slightly raised, red, scaly plaque in a skinfold
   C. blistering lesion along a dermatome
   D. crusting lesion along flexor aspects of the fingers

45. Treatment options for actinic keratoses include topical:

   A. hydrocortisone
   B. fluorouracil
   C. acyclovir
   D. doxepin

ANSWERS

40. D
41. B
42. A
43. B
44. A
45. B

DISCUSSION

As with any area of dermatology, accurate diagnosis of a condition depends on knowledge of the description of the lesion as well as its most likely site of occurrence. The most potent risk factor for any skin cancer is sun exposure; instructing patients on sun avoidance and the consistent use of high SPF sunscreen is critical.

Skin examination has the benefit of allowing the examiner to be able to detect premalignant lesions (e.g., actinic keratoses and precursor lesions to squamous cell carcinoma) as well as malignant lesions. Treatment of actinic keratoses, also known as solar keratoses, includes cryotherapy with liquid nitrogen. This causes the lesions to crust for about 2 weeks, revealing healed tissue with excellent cosmetic outcome. An alternative is the use of 1% to 5% fluorouracil creams once a day for 2 to 3 weeks until the lesions become crusted over. As an alternative, 5% fluorouracil cream can be used once a day for 1 to 2 consecutive days weekly for 7 to 10 weeks. This will yield a similar therapeutic outcome without crusting or discomfort.

The American Cancer Society proposes the "ABCD" mnemonic for assessing malignant melanoma.

A = Asymmetric with nonmatching sides
B = Borders are irregular
C = Color is not uniform; brown, black, red, white, blue
D = Diameter usually >6 mm, or the size a pencil eraser

A similar memory aid for squamous and basal cell carcinoma is as follows:

For Basal cell carcinoma ("PUT ON S"unscreen):

P = Pearly papule
U = Ulcerating
T = Telagiectasia
O = On the face, scalp, pinnae
N = Nodule
S = Slow growing

Squamous cell carcinoma—Early lesions ("NO SUN"):

N = Nodular
O = Opaque
S = Sun-exposed areas
U = Ulcerating
N = Nondistinct borders

Later lesions may also include:

    Scale
    Firm margins

Treatment of skin cancers usually involves removal of the lesion. Further therapy is guided by the histologic diagnosis.

Discussion Source

Hektor Dunphy, L. (1999). *Management Guidelines for Adult Nurse Practitioners*. Philadelphia: FA Davis. Pp. 159–162.

QUESTIONS

46. Which of the following is the most frequent cause of stasis ulcers?

    A. arterial insufficiency
    B. venous insufficiency
    C. diabetes mellitus
    D. fungal dermatitis

47. You examine the left lower extremity of a patient and find an ulcerated lesion with irregular borders and edema with brown discoloration of the surrounding tissue. The best treatment option at this time is:

    A. compression therapy
    B. referral for surgical debridement
    C. daily use of a topical antibiotic cream
    D. application of a dry, sterile dressing

48. A 70-year-old man presents with absent popliteal pulses and a cool, hairless foot with a 2-cm ulcer that has a "punched-out" appearance on the dorsum of the second toe. The appropriate next measure is to:

    A. arrange for evaluation by a vascular surgeon
    B. apply wet to dry dressings
    C. start the patient on a peripheral vasodilator
    D. advise the patient to elevate his feet 15 minutes three times a day

ANSWERS

46. B
47. A
48. A

DISCUSSION

Stasis ulcers are most commonly caused by venous insufficiency. They may also be caused far less commonly by arterial insufficiency, diabetes mellitus, and fungal infections. Because poor venous return causes lower extremity edema, which leads to decreased tissue perfusion and the resulting risk of ulcer, compression therapy is key to successful therapy. Debridement is needed only when necrotic tissue is present, and antimicrobial therapy is needed when there are signs of infection. Venous stasis ulcers usually respond well to occlusive hydroactive dressings such as Duoderm. In addition, an Unna boot can help but requires weekly changing. Regardless of the treatment chosen, venous stasis ulcers require long-term care, including good nutrition and expert wound management. Involving home help care and wound care management nursing experts greatly enhances success.

The patient in Question 48 clearly has peripheral arterial disease. The treatment of choice is revascularization of the limb to enhance circulation. This is the only treatment option that will result in resolution of the lesion (see Chapter 9 for additional information).

Discussion Source

Hektor Dunphy, L. (1999). *Management Guidelines for Adult Nurse Practitioners*. Philadelphia: FA Davis. Pp. 162–163.

QUESTIONS

49. Which of the following do you expect to find in the assessment of the person with urticaria?

    A. eosinophilia
    B. depressed sedimentation rate
    C. elevated thyroid stimulate hormone level
    D. leukopenia

50. A 24-year-old woman presents with hive-form linear lesions that form over areas where she has scratched. These resolve within a few minutes. They most likely represent:

   A. dermographism

   B. contact dermatitis

   C. angioedema

   D. allergic reaction

ANSWERS

49. A

50. A

DISCUSSION

Urticaria is a condition in which eruptions of wheals or hives occur most often in response to allergen exposure. The most common cause is a type I hypersensitivity reaction. This type of reaction is caused when IgE antibodies occupy receptor sites on mast cells. This causes a degradation of the mast cell and subsequent release of histamine, vasodilatation, mucous gland stimulation, and tissue swelling. Treatment of type I hypersensitivity includes avoidance of the provoking agent as well as antihistamines and steroids. Within the heading of type I hypersensitivity are two subgroups, atopy and anaphylaxis.

Within the atopy subgroup are a number of common clinical conditions such as allergic rhinitis, atopic dermatitis, allergic gastroenteropathy, and allergy-based asthma. Atopic diseases have a strong familial component and tend to cause localized rather than systemic reactions. The person with atopic disease is often able to identify allergy-inducing agents. Treatment for atopic disease includes avoidance of offending agents, antihistamines, corticosteroids, and mast cell stabilizers such as cromolyn sodium (Intal, Nasalcrom) and nedocromil (Tilade).

Anaphylaxis typically causes a systemic IgE-mediated reaction in response to exposure to an allergen, often a drug (e.g., penicillin) insect venom (e.g., bee sting), or food (e.g., peanuts) allergy. Anaphylaxis is characterized by widespread vasodilatation, urticaria, angioedema, and bronchospasm, creating a life-threatening condition of airway obstruction coupled with circulatory collapse. First-line treatment includes avoiding or discontinuing use of the offending agent. Simultaneously, maintaining airway patency as well as adequate circulation is critical. Angioedema and urticaria are subcutaneous anaphylactic reactions but are not life threatening unless tissue swelling impinges on the airway (see Table 3–5).

Discussion Source

Hektor Dunphy, L. (1999). *Management Guidelines for Adult Nurse Practitioners*. Philadelphia: FA Davis. Pp. 165–166.

QUESTION

51. When counseling a person who has a 2-mm verruca on the hand, you advise that:

    A. Bacteria are the most common cause of these lesions.
    B. Most lesions will resolve without therapy in 12 to 24 months.
    C. There is a significant risk for future dermatologic malignancy.
    D. Surgical excision is the treatment of choice.

ANSWER

51. B

DISCUSSION

Verruca vulgaris lesions are also known as warts. The majority of them are caused by human papillomavirus, which is passed through direct person-to-person contact. Over a 12- to 24-month period, nearly all of these lesions resolve without therapy. Surgical excision is rarely indicated. Intervention is warranted if warts interfere with function, such as with painful plantar warts on the soles of the feet, or if they are cosmetically problematic (Table 3–6).

Discussion Source

Hektor Dunphy, L. (1999). *Management Guidelines for Adult Nurse Practitioners*. Philadelphia: FA Davis. Pp. 166–168.

TABLE 3–6.
TREATMENT OPTIONS FOR WARTS

Treatment	Instruction for Use	Comments
Liquid nitrogen	Apply to achieve a thaw time of 20–45 sec Two freeze-thaw cycles may be given every 2–4 wk until lesion gone	Usually good cosmetic results. Can be painful, requires multiple treatments.
Keratolytic agents (Occlusal, Duofilm, Duoplast, others)	Apply as directed until lesions resolved	May need long-term therapy before resolution. Well tolerated. With plantar warts, pare down lesion, then apply 40% salicylic acid plaster, changing every 5 days.
Podophyllum resin (Podofilox)	Apply 3 times a week by patient for 4–6 wk	Apply 3 times a week by patient for 4–6 wk.
Tretinoin	Apply BID to flat warts for 4–6 wk	Needs consistent treatment for optimal results.
Laser therapy	Used to dissect lesions	Needs 4–6 wk to granulate tissue. Best reserved for treatment-resistant warts.

Reference: Adapted from Hektor Dunphy, L. (1999). *Management Guidelines for Adult Nurse Practitioners.* Philadelphia: FA Davis. Pp. 166–168.

4

CHAPTER

Head and Neck
Disorders

QUESTIONS

1. A 74-year-old woman has hypertension that is normally well controlled by hydrochlorothiazide. She presents with a 3-day history of unilateral throbbing headache with difficulty chewing because of pain. On physical examination, you find a tender, noncompressible temporal artery. Blood pressure (BP) = 170/98, apical pulse (AP) = 98, and respiratory rate (RR) = 22, and she is visibly uncomfortable. The most likely diagnosis is:

   A. giant cell arteritis
   B. impending transient ischemic attack
   C. migraine headache
   D. temporal mandibular joint dysfunction

2. Diagnostic tests for the patient in Question 1 should include:

   A. head computed tomography (CT) with contrast
   B. magnetic resonance imaging (MRI)
   C. ultrasound of the temporal artery
   D. sedimentation rate

3. Therapeutic interventions for the patient in Question 1 should include:

   A. steroids for a number of months
   B. addition of nisoldipine to her antihypertensive regimen
   C. warfarin therapy
   D. carbamazepine

4. Concomitant disease seen with giant cell arteritis includes:

   A. polymyalgia rheumatica
   B. pancreatitis
   C. psoriatic arthritis
   D. Reiter's syndrome

5. One of the most serious complications of giant cell arteritis is:

A. hemiparesis
B. arthritis
C. blindness
D. uveitis

ANSWERS

1. A
2. D
3. A
4. A
5. C

DISCUSSION

Giant cell or temporal arteritis is most common in patients who are 50 to 85 years old; average age at onset is 70 years. The headache is classically described as unilateral, surrounding the affected artery, and distressing.

Giant cell arteritis is a systemic disease affecting medium- and large-sized vessels. It also causes inflammation of the temporal artery because extracranial branches of the carotid artery are often involved; this is often a site of tenderness or a nodular, pulseless vessel. However, the temporal artery may be normal. Giant cell arteritis and polymyalgia rheumatica may represent two parts of a spectrum of disease and are often found together.

Apart from relieving pain, treatment of giant cell arteritis helps minimize the risk of blindness, which is the most serious complication of the disease. As soon as the diagnosis is made, steroid therapy should be initiated; this therapy typically lasts 6 months to 2 years.

In the absence of symptoms of polymyalgia rheumatica, diagnosis of giant cell arteritis includes temporal artery biopsy and sedimentation rate. At least 3 to 5 cm of artery is needed because the disease frequently skips portions of the vessel. Sedimentation rate, although it is a nonspecific test of inflammation, is usually markedly elevated.

The blood pressure of the patient in Question 1 is probably elevated because of pain response. Analgesia should be given and then BP response should be noted again. Adding a second antihypertensive agent to this patient's treatment ignores the most likely underlying cause of her BP elevation.

Discussion Sources

Hektor Dunphy, L. (1999). *Management Guidelines for Adult Nurse Practitioners*. Philadelphia: FA Davis. Pp. 175–176.
Hellman, D., Stone, J. (1999). Arthritis and musculoskeletal disorder. In Tierney, L., McPhee, S., & Papadakis, M. *Current Diagnosis and Treatment* (38th ed.). Stamford, CT: Appleton & Lange. Pp. 786–837.

QUESTIONS

6. An 88-year-old community-dwelling man who lives alone has limited mobility because of osteoarthritis. Since his last visit 2 months ago, he has lost 5% of his body weight and has developed angular chelitis. You expect to find the following on examination:

   A. fissuring and cracking at the corners of the mouth
   B. marked erythema of the hard and soft palate
   C. white plaques on the lateral borders of the buccal mucosa
   D. raised, painless lesions on the gingiva

7. First-line therapy for angular chelitis therapy includes the use of:

   A. metronidazole gel
   B. hydrocortisone cream
   C. topical nystatin
   D. oral ketoconazole

ANSWERS

6. A
7. C

DISCUSSION

A variety of oral infections are caused by *Candida* species, including angular chelitis. The primary risk factors for oral candidiasis is immunocompromise, whether caused by advanced age and apparent malnutrition (as with the patient in Question 6) or as seen in HIV infection.

Topical antifungals such as nystatin offer a reasonable first-line treatment for oral candidiasis. With particularly recalcitrant conditions and failure of topical therapy, systemic antifungals may be needed. Treatment of the underlying condition is critical.

Discussion Source

Hektor Dunphy, L. (1999). *Management Guidelines for Adult Nurse Practitioners*. Philadelphia: FA Davis. Pp. 177–179.

QUESTIONS

8. A 19-year-old man presents with conjunctivitis. He complains of a red, irritated right eye for the past 48 hours with an eyelid that was "stuck together" this morning when he awoke. This is most consistent with conjunctival inflammation caused by a(n):

   A. bacteria
   B. virus
   C. allergen
   D. injury

9. A 19-year-old woman presents with conjunctivitis. She complains of bilaterally itchy, red eyes with tearing that occurs intermittently throughout the year and is often accompanied by clear nasal discharge. This is most consistent with conjunctival inflammation caused by a(n):

   A. bacteria
   B. virus
   C. allergen
   D. injury

10. Common causative organisms of acute bacterial conjunctivitis include all of the following except:

    A. *Staphylococcus aureus*
    B. *Haemophilus influenzae*
    C. *Streptococcus pneumoniae*
    D. *Pseudomonas aeruginosa*

ANSWERS

8. A
9. C
10. D

DISCUSSION

Although both of these young adults have conjunctivitis, the causes differ. Because therapy in conjunctivitis is in part aimed at eradicating or eliminating the underlying causes, accurate diagnosis is critical. The patient in Question 8 requires antimicrobial therapy, but the patient in Question 9 will benefit from therapy focused on identifying and limiting exposure to specific allergens as well as the appropriate use of antiallergic agents.

Discussion Source

Hektor Dunphy, L. (1999). *Management Guidelines for Adult Nurse Practitioners*. Philadelphia: FA Davis. Pp. 180–181.

QUESTIONS

11. Anterior epistaxis is usually caused by:

    A. hypertension
    B. bleeding disorders
    C. localized nasal mucosa trauma
    D. foreign bodies

12. First-line intervention for anterior epistaxis includes:

    A. nasal packing
    B. application of topical thrombin
    C. firm pressure to the area superior to the nasal alar cartilage
    D. chemical cauterization

ANSWERS

11. C
12. C

DISCUSSION

Anterior epistaxis is usually the result of localized nasal mucosa dryness and trauma and is rarely a result of other causes. Most episodes can be easily managed with simple pressure. If this is ineffective, second-line therapies include nasal packing and cautery. If epistaxis is seen in the presence of a bleeding disorder, topical thrombin should be used.

Discussion Source

Hektor Dunphy, L. (1999). *Management Guidelines for Adult Nurse Practitioners*. Philadelphia: FA Davis. Pp. 183–185.

QUESTION

13. A 58-year-old woman presents with a sudden left-sided headache that is worse in her left eye. Her vision is blurred, and the left pupil is slightly dilated and poorly reactive. The left conjunctiva is markedly injected and the eyeball is firm. The most likely diagnosis is:

    A. unilateral herpetic conjunctivitis
    B. open-angle glaucoma
    C. angle-closure glaucoma
    D. acute iritis

ANSWER

13. C

DISCUSSION

The patient has the triad of an ophthalmologic emergency; a painful, red eye with a visual disturbance. In the case of angle-closure glaucoma, blindness ensues in 3 to 5 days without treatment. Prompt referral to expert ophthalmologic care focused on relieving her acute intraocular pressure is needed. Open-angle glaucoma is a slowly progressive disease that seldom produces symptoms. In acute iritis, another cause of a dully painful red eye with visual change, the pupil is usually constricted and nonreactive.

Discussion Source

Hektor Dunphy, L. (1999). *Management Guidelines for Adult Nurse Practitioners*. Philadelphia: FA Davis. Pp. 186–188.

QUESTIONS

14. Which of the following is a common vision problem in the person with open-angle glaucoma?

    A. peripheral vision loss
    B. blurring of near vision
    C. difficulty with distant vision
    D. need for increased illumination

15. Which of the following is most likely to be found on the funduscopic examination in a patient with angle-closure glaucoma?

    A. excessive cupping of the optic disk
    B. arteriovenous nicking
    C. papilledema
    D. flame-shaped hemorrhages

ANSWERS

14. A
15. A

DISCUSSION

A gradual-onset peripheral vision loss is most specific for glaucoma. Although all of these changes may be seen in patients with advanced open-angle glaucoma, changes in near vision are common as part of the aging process because of hardening of the lens (i.e., presbyopia) and the need for increased illumination. New onset of difficulty with distance vision can be found in patients with cataracts.

Glaucoma, whether open angle or angle closure, is primarily a problem with excessive intraocular pressure, or pressure in front of the optic disk and physiologic cup. As a result, the optic disk and cup are "pushed in," creating the classic finding often called *glaucomatous cupping*. Papilledema, in which the optic disk bulges and the margins are blurred, is seen when there is excessive pressure behind the eye, as in increased intracranial pressure (Fig. 4–1).

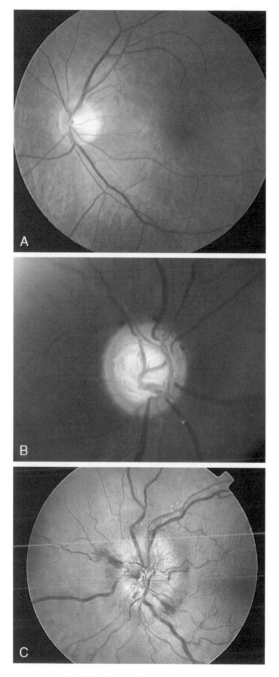

FIG. 4–1. Normal optic disk (A). Optical findings in glaucoma (B). Cupped optic disk in papilledema (C).

Discussion Source

Hektor Dunphy, L. (1999). *Management Guidelines for Adult Nurse Practitioners*. Philadelphia: FA Davis. Pp. 186–188, 192–193.

QUESTION

16. A 17-year-old woman presents with a "pimple" on her right eyelid. Examination reveals a 2-mm pustule on the lateral border of the right eyelid margin. This is most consistent with a:

    A. chalazion
    B. hordeolum
    C. blepharitis
    D. cellulitis

ANSWER

16. B

DISCUSSION

A hordeolum is often called a stye and is usually caused by a staphylococcal infection of a hair follicle on the eyelid. Blepharitis and chalazion are both inflammatory eyelid conditions that may not involve infection. Because treatment regimens for each of these differ significantly, accurate diagnosis is critical. Cellulitis is a serious complication of a hordeolum and is evidenced by widespread redness and edema over the eyelid.

Treatment for a simple hordeolum, or stye, includes warm compresses to the affected eye for 10 minutes, 10 to 15 minutes a day. Erythromycin ophthalmic ointment along the eyelash margin three times a day may accelerate healing. Ophthalmic consultation should be obtained for patients with cellulitis involving the eyelid. Because *S. aureus* is the most common pathogen, treatment options include the use of an antibiotic with gram positive coverage and beta-lactamase stability such as dicloxacillin or a first-generation cephalosporin.

Discussion Sources

Gilbert, D., Moellering, R., Sande, M. (1998). *The Sanford Guide to Antimicrobial Therapy* (28th ed.). Vienna, VA: Antimicrobial Therapy, Inc. P. 8.

Hektor Dunphy, L. (1999). *Management Guidelines for Adult Nurse Practitioners*. Philadelphia: FA Davis. Pp. 191–192.

QUESTIONS

17. Which of the following is true concerning Ménière's disease?

    A. Neuroimaging helps locate the offending cochlear lesion.
    B. Associated high-frequency hearing loss is common.
    C. It is largely a diagnosis of exclusion.
    D. Tinnitus is rarely reported.

18. Prevention and prophylaxis in Ménière's disease includes all of the following except:

    A. avoiding ototoxic drugs
    B. protecting the ears from loud noise
    C. limiting sodium intake
    D. restricting fluid intake

ANSWERS

17. C
18. D

DISCUSSION

Ménière's disease is largely a diagnosis of exclusion: diagnosis is made after other possible causes for the recurrent and often debilitating symptoms of dizziness, tinnitus, and low-frequency hearing loss occur. A distinct causative lesion cannot be identified. It is more common and repeat attacks are more frequent in those with use of otoxic drugs and exposure to loud noise. Limiting sodium intake, although encouraging adequate hydration, may help prevent future episodes.

Discussion Source

Hektor Dunphy, L. (1999). *Management Guidelines for Adult Nurse Practitioners*. Philadelphia: FA Davis. Pp. 193–196.

QUESTIONS

19. You inspect the oral cavity of a 69-year-old man who has a 100 pack-year cigarette smoking history. You find a lesion suspicious for malignancy and describe it as:

    A. raised, red, and painful
    B. a denuded patch with a removable white coating
    C. an ulcerated lesion with indurated margins
    D. a vesicular-form lesion with macerated margins

20. A firm, painless, relatively fixed submandibular node will most likely be seen in the diagnosis of:

    A. herpes simplex
    B. acute otitis media
    C. bacterial pharyngitis
    D. oral cancer

ANSWERS

19. C
20. D

DISCUSSION

Oral cancer, most often squamous cell cancer, is usually characterized by a relatively painless, firm ulceration or raised lesion. Risk factors for oral cancer include tobacco and alcohol abuse. In addition, the lymphadenopathy associated with oral cancer consists of relatively immobile nodes that are not tender when palpated. Self-limiting oral lesions such as herpes simplex, oral candidiasis, and aphthous stomatitis usually cause discomfort. With infection, the associated lymphadenopathy that follows drainage tracts is characterized by tenderness and mobility.

Discussion Source

Hektor Dunphy, L. (1999). *Management Guidelines for Adult Nurse Practitioners*. Philadelphia: FA Davis. Pp. 196–198.

QUESTIONS

21. A 45-year-old man has external otitis. Likely causative pathogens include all of the following except:

    A. fungal agents
    B. *Pseudomonas aeruginosa*
    C. *Staphylococcus aureus*
    D. *Moraxella catarrhalis*

22. Appropriate oral antimicrobial therapy for external otitis includes the:

    A. macrolides
    B. cephalosporins
    C. fluoroquinolones
    D. penicillins

ANSWERS

21. D
22. C

DISCUSSION

External otitis can be caused by a number of infectious agents. However, *Pseudomonas aeruginosa* is the most common causative agent and the most likely organism in refractory otitis externa or auricular cellulitis. Effective topical therapies include Cortisporin otic suspension neomycin and hydro-cortisone solution and VoSol HC 2% (2% nonaqueous acetic acid and hydrocortisone), but the preferred oral antipseudomonal therapy is ciprofloxacin. Fluoroquinolone otitic drops are also available and are highly effective in treating external otitis.

Discussion Source

Hektor Dunphy, L. (1999). *Management Guidelines for Adult Nurse Practitioners*. Philadelphia: FA Davis. P. 200.

QUESTIONS

23. A 25-year-old woman has a 3-day history of left ear pain after a week of upper respiratory infection (URI) symptoms. On physical examination, you find that she has acute otitis media. She is allergic to penicillin (it causes a hive-form reaction). Likely causative organisms in otitis media include:

    A. select gram-positive and -negative bacteria
    B. gram-negative bacteria and pathogenic viruses
    C. rhinovirus and *Staphylococcus aureus*
    D. predominantly beta lactamase-producing organisms

24. Expected findings in acute otitis media include:

    A. prominent bony landmarks
    B. tympanic membrane immobility
    C. itchiness and crackling in the affected ear
    D. submental lymphadenopathy

25. Which of the following represents the best choice of clinical agents for the patient in Question 23?

    A. ciprofloxacin
    B. clarithromycin
    C. amoxicillin
    D. cefixime

26. A reasonable treatment option for recurrent otitis media that does not respond to amoxicillin therapy is:

    A. cefixime
    B. erythromycin
    C. cephalexin
    D. sulfisoxazole

ANSWERS

23. A
24. B
25. B
26. A

DISCUSSION

The most common causative organisms in otitis media are *S. pneumoniae*, *H. influenzae*, *M. catarrhalis*, and various rhinoviruses. Ordinarily, amoxicillin is the antibiotic of choice. However, this patient has a significant penicillin allergy. Thus, an alternative product must be chosen, such as clarithromycin (Table 4–1).

Tympanic membrane immobility is the hallmark of acute otitis media (AOM). Itching and crackling in the ear is common in patients with AOM as well as in those with serous otitis, also known as otitis media with effusion. The bony landmarks usually appear prominent when the tympanic membrane is retracted, a condition usually seen with Eustachian tube dysfunction that may not be present in patients with AOM. The submental node is not in the drainage tract of the middle ear and therefore is not enlarged in patients with AOM. Rather, the nodes within the anterior cervical chain on the ipsilateral side of the infection are often enlarged and painful.

The organisms that cause recurrent otitis media are the same ones that cause acute disease. If amoxicillin fails to eradicate the infection, the issue of a predominant beta-lactamase–producing organism such as *H. influenzae* or *M. catarrhalis* should be considered. As a result, it is necessary to choose a product such as cefixime, a third-generation cephalosporin that is beta-lactamase stable.

Discussion Source

Hektor Dunphy, L. (1999). *Management Guidelines for Adult Nurse Practitioners*. Philadelphia: FA Davis. Pp. 200–205.

QUESTIONS

27. An 18-year-old woman has a chief complaint of a "sore throat and swollen glands" for the past 3 days. Her physical examination includes a temperature of 101°F, exudative pharyngitis, and tender anterior cervical lymphadenopathy. Right and left upper quadrant abdominal tenderness is absent. The most likely diagnosis is:

    A. *Streptococcus pyogenes* pharyngitis
    B. infectious mononucleosis
    C. viral pharyngitis
    D. Vincent's infection

TABLE 4–1.
RECOMMENDATIONS FOR TREATING COMMON
BACTERIAL EAR, EYE, SINUS, AND PHARYNX INFECTIONS

Site of Infection	Common Pathogens	Recommended Antibiotic Treatments
External otitis	*Pseudomonas* spp., *Proteus* spp.	Polymixin B, neomycin, hydrocortisone ear drops, Fluoroquinolone otic drops
Malignant otitis externa	*Pseudomonas* spp.	Oral ciprofloxacin for early disease suitable for outpatient therapy
Acute otitis media	Pneumococci, *H. influenzae* (nontypable), *M. catarrhalis,* viral	Primary: Amoxicillin, trimethoprim-sulfa, amoxicillin with clavulanate (Augmentin), second-generation cephalosporin (Cefprozil [Cefzil], cefpodoxime [Vantin], cefuroxime [Ceftin]), third-generation cephalosporin (cefixime [Suprax], cefibutien [Cedax]), single-dose intramuscular ceftriaxone Alternative: Azithromycin (Zithromax), clarithromycin (Bioxin), trimethoprim-sulfamethoxasole (Bactrim)
Acute bacterial rhinosinusitis	Pneumococci, *H. influenzae* (nontypable), *M. catarrhalis,* Group A streptococci, anaerobes, *S. aureus,* viral	Primary: Amoxicillin with clavulanate (Augmentin), second-generation cephalosporin (Cefprozil [Cefzil], cefpodoxime [Vantin], cefuroxime [Ceftin]), trimethoprim-sulfa, third-generation cephalosporin (cefixime [Suprax], cefibutien [Cedax]), single-dose intramuscular ceftriaxone Alternative: Clarithromycin (Biaxin), azithromycin (Zithromax)

(continued)

TABLE 4-1. (continued)

Site of Infection	Common Pathogens	Recommended Antibiotic Treatments
Recurrent, persistent, prolonged otitis media	Pneumococci, *H. influenzae* (non-typable), *M. catarrhalis*, viral	Consider resistant organism Amoxicillin with clavulanate (Augmentin), second-generation cephalosporin (cefuroxime [Ceftin]), third-generation cephalosporin (cefixime [Suprax])
Exudative pharyngitis	Group A, C, G streptococci	Primary: Penicillin V orally or benzathine penicillin intra-muscularly Alternative: Erythromycin or second-generation cephalosporin, azithromycin, clarith-romycin
Nongonococcal bacterial conjunctivitis	*S. aureus, S. pneumoniae, H. influenzae*	Primary: Ophthalmologic erythromycin, bacitracin (Polymixin B) Alternative: Tobramycin, ciprofloxacin, Polymixin-trimethoprin

Reference: Gilbert, D., Moellering, R., Sande, M. (1998). *The Sanford Guide to Antimicrobial Therapy* (28th ed.). Vienna, VA: Antimicrobial Therapy, Inc. P. 8.

28. The next action in providing care for this patient should be:

    A. provide advice on using over-the-counter analgesic agents
    B. initiate penicillin therapy
    C. obtain a throat culture and inform the patient that you will contact her about therapy when the results are available
    D. use salt water gargles

29. Treatment options for streptococcal pharyngitis for a patient with penicillin allergy include all of the following except:

    A. azithromycin
    B. trimethoprim-sulfa
    C. clarithromycin
    D. erythromycin

ANSWERS

27. A
28. B
29. B

DISCUSSION

The examination of the patient in Question 27 is highly suggestive of *S. pyogenes* pharyngitis. Antimicrobial therapy should be initiated immediately. Although analgesic therapy is important, antistreptococcal therapy to *S. pharyngitis* infection is focused on this particular disease.

The macrolides offer an effective treatment option for patients allergic to penicillin who have streptococcus pharyngitis because there is no noted crossover allergy. Approximately 8% of those with penicillin allergy also have problems with the cephalosporins, a group of medications to consider as a treatment alternative for those with *S. pyogenes* infection.

Discussion Source

Hektor Dunphy, L. (1999). *Management Guidelines for Adult Nurse Practitioners*. Philadelphia: FA Davis. Pp. 207–209.

QUESTION

30. When giving advice to a patient who plans to use zinc therapy, which of the following represents the most accurate information?

    A. Zinc tablets taken daily for the duration of the cold season will help you in avoiding catching colds.
    B. Zinc should be taken in lozenge form at the first sign of URI symptoms.
    C. High-dose zinc therapy helps stimulate lymphocyte production.
    D. The product is most effective if taken when symptoms are most severe.

ANSWER

30. B

DISCUSSION

Zinc gluconate lozenges can be effective in limiting the length and severity of URIs when taken at the first signs and symptoms of a cold. Using zinc at other times has not been shown to be helpful.

Discussion Source

Uphold, C., Johns, T. (1999). Upper respiratory disorders. In Youngkin, E. Sawin, K., Kissinger, J., & Israel, D. *Pharmacotherapeutics: A Primary Care Clinical Guide* Norwalk, CT: Appleton & Lange. Pp. 369–392.

QUESTIONS

31. A 25-year-old woman who has seasonal allergic rhinitis likes to spend time outdoors. She asks you when the pollen count is likely to be the lowest. You respond:

    A. early in the morning
    B. during breezy times of the day
    C. after a rain shower
    D. when the sky is overcast

32. You prescribe nasal steroid spray for a patient with allergic rhinitis. What is the anticipated onset of symptom relief with its use?

    A. immediately with the first spray
    B. 1 to 2 days
    C. 1 to 2 weeks
    D. about 1 month

33. Which of the following medications is most appropriate for allergic rhinitis therapy in an acutely symptomatic 24-year-old machine operator?

    A. nasal cromolyn (Nasalcrom)
    B. diphenhydramine (Benadryl)
    C. flunisolide nasal spray (Nasarel)
    D. loratadine (Claritin)

34. Antihistamines work primarily through:

    A. vasoconstriction
    B. action on the histamine$_1$ (H$_1$) receptor sites
    C. inflammatory mediation
    D. peripheral vasodilatation

35. Decongestants work primarily through:

  A. vasoconstriction
  B. action on the H_1 receptor sites
  C. inflammatory mediation
  D. peripheral vasodilatation

ANSWERS

31. C
32. C
33. D
34. B
35. A

DISCUSSION

The most important component of allergic rhinitis therapy is avoidance of the allergen. Pollen counts are generally the highest early in the morning because these substances are released during the night. After a rain shower, the air is relatively cleansed of the offending agent.

Because the mechanism of action of steroid nasal spray is prevention of production of inflammatory substances, steroid nasal sprays are highly effective at preventing, but not acutely controlling, symptoms of allergic rhinitis. Therefore, at least 1–2 weeks of use is needed before symptom relief is achieved. However, antihistamines prevent action of formed histamine, a potent inflammatory mediator, and therefore can be used to control acute allergic symptoms. A nonsedating antihistamine such as loratadine (Claritin) is the best choice for active adults. Diphenhydramine (Benadryl) is a rapidly-acting sedating antihistamine. Both flunisolide and nasal cromolyn work only to help prevent, not to treat, allergic symptoms. All antihistamines work by blocking H_1 receptor sites. Decongestants act as vasoconstrictors, thus opening edematous nasal passages (Table 4–2).

Discussion Source

Hektor Dunphy, L. (1999). *Management Guidelines for Adult Nurse Practitioners*. Philadelphia: FA Davis. Pp. 209–214.

QUESTIONS

36. The most specific finding for acute bacterial rhinosinusitis is:

  A. purulent drainage from a nasal turbinate
  B. mild midfacial fullness and tenderness
  C. preauricular lymphadenopathy
  D. marked eyelid edema

37. The most common causative pathogen in ABRS is:

  A. *Mycoplasma pneumoniae*
  B. *S. pneumoniae*
  C. *M. catarrhalis*
  D. *H. influenza*

38. Which of the following is not consistent with the diagnosis of ABRS?

  A. nasal congestion responsive to decongestant use
  B. maxillary toothache
  C. URI symptoms persisting more than 7 to 10 days
  D. colored nasal discharge

39. The most appropriate pharmacologic intervention for treating ABRS is:

  A. erythromycin
  B. amoxicillin with clavulanate
  C. cephalexin
  D. ciprofloxacin

ANSWERS

36. A
37. B
38. A
39. B

TABLE 4–2.
MEDICATIONS USED IN TREATING ALLERGIC DISORDERS

Medications	Mechanism of Action	Comments
Antihistamines	Antagonize H$_1$ receptor sites	First-generation oral products (Diphenhydramine [Benadryl], chlorpheniramine [Chlor Trimeton])
		Cross blood-brain barrier, causing sedation
		Anticholinergic activity causes some drying of secretions
		Second-generation oral products (Loratadine [Claritin], cetirizine [Zyrtec], fexofenadine [Allegra])
		Little transfer across blood brain barrier, lower rates of sedation, less anticholinergic effect
		Less anticholinergic effect
		Prevents action of formed histamine, therefore, helpful in acute allergic reactions
		Topical products also available
Cromolyn sodium (Nasalcrom, Intal)	Halts degradation of mast cells and release of histamine and other inflammatory mediators (mast cell stabilizer)	Prevents rather than treats allergic reactions
		Need consistent use to be helpful
		Used in inhaled form (nasal spray, MDI)
Topical corticosteroids (nasal sprays, inhaled via MDI)	Inhibit eosinophilic action and other inflammatory mediators	Prevent rather than treat allergic reactions
		Need consistent use to be helpful

(continued)

TABLE 4–2. (continued)

Medications	Mechanism of Action	Comments
Epinephrine	Alpha, beta$_1$, beta$_2$ agonists; potent vasoconstrictor, cardiac stimulant, bronchodilator	Initial therapy for anaphylaxis because of its multiple modes of reversing airway and circulatory dysfunction Anaphylaxis usually responds quickly to 0.3 to 0.5 mL subcutaneously (SC) of 1:1000 solution Use with caution in presence of cardiac disease
Ipratropium bromide (Atrovent nasal spray)	Reduces nasal secretions in URIs and allergic rhinitis	Not a systemic drug Well tolerated Does not alter course of URIs or allergies
Decongestants (oral, topical via nasal spray)	Alpha agonist, vaso-constrictor	May cause increase in BP and heart rate when high-dose oral products are used Short-term use (< 5 days) of nasal spray safe with little sequelae

DISCUSSION

Acute bacterial rhinosinusitis is a clinical condition caused by an inflammation of the lining of the membranes of the paranasal sinuses. Risk factors include any condition that alters the normal cleansing mechanism of the sinuses, including viral infection, allergies, tobacco use and abnormalities in sinus structure. Cigarette smoking disturbs normal sinus mucocilliary action and drainage, causing secretions to pool and increasing risk of superimposed bacterial infection. In addition, viral URI causes similar dysfunction, thus increasing ABRS risk. The observation of purulent discharge from one of the nasal turbinates is a highly sensitive finding in ABRS. Midfacial fullness is common in patients with uncomplicated URI, and anterior cervical lymphadenopathy is often found in a number of infectious and inflammatory conditions involving the head and pharynx. Marked eyelid edema is found only when the infection has extended beyond the sinuses and an orbital cellulitis has formed a potentially life-threatening complication of ABRS.

Although *S. pneumoniae* is the most common pathogen implicated in ABRS, *H. influenzae* and *M. catarrhalis* rank as the second and third most often implicated. The latter two pathogens have significant rates of beta lactamase production, rendering amoxicillin ineffective. The choice of an antimicrobial agent for a patient with this condition must be one that covers both these gram-positive and -negative organisms and resists inactivation by beta lactamase. Reflecting this, amoxicillin with clavulanate (Augmentin), cefuroxime axetil (Ceftin), or trimethoprin-sulfamethoxazole (Bactrim) are recommended as first-line therapy, with cefprozil (Cefzil), cefpodoxime (Vantin), or clarithromycin (Braxin) as second-line treatment options (see Table 4–1).

Discussion Sources

Gilbert, D., Moellering, R., Sande, M. (1998). *The Sanford Guide to Antimicrobial Therapy* (28th ed.). Vienna, VA: Antimicrobial Therapy, Inc. P. 8.
Hektor Dunphy, L. (1999). *Management Guidelines for Adult Nurse Practitioners*. Philadelphia: FA Davis. Pp. 215–218.

QUESTION

40. Which of the following best describes hearing loss associated with presbyacusis?

 A. rapidly progressing and often asymmetric in all frequencies

 B. slowly progressive, usually symmetric, and predominately high frequency

 C. variable in progress, usually unilateral, with midrange frequencies

 D. primarily conductive and bilateral with slow progress

ANSWER

40. B

DISCUSSION

Presbyacusis is a progressive, fairly symmetric, high-frequency, age-related sensory hearing loss likely caused by cochlear deterioration. Speech discrimination is usually the primary problem.

Discussion Source

Hektor Dunphy, L. (1999). *Management Guidelines for Adult Nurse Practitioners*. Philadelphia: FA Davis. Pp. 74–75.

QUESTIONS

41. A 78-year-old woman has early bilateral senile cataracts. Which of the following situations would likely pose the greatest difficulty?

    A. reading the newspaper
    B. distinguishing between the primary colors
    C. following extraocular movements
    D. reading road signs while driving

42. Which of the following is consistent with the visual problems associated with presbyopia?

    A. bilateral peripheral vision loss
    B. blurring of near vision
    C. difficulty with distant vision
    D. loss of central visual field

43. Which of the following is consistent with the visual problems associated with macular degeneration?

    A. bilateral peripheral vision loss
    B. blurring of near vision
    C. difficulty with distant vision
    D. loss of central vision field

44. All of the following are consistent with normal age-related vision changes except:

    A. need for increased illumination
    B. increasing sensitivity to glare
    C. washing out of colors
    D. gradual loss of peripheral vision

ANSWERS

41. D
42. B
43. D
44. D

DISCUSSION

Distance vision poses the greatest problem for individuals with senile cataracts. As the lens becomes more opaque, near vision also deteriorates. Other visual changes of age-related cataracts include loss of ability to distinguish contrasts and progressive dimming of vision. Close vision is usually retained, and there are occasional improvements in reading ability.

Presbyopia is age-related vision changes caused by a progressive hardening of the lens. Patients most often complain of close vision problems, usually first manifested by difficulty with reading smaller print. Other normal age-related vision changes include a progressive yellowing of the lens and decreased flexibility of the sclera, in part leading to the washing out of colors, difficulty seeing under low illumination, and increased sensitivity to glare.

Macular degeneration is the most common cause of blindness and vision loss in the elderly. Vision changes seen in macular degeneration include loss of the central vision field. This disease is more often seen in women of European descent. A history of cigarette smoking and a family history of the disease are often found as well. Recently, a history of excessive sun exposure has been implicated as a risk factor for macular degeneration. The ophthalmologic examination reveals hard drusen or yellow deposits in the macular area. Soft drusen may also be seen. These appear larger, paler, and less distinct.

Discussion Sources

Hektor Dunphy, L. (1999). *Management Guidelines for Adult Nurse Practitioners*. Philadelphia: FA Davis. P. 9.
Riordan-Eva, P., Vaughan, D. (1999). Eye. In Tierney, L., McPhee, S., & Papadakis, M. *Current Diagnosis and Treatment* (38th ed.). Stamford, CT: Appleton & Lange. Pp. 181–212.

5
CHAPTER

Chest
Disorders

QUESTIONS

1. Angina pectoris is most often caused by:

    A. intracoronary thrombus
    B. ventricular hypertrophy
    C. atherosclerosis
    D. aortic valve incompetence

2. Which of the following is most consistent with a person presenting with unstable angina pectoris?

    A. a 5-minute episode of chest tightness brought on by stair climbing and relieved by rest
    B. a severe, searing pain that penetrates the chest and lasts about 30 seconds
    C. chest pressure lasting 20 minutes that occurs at rest
    D. "heartburn" promptly relieved by position change

3. In assessing a woman at risk for coronary artery disease, the NP considers that the patient will likely present:

    A. in a manner similar to a man with equivalent disease
    B. at the same age as a man with similar health problems
    C. more commonly with angina and less commonly with acute myocardial infarction (MI)
    D. less commonly with congestive heart failure (CHF)

4. The cardiac finding most commonly associated with unstable angina is:

    A. physiologic split S_2
    B. S_4
    C. opening snap
    D. summation gallop

5. Which of the following changes on the 12-lead electrocardiogram (ECG) do you expect to find in a patient with myocardial ischemia?

   A. ST-segment elevation
   B. R wave > 25 mm
   C. T-wave inversion
   D. deep Q wave

6. Beta adrenergic antagonists are used in angina pectoris therapy because of their ability to:

   A. reverse obstruction-fixed vessel lesions
   B. reduce myocardial oxygen demand
   C. enhance myocardial vessel tone
   D. stabilize cardiac rhythm

7. Nitrates are used in angina pectoris therapy because of their ability to:

   A. reverse fixed vessel obstruction
   B. reduce myocardial oxygen demand
   C. cause vasodilatation
   D. stabilize cardiac rhythm

8. Which of the following is most consistent with a patient presenting with acute myocardial infarction?

   A. a 5-minute episode of chest tightness brought on by stair climbing
   B. a severe, localized pain that penetrates the chest and lasts about 3 hours
   C. chest pressure lasting 20 minutes that occurs at rest
   D. retrosternal diffuse pain for 30 minutes accompanied by diaphoresis

9. Which of the following changes on the 12-lead ECG would you expect to find in a patient with MI?

   A. 2-mm ST-segment elevation
   B. R wave > 25 mm
   C. T-wave inversion
   D. deep Q waves

10. Which of the following changes on the 12-lead ECG would you expect to find in a patient with myocardial injury?

    A. 2-mm ST-segment elevation
    B. S wave > 10 mm
    C. T-wave inversion
    D. deep Q waves

11. Thrombolytic therapy is indicated in patients with chest pain and ECG changes such as:

    A. 1-mm ST-segment depression in leads 1 and 3
    B. physiologic Q waves in aVF and V5–6
    C. 2-mm ST-segment elevation in V1–4
    D. T-wave inversion in aVl and aVR

12. Which of the following is the most sensitive marker for myocardial damage?

    A. AST
    B. CPK
    C. cTnI
    D. LDH

13. All of the following should be prescribed within 24 hours of MI except:

    A. aspirin
    B. atenolol
    C. lisinopril
    D. nisoldipine

14. Which of the following is an absolute contraindication to the use of thrombolytic therapy?

    A. history of hemorrhagic stroke
    B. blood pressure (BP) = 160/100 at presentation
    C. current use of warfarin
    D. active peptic ulcer disease

15. A 64-year-old man who had an MI 2 years ago has high BP and diabetes mellitus. His fasting lipid profile was obtained after an appropriate diet for 8 months. High-density lipoprotein (HDL) = 38 mg/dL; low-density lipoprotein (LDL) = 140 mg/dL; triglycerides = 180 mg/dL. Which of the following is the most appropriate advice?

    A. No further intervention is needed.
    B. This lipid profile should be repeated in 6 months.

C. His LDL goal should be lower than 100 mg/dL.

D. His triglyceride level is acceptable.

ANSWERS

1. C
2. C
3. C
4. B
5. C
6. B
7. C
8. D
9. D
10. A
11. C
12. C
13. D
14. A
15. C

DISCUSSION

Angina pectoris, most often caused by atherosclerosis, is the clinical manifestation of myocardial ischemia and a result of imbalance in the ability to supply the myocardium with sufficient oxygen to meet its demands. Patterns of symptom provocation are usually predictable (stable), with exertion often causing discomfort promptly relieved with rest or use of sublingual nitroglycerin, or both. Unstable angina is defined as a new onset of rest symptoms or worsening symptoms with previously provoking activities. Treatment of angina pectoris includes reduction of cardiovascular disease risk factors. In addition, beta adrenergic blockers are among first-line therapy because these agents reduce myocardial workload through lowering heart rate and stroke volume. Nitrates are used to enhance myocardial perfusion through peripheral and central vasodilatation.

The S_4 heart sound is often heard with myocardial ischemia and poorly controlled angina pectoris. This sound of poor myocardial relaxation (compliance), diastolic dysfunction, may potentially cause decreased cardiac output. The S_3 heart sound is the sound of poor myocardial contractility, systolic dysfunction, and usually leads to decreased cardiac output.

Women usually have significantly older onset of coronary heart disease and are likely to present differently from men. For example, dyspnea may be an anginal equivalent in older women. Women usually present first with angina pectoris that may lead to MI. Men often have their first manifestation of coronary heart disease in the form of MI.

Myocardial infarction most commonly occurs when an atherosclerotic plaque ruptures, leading to the formation of an occlusive thrombus. Coronary artery spasm may also occur, adding to the vessel obstruction. The patient with a suspected MI needs to be assessed promptly and accurately because thrombolytic therapy should be initiated early in the process to limit myocardial damage. The 12-lead ECG should be assessed for changes consistent with myocardial ischemia, injury, and infarction (Fig. 5–1).

Seventy-five percent of patients admitted for MI are ruled out for this condition. At the same time, 25% of all MIs are silent. In order to reduce unneeded hospitalization and detect asymptomatic MI, diagnostic tests that are highly sensitive and specific for myocardial damage are needed.

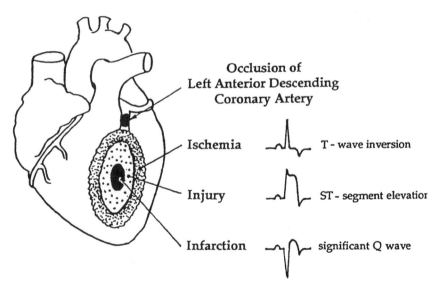

FIG. 5–1. ECG changes of acute MI. In this example, occlusion of the left anterior descending coronary artery results in ischemia, injury, and infarction of heart muscle. ECG evidence of tissue damage is reflected in the T wave, ST segment, and initial QRS deflection (a significant Q wave develops). (Adapted from Lipman, B.C., and Lipman, B.S. [1987]. ECG Pocket Guide [p. 98]. Chicago: Yearbook Medical Publishers.)

Creatinine phosphokinase (CK) isoenzyme MB has long been used as a serum marker of myocardial damage. It increases within 6 to 12 hours of MI, begins to decrease within 24 to 48 hours and usually returns to normal in about 60 hours. As CK-MB clears quickly, its use in late detection of MI is limited. In addition, false-positive and false-negative results are noted.

Troponin is a regulatory protein of the myofibril with three major subtypes, C, I, and T. Subtypes troponin I (cTnI) and troponin T (cTnT) are released in presence of myocardial damage. Both increase rapidly within first 12 hours after MI, with cTnT typically remaining elevated for about 168 hours, where as cTnI remains elevated for about 192 hours. cTnI is the more cardiac-specific measure and is sensitive for small-volume myocardial damage. cTnT can be elevated in chronic renal failure, muscle trauma, and rhabdomyolysis. Troponin I is more sensitive and specific than ECG and CK-MB in diagnosing unstable angina and non-Q-wave MI. In addition, cTnI results are available quickly through a rapid assay test.

Protracted elevation of cTnI after MI or unstable angina may be a predictor of increased mortality. Angina patients without documented MI had significantly higher risk of death within 42 days if cTnI is persistently elevated.

The American Heart Association (AHA) has published Guidelines for the Management of Patients with Acute Myocardial Infarction. Developed from consensus of nursing and medical experts as well as evidence-based health care, the AHA recommends the following for patients with suspected MI:

- Community systems, including primary care sites, should work together to ensure prompt initial care of patients with suspected MI. After a patient enters care in the emergency department (ED), initial evaluation should occur within 10 minutes.
- The following care should be provided immediately: oxygen via nasal prongs, sublingual nitroglycerin (unless systolic BP is less than 90 mm Hg, heart rate is less than 50 or greater than 100 bpm), adequate analgesia with morphine sulfate or meperidine, and aspirin 160 to 325 mg orally. Other antiplatlet agents such as dipyridmole, ticlopidine or clopidogrel may be used if aspirin allergy is present or if there is no response to aspirin.
- A 12-lead ECG should be performed promptly, looking for greater than 1-mm ST-segment elevation in contiguous leads. The presence of these changes usually indicates acute coronary artery occlusion, usually from thrombosis. In addition, clinically signifi-

cant ST-segment elevation largely dictates reperfusion therapy with the use of thrombolytic therapy or primary percutaneous transluminal coronary angioplasty (PTCA). These therapies have the best effect on clinical outcomes if used within 6 hours after onset of chest pain but may be helpful as much as 7 to 12 hours or more after MI symptoms begin. When thrombolysis is used, heparin is usually given for 48 hours to ensure continued vessel patency.

• Before giving a product such as tPA or streptokinase, the prescriber must be aware of absolute and relative contraindication for thrombolytic therapy. Absolute contraindications include previous history or hemorrhagic stroke at any time or stroke within 1 year, known intracranial neoplasm, active internal bleeding, or suspected aortic dissection. Relative contraindications for the use of thrombolytic therapy include uncontrolled hypertension on presentation (BP > 180/110 mm Hg), current use of anticoagulants in therapeutic doses (INR-International Normalized Ratio 2 to 3), trauma within the past 2 to 4 weeks, pregnancy, active peptic ulcer disease, and recent internal bleeding. With streptokinase and anistreplase use, prior exposure within the past 5 days to 2 years, or prior allergic reaction to either agent dictates caution. Percutaneous transluminal coronary angioplasty (PTCA) may be considered an alternative to thrombolytic therapy in certain circumstances.

• If left bundle branch block is present on ECG and the clinical scenario is consistent with acute MI, standard acute MI care should be offered. Patients with presentation suggestive of MI but without ST-segment changes should not receive thrombolysis. These patients should be hospitalized and placed on continuous ECG monitoring for rhythm disturbances; those that are noted should be appropriately treated. Serial 12-lead ECGs should be obtained and results correlated with clinical measures of myocardial necrosis such as CPK or CK isoenzymes and troponin. Aspirin therapy should be continued, and consideration should be given to heparin use in the presence of a large anterior MI or left ventricular (LV) mural thrombus because of increased risk of embolic stroke.

• If no contraindications are present, beta blocker therapy and angiotensin-converting enzyme (ACE) inhibitor therapy should be initiated promptly because the use of these products is associated with reduced mortality and morbidity after MI. beta blocker therapy should be continued indefinitely; ACE inhibitor use is most appropriate for those with LV dysfunction characterized by systolic ejection fraction of less than 40% or in the presence of CHF.

- Before hospital discharge, patients should undergo standard exercise testing to assess functional capacity, efficacy of current medical regimen, and risk stratification for subsequent cardiac events.
- Ongoing care includes a goal of reducing LDL cholesterol to less than 100 mg/dL and using diet, exercise and, if needed, drug therapy. This is in keeping with an overall plan to reduce or eliminate all cardiac risk factors, including inactivity, smoking, and obesity (Tables 5–1 and 5–2).

Discussion Sources

American College of Cardiology/American Heart Association Task Force on Practice Guidelines, Committee on Management of Acute Myocardial Infarction. Available at http://www.americanheart.org/Scientific/Statements/1999/hc3499.html
Hektor Dunphy, L. (1999). *Management Guidelines for Adult Nurse Practitioners*. Philadelphia: FA Davis. Pp. 260–264.

TABLE 5–1. ADULT TREATMENT PANEL III LIPID AND LIPOPROTEIN CLASSIFICATION		
HDL-C (mg/dL)	< 40	Low
	≥ 60	High
TC (mg/dL)	< 200	Desirable
	200–239	Borderline high
	≥ 240	High
LDL Cholesterol (mg/dL)	< 100	Optimal
	100–129	Near optimal
	130–159	Borderline high
	160–189	High
	≥ 190	Very high

Reference: National Cholesterol Education Program Adult Treatment Panel III (ATP III) Guidelines [On-line]. Available at www.nhlbi.nih.gov/ncep.

TABLE 5–2. RISK CATEGORIES THAT MODIFY LDL-CHOLESTEROL GOALS	
Risk Category	**LDL Goal**
CHD and CHD risk equivalents	< 100 mg/dl
Multiple (2+) risk factors	< 130 mg/dl
Zero to one risk factor	< 160 mg/dl

Reference: National Cholesterol Education Program Adult Treatment Panel III (ATP III) Guidelines [On-line]. Available at www.nhlbi.nih.gov/ncep.

QUESTIONS

16. Which of the following best describes asthma?

   A. intermittent airway inflammation with occasional bronchospasm
   B. a disease of bronchospasm leading to airway inflammation
   C. chronic airway inflammation with superimposed bronchospasm
   D. relatively fixed airway constriction

17. The patient you are evaluating is having an asthma attack. You have assessed that his condition is appropriate for office treatment. You expect to find the following on physical examination:

   A. tripod posture
   B. inspiratory crackles
   C. increased vocal fremitus
   D. hyperresonance to percussion

18. A 44-year-old man has a long-standing history of asthma that is normally well controlled with beclomethasone via metered-dose inhaler 4 puffs twice a day and the use of albuterol 1 to 2 times a week as needed for wheezing. Three days ago, he developed a sore throat, clear nasal discharge, body aches, and a dry cough. In the past 24

hours, he has had intermittent wheezing, necessitating the use of albuterol 2 puffs every 3 hours with partial relief. Your next most appropriate action is to obtain a:

A. chest radiograph
B. sputum Gram stain
C. peak flow measurement
D. white blood cell (WBC) differential

19. You examine a 24-year-old woman who has acute asthma flare-ups. She is using fluticasone and albuterol as directed and continues to have difficulty with coughing and wheezing. Her peak expiratory flow (PEF) is 55% of predicted. Her medication regimen should be adjusted to include:

A. theophylline
B. salmeterol (Servent)
C. Prednisone
D. zafirlukast (Accolate)

20. Which of the following is most likely to be reported on a chest radiograph of a person during an acute asthma attack?

A. hyperinflation
B. atelectasis
C. consolidation
D. Kerley B signs

21. A 36-year-old man with asthma also needs antihypertensive therapy. Which product would you avoid prescribing?

A. hydrochlorothiazide
B. propanolol
C. nicardipine
D. enalapril

ANSWERS

16. C
17. D
18. C
19. C
20. A
21. B

TABLE 5-3.
STEPWISE APPROACH FOR MANAGING ASTHMA IN ADULTS AND CHILDREN OLDER THAN AGE 5 YEARS

Goals of Asthma Treatment

- Prevent chronic and troublesome symptoms (e.g., coughing or breathlessness in the night, in the early morning, or after exertion)
- Maintain (near) "normal" pulmonary function
- Maintain normal activity levels (including exercise and other physical activity)
- Prevent recurrent exacerbations of asthma and minimize the need for emergency department visits or hospitalizations
- Provide optimal pharmacotherapy with minimal or no adverse effects
- Meet patients' and families' expectation of and satisfaction with asthma care

Classification of Severity: Clinical Features Before Treatment*

	Symptoms**	Nighttime Symptoms	Lung Function
STEP 4 Severe Persistent	• Continual symptoms • Limited physical activity • Frequent exacerbations	Frequent	• FEV$_1$ or PEF ≤60% predicted • PEF variability >30%

	Symptoms	Nighttime Symptoms	Lung Function
STEP 3 Moderate Persistent	• Daily symptoms • Daily use of inhaled short-acting beta$_2$ agonist • Exacerbations affect activity • Exacerbations ≥2 times a week; may last days	>1 time a week	• FEV$_1$ or PEF >60% ≤80% predicted • PEF variability >30%
STEP 2 Mild Persistent	• Symptoms >2 times a week but <1 time a day • Exacerbations may affect activity	>2 times a month	• FEV$_1$ or PEF ≥80% predicted • PEF variability 20–30%
STEP 1 Mild Intermittent	• Symptoms ≤2 times a week • Asymptomatic and normal PEF between exacerbations • Exacerbations brief (from a few hours to a few days); intensity may vary	≤2 times a month	• FEV$_1$ or PEF ≥80% predicted • PEF variability <20%

*The presence of one of the features of severity is sufficient to place a patient in that category. An individual should be assigned to the most severe grade in which any feature occurs. The characteristics noted in this figure are general and may overlap because asthma is highly variable. Furthermore, an individual's classification may change over time.

**Patients at any level of severity can have mild, moderate, or severe exacerbations. Some patients with intermittent asthma experience severe and life-threatening exacerbations separated by long periods of normal lung function and no symptoms.

National Asthma Education & Prevention Program. Expert Panel Report 2: Guidelines for the Diagnosis and Management of Asthma National Institute of Health Pub. No 97-4051. Bethesda, MD, 1997.

(continued)

TABLE 5-3. (continued)

	Long-Term Control	Quick Relief	Education
	Preferred treatments are in bold print.		
STEP 4 Severe Persistent	Daily medications: • **Anti-inflammatory: inhaled corticosteroid (high dose)** and • Long-acting bronchodilator: either long-acting inhaled beta$_2$ agonist, sustained-release theophylline, or long-acting beta$_2$ agonist tablets AND • Corticosteroid tablets or syrup long term (2 mg/kg/day, generally do not exceed 60 mg/day).	• Short-acting bronchodilator: **inhaled beta$_2$ agonists** as needed for symptoms. • Intensity of treatment will depend on severity of exacerbation; see "Managing Exacerbations of Asthma." • Use of short-acting inhaled beta$_2$ agonists on a daily basis, or increasing use, indicates the need for additional long-term-control therapy.	Steps 2 and 3 actions plus: • Refer to individual education/counseling

STEP 3
Moderate Persistent
	Daily medication:
	• Either
	  — **Anti-inflammatory: in-**
	    haled corticosteroid
	    (medium dose) OR
	  — Inhaled corticosteroid (low-
	    medium dose) and add a
	    long-acting bronchodilator,
	    especially for nighttime
	    symptoms: either **long-**
	    acting inhaled beta$_2$
	    agonist, sustained-release
	    theophylline, or long-acting
	    beta$_2$ agonist tablets.
	• If needed
	  — Anti-inflammatory: inhaled
	    corticosteroids (medium-
	    high dose) AND
	  — Long-acting bronchodilator,
	    especially for nighttime
	    symptoms; either **long-**
	    acting inhaled beta$_2$ ago-
	    nist, sustained-release
	    theophylline, or long-acting
	    beta$_2$ agonist tablets.
		• Short-acting bronchodilator:
		  inhaled beta$_2$ agonists as
		  needed for symptoms.
		• Intensity of treatment will de-
		  pend on severity of exacerba-
		  tion; see "Managing Exacer-
		  bations of Asthma."
		• Use of short-acting inhaled
		  beta$_2$ agonists on a daily ba-
		  sis, or increasing use, indi-
		  cates the need for additional
		  long-term-control therapy.
			Step 1 actions plus:
			• Teach self-monitoring
			• Refer to group education if
			  available
			• Review and update self-
			  management plan

(continued)

TABLE 5–3. (continued)

Preferred treatments are in bold print.

	Long-Term Control	Quick Relief	Education
STEP 2 Mild Persistent	Daily medication: • **Anti-inflammatory**: either **inhaled corticosteroid** (low doses) or **cromolyn or nedocromil** (children usually begin with a trial of cromolyn or nedocromil). • Sustained-release theophylline to serum concentration of 5-15 µg/mL is an alternative. Leukotriene modifier may also be considered for patients ≥ 12 years of age, although their position in therapy is not fully established.	• Short-acting bronchodilator: **inhaled beta₂ agonists** as needed for symptoms. • Intensity of treatment will depend on severity of exacerbation; see "Managing Exacerbations of Asthma." • Use of short-acting inhaled beta₂ agonists on a daily basis, or increasing use, indicates the need for additional long-term-control therapy.	Step 1 actions plus: • Teach self-monitoring • Refer to group education if available • Review and update self-management plan
STEP 1 Mild Intermittent	• No daily medication needed.	• Short-acting bronchodilator: **inhaled beta₂ agonists** as needed for symptoms. • Intensity of treatment will depend on severity of exacerbation; see "Managing Exacerbations of Asthma."	• Teach basic facts about asthma • Teach inhaler/spacer/holding chamber technique • Discuss roles of medications • Develop self-management plan

- Use of short-acting inhaled beta$_2$ agonists more than 2 times a week may indicate the need to initiate long-term-control therapy.

- Develop action plan for when and how to take rescue actions
- Discuss appropriate environmental control measures to avoid exposure to known allergens and irritants. (See component 4.)

Step down
Review treatment every 1 to 6 months; a gradual stepwise reduction in treatment may be possible.

Step up
If control is not maintained, consider step up. First, review patient medication technique, adherence, and environmental control (avoidance of allergens or other factors that contribute to asthma severity).

Notes:
- The stepwise approach presents general guidelines to assist clinical decision making; it is not intended to be a specific prescription. Asthma is highly variable; clinicians should tailor specific medication plans to the needs and circumstances of individual patients.
- Gain control as quickly as possible; then decrease treatment to the least medication necessary to maintain control. Gaining control may be accomplished either by starting treatment at the step most appropriate to the initial severity of the condition or by starting at a higher level of therapy (e.g., a course of systemic corticosteroids or higher dose of inhaled corticosteroids).
- A rescue course of systemic corticosteroid may be needed at any time and at any step.
- Some patients with intermittent asthma experience severe and life-threatening exacerbations separated by long periods of normal lung function and no symptoms. This may be especially common with exacerbations provoked by respiratory infections. A short course of systemic corticosteroids is recommended.
- At each step, patients should control their environment to avoid or control factors that make their asthma worse (e.g., allergens, irritants); this requires specific diagnosis and education.
- Referral to an asthma specialist for consultation or comanagement is recommended if there are difficulties achieving or maintaining control of asthma or if the patient requires step 4 care. Referral may be considered if the patient requires step 3 care (see also component 1—Initial Assessment and Diagnosis).

DISCUSSION

Asthma is predominantly a disease of inflammation with superimposed bronchospasm. This leads to air trapping. As such, the normally resonant thorax becomes hyperresonant, and hyperinflation is seen on chest radiographs.

The backbone of mild, moderate, or severe asthma therapy is the use of an inflammatory controller drug such as an inhaled corticosteroids, or mast cell stabilizers such as nedocromil or cromolyn. According to the National Asthma Education and Prevention Program, additional but acceptable anti-inflammatory options include leukotriene modifiers. These include leukotriene antagonists such as zafirlukast (Accolate), montelukast (Singulair), and the leukotriene inhibitor zileuton (Zyflo). Rescue medications that relieve acute superimposed bronchospasm include short-acting beta$_2$ agonists. When acute asthma flare-up is present and PEF is 50% to 80% of predicted, rapidly acting anti-inflammatory therapy with oral corticosteroids is needed. Adding more bronchodilators, such as theophylline and salmeterol, does not reverse the cause of the bronchospasm. The leukotriene antagonists such as zafirlukast (Accolate) can be helpful in preventing, but not acutely treating, inflammation (Table 5–4.)

Here are memory aids you may find useful as you develop a plan of care for patients with asthma:

- Antagonists are drugs that block activity of a receptor site; agonists stimulate activity of a receptor site.
- β_1 receptors predominate in the heart; the β_2 receptors predominate in the lungs. Whereas cardioselective beta blockers such as metoprolol focus activity in the heart, mixed or noncardioselective beta$_1$ and beta$_2$ blockers such as propanolol antagonize activity at receptors in the heart and lungs. (One easy way to remember: you have beta$_1$ receptors in your 1 heart [β_1] and beta$_2$ receptors in your 2 lungs [β_2].)
- Corticosteroids have an -one or -ide suffix. Fluticasone (Flovent), prednisone, and flunisolide (Aerobid) are examples of steroids used in the treatment of asthma.
- Beta$_2$ agonists have a -terol suffix. Medication such as albuterol stimulate beta$_2$ receptor sites and cause bronchodilation.
- Beta adrenergic antagonists (beta blockers) block adrenergic (adrenaline-like) activity. Examples include medication with the -lol suffix, such as atenolol and propanolol.
- Using beta blockers, particularly a nonselective agent such as propanolol, in the presence of asthma can precipitate bronchospasm.

TABLE 5–4.
MEDICATIONS USED FOR TREATING PATIENTS
WITH ASTHMA AND CHRONIC OBSTRUCTIVE PULMONARY DISEASE

Medication	Mechanism of Action	Comments
Albuterol (Ventolin, Proventil), pibuterol (Maxair), salmeterol (Servent)	Beta$_2$ agonist; bronchodilation through stimulation of beta$_2$ receptor site	Albuterol and pibuterol Onset of action, 15 minutes • Duration of action, 4–6 hours • First-line rescue drugs for treating acute bronchospasm Salmeterol • Onset of action, 1 hour • Duration of action, 12 hours • Indicated for prevention rather than treatment of bronchospasm • Patient should also have short-acting beta$_2$ agonist as rescue drug
Antihistamines	Antagonize H$_1$ receptor sites Prevents action of formed histamine	First-generation products (diphenhydramine [Benadryl], chlorpheniramine [Chlortrimeton]) • Cross blood-brain barrier, causing sedation • Anticholinergic activity causes some drying of secretions Second-generation products (loratadine [Claritin], cetirizine [Zyrtec], fexofenadine [Allegra]) • Little transfer across blood-brain barrier; low rates of sedation • Less anticholinergic effect; adjunct in asthma complicated by allergic rhinitis

(continued)

TABLE 5–4. (continued)

Medication	Mechanism of Action	Comments
Cromolyn sodium (Intal, Nasal-crom), nedocromil (Tilade)	Halts degradation of mast cells and release of histamine and other inflammatory mediators (mast cell stabilizer)	Prevents rather than treats allergic reactions Need consistent use to be helpful First-line asthma controller drug in children
Theophylline (TheoDur, Theo-24)	Bronchodilator improved respiratory muscle function	Narrow therapuetic index. Many drug-drug interactions
Leukotriene modifiers • Antagonist such as zafirlukast (Accolate), montelukast (Singulair) • Inhibitor such as zileuton (Zylfo)	Prevents inflammation through minimizing effects of leukotrienes, an important part of the inflammatory cascade	Likely as effective as low-dose inhaled steroids. May be added to inhaled anti-inflammatory agents to enhance asthma control
Inhaled corticosteroids	Inhibit eosinophilic action and other inflammatory mediators, potentate effects of $beta_2$ agonists	Prevents rather than treats inflammation Need consistent use to be helpful

Drug	Action	Comments
Epinephrine	Alpha, beta$_1$, beta$_2$ agonists; potent vasoconstrictor, cardiac stimulant, bronchodilator	Initial therapy for anaphylaxis because of its multiple modes of reversing airway and circulatory dysfunction Anaphylaxis usually responds quickly to 0.3–0.5 mL subcutaneously of 1:1000 solution Use with caution in presence of cardiac disease
Ipratropium bromide (Atrovent)	Bronchodilator	Not a systemic drug Well tolerated First-line therapy in COPD
Oral corticosteroids	Inhibit eosinophilic action and other inflammatory mediators	Indicated in treatment of acute asthma flare-ups to reduce inflammation In higher dose and with longer therapy (> 2 weeks), adrenal suppression may occur No taper needed if use is short term (< 10 days) and at lower dose (prednisone 40–60 mg/d) Potential for causing gastropathy

References: National Asthma Education and Prevention Program. *Expert panel 2: Guidelines for Diagnosis and Management of Asthma*. National Institute of Health Publication No. 97–4051. Bethesda, MD 1997.
Uphold, C., Johns, T. (1999). Upper respiratory disorders. In Youngkin, E., Savin, K., Kissinger, J., & Israel, D. *Pharmacotherapeutics*. Stamford, CT: Appleton & Lange. Pp. 369–392.

Discussion Source

Hektor Dunphy, L. (1999). *Management Guidelines for Adult Nurse Practitioners*. Philadelphia: FA Davis. Pp. 227–231.

QUESTIONS

22. What is the desired therapeutic action of ipratropium bromide (Atrovent) when used in treating chronic obstructive pulmonary disease (COPD)?

    A. increase mucocilliary clearance
    B. reduce alveolar volume
    C. bronchodilator effect
    D. mucolytic agent

23. What is the desired therapeutic action of corticosteroids when used in treating COPD?

    A. reversal of fixed airway obstruction
    B. improvement of central respiratory drive
    C. reduction of inflammation
    D. mucolytic agent

24. Which is most consistent with the diagnosis of COPD?

    A. $FEV_1/FVC < .70$
    B. Dyspnea on exhalation
    C. elevated diaphragms noted on x-ray
    D. polycythemia noted on CBC

25. Which of the following characteristics is found in the early stages of chronic bronchitis?

    A. enlargement of air spaces distal to the terminal bronchiole
    B. excessive mucus production
    C. alveolar fibrosis
    D. dyspnea at rest

26. Which of the following characteristics is typically found in patients with emphysema?

    A. alpha$_1$ antiprotease deficiency
    B. enlargement of air spaces distal to the terminal bronchiole
    C. alveolar fibrosis
    D. hypertrophy of the larger airways

27. Which of the following pathogens is often found in the sputum during an acute exacerbation of chronic bronchitis?

    A. *Klebsiella pneumoniae*
    B. *Streptococcus pyogenes*
    C. *Haemophilus influenzae*
    D. *Staphylococcus aureus*

ANSWERS

22. C
23. C
24. A
25. B
26. B
27. C

DISCUSSION

Chronic obstructive pulmonary disease is an airflow disease caused by the presence of both chronic bronchitis and emphysema and results in a decrease in FEV$_1$/FVC ratio. The diagnosis of chronic bronchitis is made clinically, with the patient reporting the presence of excessive mucus production for 3 or more months per year for at least 2 consecutive years in the absence of other causes. Emphysema is characterized by permanent enlargement of the air spaces distal to the terminal bronchiole without fibrosis.

Patients with COPD typically present for care in the fifth and sixth decades of life after having some symptoms, particularly excessive sputum production and dyspnea on exertion, for more than a decade. Late in the disease, dyspnea at rest may be reported.

Because 80% of all COPD can be directly attributed to tobacco use, smoking cessation is the goal. In spite of symptoms, many patients continue to smoke. Raising the issue of smoking cessation with every visit and offering assistance is an important part of the ongoing care of the person with COPD.

An acute exacerbation of COPD can be triggered by a number of factors. *H. influenzae, S. pneumoniae,* or *M. catarrhalis* are often found in the sputum, leading to the hypothesis that the flare-up is caused by bacterial infection. However, this may represent a chronic colonization or carrier state of the airways.

Ipratropium bromide (Atrovent) is an anticholinergic agent considered the backbone of pharmacologic therapy for patients with COPD. An atropine analogue, ipratropium acts as a muscarinic antagonist. Muscarinic receptor sites are located in organs innervated by the parasympathetic nervous system. When these sites are stimulated, bronchoconstriction occurs. Ipratropium acts as a bronchodilator but has no sympathomimetic effects or action at beta$_2$ receptors sites such as with albuterol. In contrast to albuterol, ipratropium has a long onset of action (> 1 hour) and is best used to avoid rather than treat the bronchospasm associated with COPD. In addition, ipratropium may help reduce the volume of secretions produced in COPD. If a patient with COPD continues to have symptoms despite consistent use of a full therapeutic dose of ipratropium, a beta$_2$ agonist should be added to provide additional bronchodilation using another mechanism of action.

Theophylline, which has mild bronchodilating and anti-inflammatory action, is used as a third-line agent in treating COPD. Corticosteroids are also used to reduce airway inflammation (see Table 5-4).

Discussion Source

Hektor Dunphy, L. (1999). *Management Guidelines for Adult Nurse Practitioners.* Philadelphia: FA Davis. Pp. 239–245.

QUESTIONS

28. Which of the following is among the most common causes of congestive heart failure (CHF)?

    A. increased sodium intake

    B. pneumonia

    C. hypertensive heart disease

    D. anemia

29. You examine an 82-year-old woman who has a history of CHF. She is in the office because of increasing shortness of breath. When auscultating her heart, you note a tachycardia with a rate of 104 bpm and an extra heart sound early in diastole. This most likely represents:

    A. summation gallop
    B. S_3 heart sound
    C. opening snap
    D. S_4 heart sound

30. You examine a 65-year-old man with dilated cardiomyopathy and CHF. On examination, you expect to find all of the following except:

    A. jugular venous distention
    B. tenderness on right upper abdominal quadrant palpation
    C. point of maximum impulse (PMI) at the fifth intercostal space midclavicular line
    D. peripheral edema

31. The cornerstone(s) of drug therapy in congestive heart failure is/are:

    A. thiazide diuretics
    B. ACE inhibitors
    C. digoxin
    D. loop diuretics

32. Patients reporting digoxin toxicity are most likely to include:

    A. anorexia
    B. disturbance in color perception
    C. blurred vision
    D. diarrhea

33. ECG findings in a patient who is taking digoxin in a therapeutic dose typically includes:

    A. shortened PR interval
    B. slightly depressed, cupped ST segments
    C. widened QRS
    D. tall T-waves

34. ECG findings in a patient with digoxin toxicity will most likely include:

   A. atrioventricular (AV) heart block
   B. T-wave inversion
   C. sinus tachycardia
   D. pointed P waves

35. Among the most commonly found adverse reactions to angiotensin-converting enzyme inhibitor ACEI therapy is

   A. hypotension
   B. renal insufficiency
   C. hyperkalemia
   D. proteinuria

36. The rationale for using beta blocker therapy in treating a patient with CHF is to:

   A. increase myocardial contractility
   B. reduce the effects of circulation catecholamines
   C. relieve concomitant angina
   D. stabilize cardiac rhythm

37. In prescribing salmeterol, you advise the patient that it has:

   A. anti-inflammatory activity
   B. a rapid onset of action
   C. a 12-hour duration of action
   D. anticholinergic effect

ANSWERS

28. C
29. B
30. C
31. B
32. A
33. B
34. A
35. A
36. B
37. C

DISCUSSION

Congestive heart failure occurs as a result of altered cardiac function that leads to inadequate cardiac output and a resulting inability to meet the oxygen and metabolic demands of the body. Hypertensive heart disease and atherosclerosis are the leading causes of CHF. Less common causes include pneumonia (as a result of increased right-sided heart workload), anemia (because of the resulting decreased oxygen-carrying capability of the blood), and increased sodium intake (because of the resultant increase in circulating volume).

The cornerstone of therapy for patients with CHF is the use of angiotensin-converting enzyme inhibitors (ACEIs) because these agents cause central and peripheral vasodilatation, resulting in a reduction in cardiac workload and improvement in cardiac output. Angiotensin receptor blockers (ARB; -sartan suffix drugs) can also be used as an ACEI substitute. Diuretics and digoxin are both second-line therapies.

Digoxin has a positive inotropic effect and slows conduction through the AV node. A prolongation of the PR interval and cupping of the ST segment are typically seen in ECGs of patients taking a therapeutic dose of digoxin. With digoxin toxicity, a number of cardiac effects can be seen; AV block is the most common. Anorexia is the most common patient report during digoxin toxicity. Visual changes are rarely reported.

Although ACEIs and ARBs are the cornerstone of CHF therapy, their use can be associated with adverse effects. Most common is hypotension, particularly when one of these agents is prescribed for a person who is currently taking a diuretic or vasodilator. In order to avoid this, ACEI or ARB therapy should be started at low doses and slowly increased to achieve a therapeutic response. Renal insufficiency can be precipitated by ACEI or ARB therapy; this usually only occurs in the presence of renal artery stenosis or underlying renal disease. Whereas hyperkalemia with ACEI or ARB use is usually seen only with concurrent use of a potassium-sparing diuretic, proteinuria is rarely seen (Table 5–5).

The S_3 heart sound is heard in patients with CHF as well as in those with myocardial ischemia. This is the sound of poor myocardial contractility and systolic dysfunction. The S_4 heart sound may also be heard but is less common. This is the sound of poor myocardial relaxation (compliance), diastolic dysfunction, and potentially decreasing cardiac output. The PMI is normally at the fifth intercostal space (ICS), midclavicular line (MCL). It is shifted laterally and perhaps over more than one ICS in the presence of dilated cardiomyopathy and its resultant increase in cardiac size.

TABLE 5-5.
CONGESTIVE HEART FAILURE THERAPY

Therapy	Mechanism of Action	Comment
Diuretics	Volume depletion	Provide symptomatic relief Excessive diuresis may lead to excessive neurohumoral activation Should be used in conjunction with ACEIs or ARBs
Angiotensin converting enzyme inhibitors (ACEIs)	Block conversion of angiotensin I to angiotensin II, a potent vasoconstrictor Decreases sodium retention	May cause hypotension when given to volume-constricted patients ACEI use with a potassium-sparing diuretic may lead to hyperkalemia May cause cough
Angiotensin II receptor blockers (ARB)	Block activity of angiotensin II, a potent vaso-constrictor Decrease sodium retention	May cause hypotension when given to volume-constricted patients ARB use with a potassium-sparing diuretic may lead to hyperkalemia Does not cause cough
Beta blocker	Reduction in neuro-humoral effect, lower levels of circulation catecholamines	Improved longevity and quality of life with beta blocker use despite possible negative inotropic effects Carvedilol is a beta blocker with vasodilating qualities approved for the treatment of CHF
Digoxin	Positive inotrope	Use should be limited to those with CHF who continue to be symptomatic in spite of adequate ACEI or ARB therapy
Spironolactone (Al dactone)	Aldosterone inhibitor and K + -potassium sparing diuretic	Improved function and reduced hospitalization noted with use. Unlikely to cause hyperkalemia when used in low dose in conjunction with ACEI or ARB

References: Sellers, J., Brubaker, M. (1999). Cardiovascular disorders. In Youngkin, Savin, Kissinger, and Israel. *Pharmacotherapeutics.* Stamford, CT: Appleton & Lange. Pp. 309–368.

Discussion Source

Hektor Dunphy, L. (1999). *Management Guidelines for Adult Nurse Practitioners*. Philadelphia: FA Davis. Pp. 245–248.

QUESTIONS

38. You examine a 38-year-old obese woman who has presented for an initial examination Pap test. She has no complaint. Her BP is 144/98 mm Hg bilaterally. The rest of her physical examination is unremarkable. Your next best action is to:

    A. initiate antihypertensive therapy
    B. arrange for two additional BP measurements during the next two weeks
    C. order a BUN, Cr, K+, and urinalysis
    D. advise her to reduce her sodium intake

39. You see a 68-year-old woman who has systolic hypertension that is currently treated with nisoldipine. Her BP is usually within a satisfactory range. Today she presents with a 3-lb weight gain and BP of 152/85 mm Hg. The rest of her history and examination is unremarkable. Your next best action is to:

    A. prescribe low-dose captopril
    B. have her return for a BP check in 1 week
    C. obtain a BUN, Cr, K+ and urinalysis
    D. review dietary sodium, fat, and caloric reduction

40. You examine an elderly woman with long-standing, poorly controlled hypertension. When evaluating her for hypertensive end-organ damage, you look for evidence of:

    A. lipid abnormalities
    B. hyperinsulinemia and insulin resistance
    C. LV hypertrophy
    D. clotting disorders

41. A 62-year-old woman of African ancestry presents with BP of 150/102 mm Hg on three separate occasions. She is of normal weight and is a nonsmoker with no other health problems. Which of the following represents the best choice of an antihypertensive agent?

    A. short-acting nicardipine (Cardene)
    B. hydrochlorothiazide (Hydrodiuril)
    C. sustained-release metoprolol (Toprol XL)
    D. captopril (Capoten)

42. All of the following patients are in need of antihypertensive therapy. Who is the best candidate for long-acting beta adrenergic antagonist use?

    A. a 48-year-old woman with type 1 diabetes
    B. a 46-year-old man with a history of MI
    C. a 68-year-old woman with COPD
    D. a 44-year-old man with a history of poor adherence to medication regimens

43. Which is the most helpful pharmacologic agent for an older man with hypertension, COPD, and BPH?

    A. alpha adrenergic antagonist
    B. beta adrenergic antagonist
    C. ACE inhibitor
    D. dihydropyridine calcium channel blocker

44. Which of the following is the preferred antihypertensive choice for a 42-year-old man with type 1 diabetes mellitus?

    A. atenolol
    B. hydrochlorothiazide
    C. losartan
    D. amlodipine

45. Which of the following is the preferred antihypertensive choice for a 72-year-old man who had an MI 6 months ago?

    A. atenolol
    B. hydrochlorothiazide
    C. diltiazem
    D. amlodipine

46. Diagnostic testing for a patient with newly detected hypertension should include all of the following except:

    A. urine protein
    B. chest radiograph

C. 12-lead ECG

D. potassium

47. Which of the following should be considered for hypertensive therapy in a 66-year-old woman with CHF?

A. verapamil

B. nifedipine

C. doxazosin

D. fosinopril

ANSWERS

38. **B**
39. **D**
40. **C**
41. **B**
42. **B**
43. **A**
44. **C**
45. **A**
46. **B**
47. **D**

DISCUSSION

The goal of treating hypertension is not to establish normotensive status but rather to eliminate or minimize target organ damage. The target organs of hypertension and their most commonly hypertension-related problems are as follows.

- Eye: Hypertensive retinopathy
- Brain: Stroke, vascular dementia, hypertensive encephalopathy
- Heart: Atherosclerosis, MI, left ventricular hypertrophy (LVH), CHF
- Kidney: Renal failure

In addition, you should focus your examination on the following (see Tables 5–6 and 5–7).

Establishing the diagnosis of hypertension in adults without evidence of target organ damage consists of finding elevated BP measurements on three or more occasions. The patient in Question 38 needs to have the diagnosis of hypertension established before further diagnostics or initia-

TABLE 5–6.
PHYSICAL EXAMINATION FOR PATIENTS WITH HYPERTENSION

Physical Examination	Hypertension-Associated Finding	Comments
Height and weight, body mass index (BMI)	Obesity (BMI > 27), especially with central or truncal pattern	Strong correlation of obesity with hypertension Weight loss is one of the most powerful interventions for hypertension
Waist measurement	> 34 inches for women and 36 inches for men	Associated with higher rates of dyslipidemia, type 2 diabetes, and coronary heart disease mortality
Funduscopic examination	Hypertension retinopathy (arteriolar narrowing, arteriovenous nicking, hemorrhages, exudates, and papilledema)	Presence of hypertension retinopathy indicates long-standing poor hypertension control
Carotid arteries	Bruits	The presence of a bruit usually indicates carotid artery atherosclerosis and increased stroke risk Strong correlation between carotid and coronary artery disease
Neck veins	Distention	Found in congestive heart failure, a sequelae of hypertension
Thyroid	Enlargement and the presence of nodules	Hyperthyroidism is a cause of secondary hypertension
Cardiac apex and point of maximum impulse	PMI and apex laterally displaced, greater than one intercostal space	May indicate left ventricular hypertrophy, hypertensive cardiomyopathy

(continued)

TABLE 5–6. (continued)

Physical Examination	Hypertension-Associated Finding	Comments
Heart sounds	S_3 and S_4 heart sounds	S_4 heart sound may indicate diastolic dysfunction, most common in poorly controlled hypertension and recurrent myocardial ischemia S_3 heart sound indicates systolic dysfunction and potential for CHF
Heart murmurs	Mitral regurgitation	Present when cardiac workload and poor approximation of valve leaflets occur as a result of poor hypertension control
Lungs	Evidence of rales and bronchospasm that may indicate obstructive pulmonary disease or heart failure	May influence the choice of antihypertensive agent
Abdominal examination	Bruits, masses, and abnormal aortic pulsation, enlarged kidneys	May indicate renovascular disease, abdominal aortic aneurysm
Extremities	Absence of peripheral arterial pulsation, bruits, edema	May indicate peripheral vascular disease

Adapted from Kaplan, N. (1998). *Management of hypertension.* (7th ed.). Durant, OK: EMIS, Inc. Pp. 8–140.

tion of drug therapy. In addition, lifestyle modification should be first-line therapy and is a vital part of the ongoing care of patients with hypertension. In that, the elderly patient in Question 39 with the modest BP increase and weight gain should be encouraged to use lifestyle modification (i.e., change in diet) (Box 5–1). Although it is tempting to or-

TABLE 5–7.
CLASSIFICATION OF BLOOD PRESSURE FOR ADULTS AGE 18 YEARS AND OLDER

Classification	Blood Pressure Value
Optimal	< 120 SBP; < 80 DBP
Normal	< 130 SBP; < 85 DBP
High normal	130–139 SBP; 85–89 DBP
Stage 1	140–159 SBP; 90–99 DBP
Stage 2	160–179 SBP; 100–109 DBP
Stage 3	> 180 SBP; > 110 DBP

If blood pressure fits into two stages, assign the higher stage (Example: 138/95 mm Hg = stage 1)

Stage 4 hypertension (as reported in JNC 5) has been eliminated in favor of a broader definition of stage 3.

Adapted from Kaplan, N. (1998). *Management of hypertension.* (7th ed.). Durant, OK: EMIS, Inc. Pp. 8–140.

der more tests, add new medication, or simply bring her back to recheck the BP, reinforcing simple but critically important measures such as proper diet is the best way to treat this chronic and potentially life-threatening disease (Box 5–2).

According to the JNC 6 recommendation, beta adrenergic antagonist (beta blockers) and diuretics continue to be recommended as first-line, proven therapy for treating uncomplicated hypertension. These are well documented to reduce stroke and cardiovascular mortality and morbidity. However, the NP should choose antihypertensive therapy with concurrent disease or comorbid conditions in mind (Boxes 5–3 and Box 5–4). Examples of these choices in concurrent disease include the following:

- Angiotensin-converting enzyme inhibitors (i.e., drugs with the -pril suffix) and perhaps ARBs (i.e., drugs with the -sartan suffix) in the presence of heart failure and MI with systolic dysfunction (help limit myocardial remodeling); for renal insufficiency and diabetes mellitus (may assist in preserving/enhancing renal function).

BOX 5–1
LIFESTYLE MODIFICATIONS TO PREVENT OR TREAT ELEVATED BLOOD PRESSURE

- Weight reduction: Body mass index >27 closely correlated with increased blood pressure
- Alcohol: No more than 1 oz ethanol (24-oz beer, 10-oz wine, 2-oz whiskey daily)
- Regular aerobic physical activity to a moderate level of fitness: Sedentary individuals have 20% to 50% increased risk of developing hypertension; blood pressure is lowered by 30 to 45 minutes walking most days of the week
- Discontinue cigarette smoking: blood pressure increases when smoking; smoking may diminish cardiovascular disease protection offered by hypertensive therapy

References: Kaplan, N. (1998). *Management of hypertension.* (7th ed.). Durant, OK: EMIS, Inc. Pp. 8–140.

Sixth Report of the Joint National Committee on Prevention, Detection, Evaluation and Treatment of High Blood Pressure (JNC 6). (1997). Bethesda, MD: National Institutes of Health.

BOX 5–2
JNC 6 RECOMMENDATIONS FOR CHECKING BLOOD PRESSURE

- Cuff size at least 80% of upper arm, using a cuff too big rather than too small
- Have the patient rest for 5 minutes before reading
- Arm should be resting at level of the heart
- No smoking or caffeine ingestion for at least 30 minutes before blood pressure measurement
- Two readings at least 2 minutes apart should be averaged; if there is more than 5 mm Hg difference, additional readings should be obtained
- Self-measurement of blood pressure is a valuable tool because it allows ongoing monitoring of blood pressure outside of the office, as well as response to antihypertensive therapies, possibly enhancing adherence and reducing costs

References: Kaplan, N. (1998). *Management of hypertension.* (7th ed.). Durant, OK: EMIS, Inc. Pp. 8–140.

Sixth Report of the Joint National Committee on Prevention, Detection, Evaluation and Treatment of High Blood Pressure (JNC 6). (1997). Bethesda, MD: National Institutes of Health.

BOX 5-3
MAJOR RISK FACTORS FOR CARDIAC COMORBIDITY IN PATIENTS WITH HYPERTENSION

- Cigarette smoking
- Dyslipidemia
- Diabetes mellitus
- Age older than 60 years
- Men and postmenopausal women
- Family history of premature heart disease (women age < 65 years; men age < 55 years)

References: Kaplan, N. (1998). *Management of hypertension.* (7th ed.). Durant, OK: EMIS, Inc. Pp. 8–140.
Sixth Report of the Joint National Committee on Prevention, Detection, Evaluation and Treatment of High Blood Pressure (JNC 6). (1997). Bethesda, MD: National Institutes of Health.

BOX 5-4
ANTIHYPERTENSIVE MEDICATIONS THAT ARE CONTRAINDICATED OR TO BE USED WITH CAUTION IN SELECT CLINICAL CONDITIONS

- Beta blockers: In asthma and obstructive pulmonary disease because of the risk of worsening bronchospasm
- Beta blockers: In peripheral vascular disease because of the risk of worsening claudication symptoms
- High-dose diuretics: In diabetes mellitus because of risk of increasing insulin resistance and negatively affecting glucose control
- ACEI and ARB: In pregnant women because of the risk of fetal hypotension and intrauterine fetal demise
- Beta blockers (except carvedilol) and calcium channel blocker (except amlodipine, felodipine) in heart failure because of negative inotropic effects
- Shorter- to intermediate-acting calcium channel blockers, including sublingual nifedipine, because of possible risk of increased mortality

---

References: Kaplan, N. (1998). *Management of hypertension.* (7th ed.). Durant, OK: EMIS, Inc. Pp. 8–140.
Sixth Report of the Joint National Committee on Prevention, Detection, Evaluation and Treatment of High Blood Pressure (JNC 6). (1997). Bethesda, MD: National Institutes of Health.

- Beta blockers (drugs with the -lol suffix) in the presence of angina; after MIs (ability to reduce cardiac workload and enhance rhythm stability); for atrial tachycardia (blunt tachycardia response), migraine headache (nonselective), reducing the frequency and severity of headache, essential tremor (nonselective), and reducing tremor because of blockage of $beta_2$ receptor sites
- Thiazide diuretics in the presence of systolic hypertension (inexpensive and efficacious agent) and osteoporosis (helps preserve bone density)
- Long-acting dihydropyridine (DHP) calcium channel antagonist (CA) in systolic hypertension (efficacious agent)

TABLE 5–8.
DIAGNOSTIC TESTING AS PART OF THE EVALUATION OF PATIENTS WITH HYPERTENSION

Test	Indication in Hypertension
Urinalysis	Proteinuria may predate increase in BUN level by as much as a decade
CBC	Rule out anemia Bone marrow suppression that may influence choice of anti-hypertensive agent
K+, Na+	Primary hyperaldosteronism (a cause of secondary hypertension) can cause hypokalemia Certain antihypertensives can cause hyperkalemia (ACEI, ARB) or hypokalemia (diuretics)
Blood glucose	Type 2 diabetes common co-condition with hypertension Certain antihypertensive agents (thiazide diuretics, beta blockers) can cause a blood glucose elevation
Lipid profile	Hyperlipidemia is a common co-condition with hypertension Certain antihypertensive agents (thiazide diuretics, beta blockers) can cause a elevation in cholesterol
12-Lead ECG	Evidence of hypertensive target organ damage (TOD) including left ventricular hypertrophy myocardialischemia and infraction.

Adapted from Kaplan, N. (1998). *Management of hypertension.* (7th ed.). Durant, OK: EMIS, Inc. Pp. 8–140.

**BOX 5–5
FACTORS INFLUENCING ADHERENCE TO
HYPERTENSIVE THERAPY**

- Involve patient and family in care planning
- Encourage home blood pressure monitoring
- Keep the pharmacologic plan of care simple and easy to tolerate
- Assist patient in integrating all therapeutic activities (e.g., lifestyle modification, medications) into established daily routine
- Be flexible in plan adjustment and accepting of small incremental changes in patient's lifestyle
- Encourage frequent follow-up visits, including nursing visits for ongoing education and monitoring and nursing case management

---

References: Kaplan, N. (1998). *Management of hypertension.* (7th ed.). Durant, OK: EMIS, Inc. Pp. 8–140.

Sixth Report of the Joint National Committee on Prevention, Detection, Evaluation and Treatment of High Blood Pressure (JNC 6). (1997). Bethesda, MD: National Institutes of Health.

- Alpha$_1$ adrenergic antagonists (alpha blockers) in benign prostatic hyperplasia (helps with bladder emptying) (Table 5–8, Box 5–5). A recent study cautions against the use of alpha blockers as first-line or solo agents because of increased risk of stroke and heart failure.

Discussion Sources

Deshmukh, R., Smith, A., Lilly, L. (1998). Hypertension. In *Pathophysiology of Heart Disease* (2nd ed.). Baltimore: Williams & Wilkins. Pp. 267–288.
Hektor Dunphy, L. (1999). *Management Guidelines for Adult Nurse Practitioners.* Philadelphia: FA Davis. Pp. 249–255.
Kaplan, N. (1998). *Management of Hypertension.* (7th ed.). Durant, OK: EMIS, Inc. Pp. 8–140.
Massie, B. (1999). Systemic hypertension. In Tierny, L., McPhee, S. & Papadakis, M. *Current Medical Diagnosis and Treatment* (38th ed.). Norwalk, CT: Appleton & Lange. Pp. 430–452.
Sixth report of the Joint National Committee on Prevention, Detection, Evaluation and Treatment of High Blood Pressure (JNC 6). (1997). Bethesda, MD: National Institutes of Health.

QUESTIONS

48. You examine a 24-year-old woman with mitral valve prolapse (MVP). Her physical examination findings may include:

    A. pectus excavatum
    B. obesity

    C. petite stature

    D. hyperextendible joints

49. The patient in the Question 48 informs you that she has a heart murmur from her MVP. In performing her cardiac examination, you expect to find a(n):

    A. early to midsystolic, crescendo-decrescendo murmur

    B. pansystolic murmur

    C. low-pitched, diastolic rumble

    D. middle to late systolic murmur

50. When examining the patient in Questions 48 and 49, you also expect to find a(n):

    A. opening snap

    B. midsystolic click

    C. paradoxical splitting of the second heart sound

    D. S_4 heart sound

51. Intervention for patients with MVP may include:

    A. restricted activity because of low cardiac output

    B. control of fluid intake to minimize risk of volume overload

    C. routine use of beta adrenergic antagonists to control palpitations

    D. encouragement of a regular program of aerobic activity

52. When a heart valve fails to open to its normal orifice, it is:

    A. stenotic

    B. incompetent

    C. sclerotic

    D. regurgitant

53. When a heart valve fails to close properly, it is:

    A. stenotic

    B. incompetent

    C. sclerotic

    D. regurgitant

54. You are evaluating a patient who has rheumatic heart disease. When assessing her for mitral stenosis, you look for the following murmur.

    A. systolic with wide radiation over the precordium
    B. localized diastolic with little radiation
    C. diastolic with radiation to the neck
    D. systolic with radiation to the axilla

55. In evaluating mitral incompetency, you expect to find the following murmur:

    A. systolic with radiation to the axilla
    B. diastolic with little radiation
    C. diastolic with radiation to the axilla
    D. localized systolic

56. Which of the following changes on the 12-lead ECG would you expect to find in a patient with aortic stenosis (AS)?

    A. bundle branch block
    B. right-axis deviation
    C. right atrial enlargement
    D. LV hypertrophy

57. Of the following patients, who is in greatest need of endocarditis prophylaxis with dental work?

    A. a 22-year-old woman with MVP with trace mitral regurgitation (MR) noted on echocardiogram
    B. a 54-year-old woman with prosthetic aortic valve
    C. a 66-year-old man with cardiomyopathy
    D. a 58-year-old woman who had a three-vessel coronary artery bypass graft 1 year ago

58. Of the following, who is at greatest risk for developing bacterial endocarditis?

    A. a 23-year-old woman with MVP and trace MR noted on echocardiogram
    B. a 55-year-old man who had undergone three-vessel coronary artery bypass grafting
    C. a 75-year-old woman with a prosthetic aortic valve
    D. a 45-year-old man with cardiomyopathy

59. You are examining an elderly woman and find a grade 3/6 cresendo-decresendo systolic murmur with radiation to the neck. This most likely caused by:

    A. aortic stenosis (AS)
    B. aortic regurgitation (AR)
    C. anemia
    D. mitral stenosis (MS)

60. Aortic stenosis in a 15-year-old boy is most likely:

    A. a sequelae of rheumatic fever
    B. as a result of congenital defect
    C. calcific in nature
    D. found with atrial septal defect

61. A physiologic murmur has which of the following characteristics?

    A. occurs late in systole
    B. localized area of auscultation
    C. becomes softer when the patient moves from supine to standing
    D. frequently obliterates S_2

62. You are examining an 18-year-old man who is seeking a sports clearance physical examination. You note a midsystolic murmur that gets louder when he stands. This may represent:

    A. aortic stenosis (AS)
    B. hypertrophic obstructive cardiomyopathy (HOCM)
    C. a physiologic murmur
    D. Still's murmur

63. Which of the following is the American Heart Association recommended agent for endocarditis prophylaxis in patients who are allergic to penicillin?

    A. erythromycin
    B. dicloxacillin
    C. azithromycin
    D. ofloxacin

ANSWERS

48. A
49. D
50. B
51. D
52. A
53. B
54. B
55. A
56. D
57. B
58. C
59. A
60. B
61. C
62. B
63. C

DISCUSSION

Heart murmurs are the sounds of turbulent blood flow. Blood traveling through the chambers and great vessels is usually a silent event. When the flow is sufficient to generate turbulence in the wall of the heart or great vessel, a murmur occurs.

Murmurs may be benign in that the examiner simply hears the blood flowing through the heart but no cardiac structural abnormality exists. However, certain cardiac structural problems, such as valvular and myocardial disorders, can contribute to the development of a murmur (Table 5–9).

Normal heart valves allow one-way, unimpeded forward blood flow through the heart. The entire stroke output is able to pass freely during one phase of the cardiac cycle (diastole with the AV valves, systole with the others), and there is no backflow of blood. When a heart valve fails to open to its normal orifice, it is stenotic. When it fails to close appropriately, the valve is incompetent, causing regurgitation of blood to the previous chamber or vessel. Both of these events place a patient at significant risk for embolic disease.

Physiologic murmurs are found in the absence of cardiac pathology. The term implies that the reason for murmur is something other than obstruction to flow and that the murmur is present with a normal gradient across the valve. This murmur may be heard in up to 80% of thin adults or children if the cardiac examination is performed in a soundproof booth and is best heard at the left sternal border. It occurs in early to midsystole, leaving the two heart sounds intact. In addition, the person with a benign systolic ejection murmur denies cardiac symptomatology and has an otherwise normal cardiac examination, including an appropriately located PMI and full pulses. Because no cardiac pathology is present with a physiologic murmur, no endocarditis prophylaxis is needed.

Aortic stenosis (AS) is the inability of the aortic valves to open to optimum orifice. The aortic valve normally opens to 3 cm^2; AS usually does not cause significant symptoms until the valvular orifice is limited to 0.8 cm^2. The disease is characterized by a long symptom-free period with rapid clinical deterioration at the onset of symptoms, including dyspnea, syncope, chest pain, and CHF. Small pulse pressure is a characteristic of severe AS.

When AS is present in adults who are middle-aged and older, it is most often the acquired form. In the older adult, the problem is usually calcification, leading to the inability of the valve to open to its normal orifice. Valvular changes in middle-aged adults without congenital AS, is usually the sequelae of rheumatic fever and represents about 30% of valvular dysfunction seen in rheumatic heart disease.

Aortic stenosis may be present in children and younger adults and is usually caused by a congenital bicuspid (rather than tricuspid) valve or by a three-cusp valve with leaflet fusion. This defect is most often found in boys and young men and is commonly accompanied by a long-standing history of becoming excessively short of breath with increased activity such as running. The physical examination is usually normal except for the associated cardiac findings.

The heart murmur of MR arises from mitral valve incompetency or the inability of the mitral valve to close properly. This allows a retrograde flow from a high-pressure area (LV) to an area of lower pressure (left atrium [LA]). MR is most often caused by the degeneration of the mitral valve—most commonly by rheumatic fever, endocarditis, calcific annulus, rheumatic heart disease (RHD), ruptured chordae, or papillary muscle dysfunction. In MR from RHD, there is usually some degree of mitral stenosis. After the person is symptomatic, the disease progresses in a downhill course of CHF over the next 10 years.

Mitral valve prolapse is likely the most common valvular heart problem, perhaps present in 10% of the population. This degree of distress

TABLE 5–9.
DIFFERENTIAL DIAGNOSIS OF COMMON CARDIAC MURMURS IN ADULTS

When evaluating adults with a cardiac murmur:

- Ask about major symptoms of heart disease: chest pain, CHF symptoms, palpitations, syncope, activity intolerance.
- The bell of the stethoscope is most helpful for auscultating lower-pitched sounds; the diaphragm helps in those with higher pitch.
- Systolic murmurs are graded on a scale of 1 to 6, from barely audible to audible with stethoscope off the chest. Diastolic murmurs are usually graded on the same scale but abbreviated to grades 1 to 4 because these murmurs will not be loud enough to reach grades 5 and 6.
- A critical part of the evaluation of a patient with a heart murmur is the decision to offer antimicrobial prophylaxis. No prophylaxis is needed for those with benign murmurs. Please refer to the American Heart Association Guidelines for endocardial prophylaxis.

Murmur	Important Cardiac Examination Findings	Additional Findings	Comments
Physiologic (also called innocent or functional)	Grades 1 to 3/6 early to mid-systolic murmur, heard best at LSB but usually audible over precordium	No radiation beyond precordium Softens or disappears with standing, increases in intensity with activity, fever, anemia S_1, S_2 intact, normal PMI	Cause is probably flow over aortic valve May be heard in +/- 80% of thin adults if examined in a sound-proof room Patient should be asymptomatic with no report of chest pain, CHF symptoms, palpitations, syncope, activity intolerance

Aortic stenosis	Grades 1 to 4/6 harsh systolic murmur, usually crescendo-decrescendo pattern, heard best at second RICS, apex	Radiates to carotid arteries, may have diminished S_2, slow filling carotid pulse, narrow pulse pressure, loud S_4 Softens with standing The greater the degree of stenosis, the later the peak of murmur	In young adults, usually congenital bicuspid valve In older adults, usually calcific, rheumatic in nature Dizziness and syncope are ominous signs, pointing to severely decreased cardiac output
Aortic sclerosis	Grades 2 to 3/6 systolic ejection murmur heard best at second RICS	Carotid upstroke full, not delayed, no S_4, absence of symptoms	Benign thickening or calcification of aortic valve leaflets No change in valve pressure gradient Also known as "50 over 50" murmur as found in > 50% of those older than age 50
Aortic regurgitation	Grades 1 to 3/4 high-pitched blowing diastolic murmur heard best at third LICS	May be enhanced by forced expiration, leaning forward Usually with S_3, wide pulse pressure, sustained thrusting apical impulse	More common in men, usually from rheumatic heart disease but occasionally because of tertiary syphilis
Mitral stenosis	Grades 1 to 3/4 low-pitched late diastolic murmur heard best at the apex, localized Short crescendo-decrescendo rumble, like a bowling ball rolling down an alley or distant thunder	Often with opening snap, accentuated S_1 in the mitral area Enhanced by left lateral decubitus position, squat, cough, immediately post-Valsalva	Nearly all rheumatic in origin Protracted latency period, then gradual decrease in exercise tolerance leading to rapid downhill course because of low cardiac output AF common

(continued)

TABLE 5-9. (continued)

Murmur	Important Cardiac Examination Findings	Additional Findings	Comments
Mitral regurgitation	Grades 1 to 4/6 high-pitched blowing systolic murmur, often extending beyond S$_2$. Sounds like long "haaa" or "hooo" Heard best at RLSB	Radiates to axilla, often with laterally displaced PMI Decreased with standing, Valsalva maneuver Increased by squat, hand grip	Origin: Rheumatic, ischemic heart disease, endocarditis Often with other valve abnormalities (AS, MS, AR)
Mitral valve prolapse	Grades 1 to 3/6 late systolic crescendo murmur with honking quality heard best at apex Murmur follows midsystolic click	With Valsalva maneuver or standing, click moves forward into earlier systole, resulting in a longer-sounding murmur With hand grasp, squat, click moves back further into systole, resulting in a shorter murmur	Often seen with minor thoracic deformities such as pectus excavatum, straight back, shallow AP diameter Chest pain is sometimes present, but there is question as to whether MVP itself is cause.

References: Constant, J. (1999). *Bedside Cardiology.* (5th ed.). Philadelphia: Lippincott, Williams & Wilkins. Willms, J., Schneidermans, H., Algranti, P. (1994). The heart and great vessels. In *Physical Diagnosis: Bedside Evaluation of Diagnosis and Function.* Baltimore: Williams & Wilkins. Pp. 283–346.

(chest pain, dyspnea) may depend in part on the degree of MR, although some studies have failed to reveal any difference in the rates of chest pain in patients with or without MVP. Potentially the greatest threat is the rupture of chordae, usually seen only in those with connective tissue disease, especially Marfan syndrome.

The majority of patients with MVP have a benign condition in which one of the valve leaflets is unusually long and buckles or prolapses into the LA, usually occurring in midsystole. At that time, a click occurs that is followed by a short murmur caused by regurgitation of blood into the atrium. Cardiac output is usually uncompromised, and the event goes unnoticed by the patient. However, the examiner may detect this on examination. Echocardiography fails to reveal any abnormality, with simply the valve buckling followed by a small-volume MR noted. If there are no cardiac complaints and the rest of the cardiac examination, including the ECG, is within normal limits, no further evaluation is needed.

One way of describing this variation from the norm is to inform the patient that one leaflet of the mitral valve is a bit longer than usual. However, the "holder" (valve orifice) is of average size. This causes the valve to buckle a bit, just as your foot would if forced into a shoe that is one or two sizes too small. As a result, the heart makes an extra set of sounds (click and murmur) but is not diseased or damaged. MVP is often found in patients with minor thoracic deformities such as pectus excavatum, a dish-shaped concave area at T1, and scoliosis. The exact nature of this correlation of findings is not understood.

The second and much smaller group of patients with MVP has systolic displacement of one or more of the mitral leaflets into the LA alone with valve thickening and redundancy, usually accompanied by mild to moderate MR. This group typically has additional health problems such as Marfan syndrome or other connective tissue disease. There is a risk of bacterial endocarditis in this group because structural cardiac abnormality is present.

Barring other health problems, patients with MVP usually have normal cardiac output and tolerate a program of aerobic activity. This activity should be encouraged to promote health and well-being. The degree of valve prolapse is increased, thus increasing intensity of the murmur, when circulating volume is low. Maintaining a high level of fluid intake should be encouraged for patients with MVP. Treatment with a beta adrenergic agonist (beta blocker) is indicated only when symptomatic recurrent tachycardia or palpitations is an issue.

Hypertrophic obstructive cardiomyopathy (HOCM) is a disease of the cardiac muscle. The ventricular septum is thick and asymmetric, leading to potential outflow track block. Patients with HOCM often exhibit symptoms of cardiac outflow tract blockage with activity because

BOX 5-6
AMERICAN HEART ASSOCIATION GUIDELINES FOR BACTERIAL ENDOCARDITIS PROPHYLAXIS REGIMEN FOR DENTAL, ORAL, OR RESPIRATORY TRACT OR ESOPHAGEAL PROCEDURES

One hour before procedure:

- Adults: Amoxicillin 2 g 1 hour before procedure
- Children: Amoxicillin 50 mg/kg 1 hour before procedure
- A follow-up dose is no longer recommended

If allergic to amoxicillin
One hour before procedure:

- Adult: Clindamycin 600 mg; Children: 20 mg/kg <u>or</u>
- Adult: Cephalexin or cefadroxil 2g; Children: 50 mg/kg <u>or</u>
- Adult: Azithromycin or clarithromycin 500 mg; Children: 50 mg/kg
- No follow-up dose is recommended
- Erythromycin is no longer recommended

Endocarditis prophylaxis recommended for the following:
High-risk category:

- Presence of prosthetic heart valves
- Previous bacterial endocarditis
- Complex cyanotic congenital heart disease
- Surgically constructed systemic pulmonary shunts or conduits

Moderate-risk category

- Most other congenital cardiac deformities
- Rheumatic heart disease and other acquired cardiac defects, even after repair
- Hypertrophic cardiomyopathy
- Mitral valve prolapse with valvular regurgitation or thickened valves

Patients not needing prophylaxis: Risk no greater than general population

- Isolated secundum atrial septal defect
- Surgical repair of atrial septal defect, ventricular septal defect, patent dutus arteriosis without residual problems
- Mitral valve prolapse without regurgitation
- Physiologic function or innocent heart murmurs
- Previous Kawasaki's disease without valvular dysfunction
- Previous rheumatic fever without valvular dysfunction
- Those with cardiac pacemakers (intravascular and epicardial)

Reference: Dajani, AS, et al. (1997). Prevention of bacterial endocarditis: Recommendations of the American Heart Association. *JAMA* 277 (22), Pp. 1794–1801.

the hypotrophic ventricular walls better approximate with the increased force of myocardial contraction associated with exercise. Unfortunately, the presentation of HOCM may be sudden cardiac death. Idiopathic hypertropic subaortic stenosis (IHSS) is a type of cardiomyopathy. Because it is an autosomal dominant disorder, a strong family history is often present. Patients with this disorder are usually young adults with a history of dyspnea with activity, but they may also be asymptomatic.

According to the most recent AHA Guidelines for Bacterial Endocarditis Prevention, patients with prosthetic heart valves have the highest risk for endocarditis. Thus, these patients are at greatest need for endocarditis prophylaxis. Whereas the presence of cardiomyopathy places the person at moderate risk, coronary bypass grafting for these patients has no greater endocarditis risk than for the general public. MVP without significant regurgitation carries no endocarditis risk. Trace MR may be found in patients without valvular heart problems (Box 5–6).

Discussion Source

Hektor Dunphy, L. (1999). *Management Guidelines for Adult Nurse Practitioners*. Philadelphia: FA Davis. Pp. 239–283.
Dajani, AS, et. al. Prevention of bacterial endocarditis. Recommendations of the American Heart Association. *JAMA* 277 (22), Pp. 1734–1801.

QUESTIONS

64. You examine a 28-year-old woman who has emigrated from a South American country. She has documentation of receiving bacille Calmette-Guérin (BCG) vaccine as a child. With this information, you consider that:

  A. She will always have a positive tuberculin skin test (TST).
  B. Biannual chest radiographs are needed to accurately assess her health status.
  C. TST-10 mm or more induration should be considered a positive result.
  D. Isoniazid therapy should be given for 6 months before TST is undertaken.

65. A 33-year-old woman works in a small office with a man recently diagnosed with active pulmonary tuberculosis. Which of the following
best represents plan of care for this woman?

   A. She should receive isoniazid prophylaxis if her TST is ≥ 5 mm in
   induration.
   B. Because of her age, tuberculosis chemoprophylaxis is contraindicated even in the presence of a positive TST result.
   C. If the TST result is positive but the chest radiograph is normal, no
   further evaluation or treatment is needed.
   D. Further evaluation is needed only if TST is ≥ 15 mm in induration.

ANSWERS

64. C
65. A

DISCUSSION

Pulmonary tuberculosis is a chronic bacterial infection transmitted
through droplets. Most of those infected with the causative agent, *My-
cobacterium tuberculosis*, are asymptomatic. Untreated, 10% of these patients go on to develop active disease, a number that skyrockets in the
presence of HIV infection. TST with purified protein derivative (PPD) is
an effective method of screening. A positive TST result is measured in
millimeters of induration, not simply redness. Thresholds for a positive
TST result are as follows:

   • ≥ 5-mm induration in those with suspected or known HIV, close
     contact with a person with active pulmonary tuberculosis, and
     those with radiographic changes consistent with old disease
   • ≥ 10-mm induration in those with high risk such as immigrants
     from countries where tuberculosis is endemic, intravenous drug
     users, health care providers
   • ≥ 15-mm induration in all others
   • Any induration ≥ 10 mm should be considered a positive result in
     adults who received BCG vaccine as a child

Isoniazid therapy (chemoprophylaxis) to prevent the development of active pulmonary tuberculosis should be considered in asymptomatic pa-

tients with positive TST results but negative chest radiograph results. In the presence of active pulmonary tuberculosis, multiple antimicrobial therapies are given that are aimed not only at eradicating the infection but in minimizing the risk of developing a resistant pathogen. In this era of multidrug-resistant tuberculosis, it is prudent to consult with local tuberculosis experts to ascertain the local patterns of susceptibility.

Discussion Source

Hektor Dunphy, L. (1999). *Management Guidelines for Adult Nurse Practitioners*. Philadelphia: FA Davis. Pp. 273–376.

QUESTIONS

66. An 18-year-old woman has a chief complaint of cough and body aches. Otherwise her history shows nothing unusual. You conclude that she has atypical pneumonia. Assuming she has no other significant history, you prescribe:

    A. erythromycin
    B. cefpodoxime
    C. trimethoprim sulfamethoxasole
    D. penicillin

67. A 64-year-old man presents with a 48-hour history of left-sided pleuritic chest pain with splinting and congested productive cough of white sputum. This presentation is most consistent with pneumonia caused by:

    A. *Chlamydia pneumoniae*
    B. influenza virus
    C. pneumococci
    D. *Moraxella catarrhalis*

68. The physical examination of the patient in Question 67 reveals increased tactile fremitus and dullness to percussion at the right base. These findings are consistent with:

    A. an area of decreased density
    B. pneumothorax
    C. consolidation
    D. cavitation

69. This patient in question 68 should receive:

    A. azithromycin
    B. ciprofloxacin
    C. cephalexin
    D. vancomycin

70. Which of the following represents findings in an acceptable sputum specimen for Gram staining?

    A. many squamous epithelial and few WBCs
    B. three or more stained organisms
    C. few squamous epithelial and many WBCs
    D. motile bacteria with monocytes

71. You are caring for a 52-year-old smoker who has pneumonia. It is the third day of his therapy and he is without fever, is well hydrated, and is feeling somewhat better. Which of the following represents the best schedule for ordering a chest radiograph for this patient?

    A. no chest radiograph is needed as he is recovering
    B. a chest radiograph should be done today to confirm resolution of pneumonia
    C. he should have a chest radiograph done in 7–12 weeks
    D. a computed tomography scan of the thorax is needed now

ANSWERS

66. A
67. C
68. C
69. A
70. C
71. C

DISCUSSION

When assessing patients who have pneumonia, it is important to consider the causative organism. *M. pneumoniae* is the leading causative pathogen in pneumonia found in young adults and children. Pneumonia caused by *M. pneumoniae* and *C. pneumoniae* typically cause a hacking cough, headaches, myalgia, and malaise. Because fever, shaking, chills, and production of purulent sputum are found in the classic pneumonia scenario, these illnesses are often called atypical pneumonia.

The patient in Question 67 presents as a more "typical" pneumonia, with pleuritic chest pain, fever, and sputum production. *Streptococcus pneumoniae* or pneumococcus is the most common cause of community-acquired pneumonia in older adults and is the leading pathogen in fatal pneumonia.

When obtaining a sputum specimen, it is important to note whether the specimen is truly pulmonary in origin. For example, if the patient was simply able to produce "mouth spit," the specimen is abundant with oral epithelial cells with few WBCs. A specimen from the tracheobronchial tree has few squamous and many WBCs.

In cigarette smokers, a chest radiograph should be done 7–12 weeks after initiation of pneumonia therapy to check for the presence of lung cancer.

When choosing an antibiotic for treatment of community-acquired pneumonia, two sources, the *Sanford Guide to Antimicrobial Therapy* and the *Infectious Diseases Society of America*, offer treatment options (Tables 5–10, 5–11, and 5–12).

Sputum Gram staining and culture are helpful in ascertaining the pathogen in fewer than 50% of patients with community-acquired pneumonia. Empiric therapy based on presentation, age, and risk factors is

TABLE 5–10.
INFECTIOUS DISEASE SOCIETY GUIDELINES FOR TREATMENT OF COMMUNITY-ACQUIRED PNEUMONIA

Treatment Indication	Treatment
Empiric therapy	Macrolides (erythromycin, azithromycin, clarithromycin) Respiratory fluoroquinolone such as moxifloxacin, gatifloxacin, levofloxacin Doxycycline
Suspected aspiration	Amoxicillin with clavulanate
Younger adult (age 17–40 years)	Doxycycline

Adapted from Bartlett, J., Breimon, R., Moudell, L., File, T. (1998). Guidelines from The Infectious Disease Society of America. Community-acquired pneumonia in adults: Guidelines for management. *Clinical Infectious Disease.* 26. Pp. 811–836.

TABLE 5–11.
SANFORD GUIDE RECOMMENDATIONS FOR THE EMPIRIC TREATMENT OF COMMUNITY-ACQUIRED PNEUMONIA

Patient Category	Most Likely Pathogens	Suggested Regimens
Adults over age 18	No comorbidity • *M. pneumoniae, C. pneumoniae,* viral Smoker • *S. pneumoniae, H. influenzae, M. catarrhalis* Post viral bronchitis • *S. pneumonia, S. aureus* (rare) Alcohol abuse • *S. pneumoniae,* anaerobes, coliform Airway obstruction • Anaerobes Epidemic • Legionella	Primary • Azithromycin • Clarithromycin • Dirithromycin • Respiratory fluroquinolone (levofloxacin, gatifloxacin, moxifloxacin) Alternative therapies • Amoxicillin with clavulanate • Second generation cephalosporin

Source: Gilbert, D., Moellering, R., Sande, M. (1999). *The Sanford Guide to Antimicrobial Therapy* (29th ed.). Hyde Park, VT: Antimicrobial Therapy, Inc. Pp. 27–28.

TABLE 5–12.
DIFFERENTIAL DIAGNOSIS AND TREATMENT OF COMMUNITY-ACQUIRED PNEUMONIA

- Sputum Gram staining and culture will be helpful in ascertaining the pathogen in less than 50% of persons with community-acquired pneumonia (CAP). Empiric therapy based on presentation, age and risk factors is preferred.
- When a person is sick enough to require hospitalization, correlation with presentation and causative organism is less helpful.
- Pneumonia is the 6th leading cause of death in the United States and the leading cause of infectious disease death. Careful assessment of self-care ability and meticulous follow up are needed for successful outpatient treatment.
- Since nearly ⅔ of all fatal pneumonia is caused by *S. pneumoniae*, the pneumococcal organism, consistent and appropriate use of antipneumococcal vaccine should be a therapeutic goal.

Causative Pathogen and Mechanism of Transmission	Morphology, Anticipated Gram-Stain Results	Typical Age Group Affected	Patient Presentation and Anticipated Chest X-ray Findings	Effective Therapeutic Agents
Streptococcus pneumoniae, via micro-aspiration	Gram-positive diplococci	Under 5 years Older adults. Accounts for ⅔ of all fatal pneumonias	Usually typical: Fever, chills, purulent, occasional rusty sputum, evidence of consolidation; tubular breath sounds, increased vocal fremitus, dullness to percussion Atypical presentation in elder, chronically ill, immune impairment. Chest x-ray-Lobar consolidation	Prevent with pneumococcal vaccine; Macrolides (erythromycin, azithromycin, clarithromycin, dirithromycin) Respiratory fluoroquinolones (levofloxacin, gatifloxacin, moxifloxacin) Beta lactams (amox, select cephalosporins such as cefprozil, cefuroxime, cefpodoxime)

(continued)

TABLE 5-12. (continued)

Causative Pathogen and Mechanism of Transmission	Morphology, Anticipated Gram Stain Results	Typical Age Group Affected	Patient Presentation and Anticipated Chest X-ray Findings	Effective Therapeutic Agents
Mycoplasma pneumoniae, via cough transmission	Intracellular pathogen not visible with gram-stain, neutrophils and monocytes only.	Children, adults <40 years	Headache, myalgia, malaise, dry cough, crackles, occasionally bullous myringitis. Chest x-ray-Patchy infiltrates, consolidation rare.	Macrolides, (erythromycin, azithromycin, clarithromycin, dirithromycin), respiratory fluoro-quinolones (levofloxacin, - gatifloxacin, moxifloxacin)
Chlamydia pneumoniae, via cough transmission	Intracellular pathogen not visible with gramstain, neutrophils and monocytes only.	Younger adult	Sore throat, hoarseness, headache, myalgia, malaise, dry cough, crackles. Chest x-ray-Variable infiltrates, consolidation rare.	Macrolides (erythromycin, azithromycin, clarithromycin, dirithromycin), respiratory fluoro-quinolones (levofloxacin, gatifloxacin, moxifloxacin)
Klebsiella pneumoniae, via aspiration	Gram-negative rods	Immunocompromise, alcohol abuse	May be atypical due to concomitent disease Chest x-ray-Lobar infiltrate	Amoxicillin with clavulanate, select cephalosporins, respiratory fluoro-quinolones (levofloxacin, gatifloxacin, moxifloxacin)

Haemophilus influenzae, via airway colonization	Gram-negative coccobacillus	Smokers, elders	May be atypical due to concomitant disease. Chest x-ray-Lobar consolidation	Select macrolides (azithromycin, clarithromycin, dirithromycin), respiratory fluoroquinolones, (levofloxacin, gatifloxacin, moxifloxacin), amox with clavulanate, select cephalosporins, tetracyclines
Anaerobes	Mixed flora	Patients with problems with airway maintenance	May be atypical due to concomitant disease. Chest x-ray-Patchy infiltrates in dependent lung	Amoxicillin with clavulanate, clindamycin
Legionella, via aerosol inhalation	Intracellular organism not visible on gram stain. Gram stain results variable.	Elder, smoker, DM, alcohol abuse, immunocompromise, chronic illness	Fever, rigors, hypoxemia, GI upset, dry cough Chest x-ray-Lobar consolidation, patchy infiltrates	Macrolides (erythromycin, azithromycin, clarithromycin, dirithromycin), respiratory fluoroquinolones (levofloxacin, gatifloxacin, moxifloxacin)

Source: Gilbert, D., Moellering, R., Sande, M. (1999). *The Sanford Guide to Antimicrobial Therapy* (29th ed.). Hyde Park, VT: Antimicrobial Therapy, Inc. Pp. 27–28.

Chestnutt, M., Prendergast, T., Stauffer, J. (1999). Lung. In Tierney, L., McPhee, S., Papadakis, M. *Current Diagnosis and Treatment* (38th ed.). Norwalk, CT: Appleton & Lange. Pp. 255–338.

usually preferred. When a patient is sick enough to require hospitalization, correlation with presentation and causative organism is less helpful.

Pneumonia is the sixth leading cause of death in the United States and is the leading cause of infectious disease death. Careful assessment of self-care ability and meticulous follow-up care are needed for successful outpatient treatment.

Discussion Sources

Hektor Dunphy, L. (1999). *Management Guidelines for Adult Nurse Practitioners*. Philadelphia: FA Davis. Pp. 266–270.

Infectious Disease Society of America. (1998). Commonly acquired pneumonia: Guidelines for Management. *Clinical Infectious Disease* 156, 811–838.

Gilbert, D., Moellering, R., Sande, M. (1998). *The Sanford Guide to Antimicrobial Therapy* (28th ed.). Vienna, VA: Antimicrobial Therapy, Inc. Pp. 8.

6
CHAPTER

Abdominal
Disorders

QUESTIONS

1. You examine a 59-year-old man with a chief complaint of new onset of rectal pain after a bout of constipation. On examination, you note an ulcerated lesion on the posterior midline of the anus. The most likely diagnosis is:

    A. perianal fistula
    B. anal fissure
    C. external hemorrhoid
    D. Crohn's proctitis

2. Therapy for hemorrhoids includes all of the following except:

    A. weight control
    B. low-fiber diet
    C. topical hydrocortisone
    D. stool softener

ANSWERS

1. B
2. B

DISCUSSION

In anal fissure, there is an ulcer or tear of the margin of the anus. Most fissures occur posteriorly. Risk factors include constipation, diarrhea, recent childbirth, and anal intercourse or other anal insertion practices. The best treatment for anal fissure is avoidance of the condition through adequate fiber and fluid intake and avoiding constipation.

Whereas the superior hemorrhoidal veins form internal hemorrhoids, the inferior hemorrhoidal veins form external hemorrhoids. Both forms are actually normal anatomic findings but cause discomfort when there is an increase in the venous pressure and resulting dilatation and inflammation such as in childbirth, obesity, constipation, and prolonged sitting. As with anal fissure, prevention of hemorrhoidal engorgement and inflammation is the best treatment. Strategies include weight control, high fiber diet, regular exercise, and increased fluid intake. Treatment for acute hemorrhoid flare-ups includes the use of astringents and topical steroids as well as Sitz baths and analgesics. These therapies are also used in treating patients with anal fissure.

Discussion Source

Hektor Dunphy, L. (1999). *Management Guidelines for Adult Nurse Practitioners*. Philadelphia: FA Davis. Pp. 317–318, 228–290.

QUESTIONS

3. All of the following are often found in patients with the diagnosis of acute appendicitis except:

   A. epigastric pain
   B. obturator sign
   C. rebound tenderness
   D. marked febrile response

4. A 26-year-old man presents with acute abdominal pain. As part of the evaluation for appendicitis, you order a white blood cell (WBC) count with differential and anticipate the following results:

   A. total WBC, 4,500; Neuts, 35%; Bands, 2%; Lymphs, 45%
   B. total WBC, 14,000; Neuts, 55%; Bands, 3%; Lymphs, 38%
   C. total WBC, 16,500; Neuts, 66%; Bands; 8%, Lymphs; 22%
   D. total WBC, 18,100; Neuts, 55%; Bands, 3%; Lymphs, 28%

5. In evaluating a patient with suspected appendicitis, the NP considers that:

   A. The presentation may differ according to the anatomic location of the appendix.
   B. This is a common reason for acute abdominal pain in the elderly.
   C. Vomiting before onset of abdominal pain is often seen.
   D. The presentation is markedly different from that of pelvic inflammatory disease.

6. Psoas sign can be best described as abdominal pain elicited by:

    A. passive extension of the hip
    B. passive flexion and internal rotation of the hip
    C. deep palpation
    D. asking the patient to cough

7. Obturator sign can be best described as abdominal pain elicited by:

    A. passive extension of the hip
    B. passive flexion and internal rotation of the hip
    C. deep palpation
    D. asking the patient to cough

8. To support the diagnosis of acute appendicitis, you consider obtaining a(n):

    A. magnetic resonance image (MRI)
    B. computed tomography (CT) scan
    C. ultrasound
    D. flat plate of the abdomen

ANSWERS

3. **D**
4. **C**
5. **A**
6. **A**
7. **B**
8. **C**

DISCUSSION

Appendicitis is an inflammatory disease of the vermiform appendix caused by infection or obstruction. The peak age of patients with appendicitis is between 10 and 30 years; it is rather uncommon in infants and the elderly. However, in either end of the lifespan, there is often a delay in diagnosis of appendicitis because providers may not consider appendicitis a possibility.

There is no true classic presentation of appendicitis. However, vague epigastric or periumbilical pain often heralds its beginning, with the discomfort shifting to the right lower quadrant over the next 12 hours. Pain may be aggravated by walking or coughing. Nausea and vomiting are late symptoms that invariably occur a number of hours after the onset of pain; this late onset helps to differentiate appendicitis from gastroenteritis when vomiting usually proceeds abdominal cramping. The presentation of appendicitis also differs significantly according to the anatomic position of the appendix, with pain being reported in the epigastrium, flank, or groin. Obturator and psoas signs indicate inflammation of the respective muscles and strongly suggest peritoneal irritation and the diagnosis of appendicitis. Rebound tenderness indicates the likelihood of peritoneal irritation and helps with the diagnosis of acute appendicitis.

A total WBC count and differential is obtained as part of the evaluation of patients with suspected appendicitis. The most typical WBC count pattern found in this situation is the "left shift." A "left shift" is usually seen in the presence of severe bacterial infection, such as appendicitis and pneumonia. The following is typically noted:

- Leukocytosis: An elevation in the total WBC
- Neutrophilia: An elevation in the number of neutrophils in circulation. Neutrophilia is defined as more than 7000 neutrophils per mm^3. Neutrophils are also known as "polys" or "segs," both referring to the polymorph shape of the segment nucleus of this WBC.
- Bandemia: An elevation in the number of bands or young neutrophils in circulation. Usually fewer than 4% of the total WBCs in circulation are bands. When this is exceeded and the absolute band count is greater than 500 per mm^3, bandemia is present. This indicates that the body has called up as many mature neutrophils as were available in storage pool and is now accessing less mature forms. This further reinforces the seriousness of the infection. Other reasons for an increase in circulating bands include pneumonia, meningitis, septicemia, and tonsillitis.

There are other neutrophil forms that do not belong in circulation even with severe infection. These include myelocytes and metamyelocytes, immature neutrophil forms that are typically found in the granulopoiesis pool. The presence of these cells is an ominous marker for life-threatening infection and may be found in appendiceal rupture.

In addition to the WBC differential, an abdominal or transvaginal ultrasound reveals the inflamed appendix with a diagnostic accuracy of greater than 85%. CT of the abdomen is indicated only when there is a suspicion of appendiceal perforation because this study reveals periappendiceal abscess formation.

Surgical removal of the inflamed appendix is indicated via laparoscopy or laparotomy. If there is evidence of rupture with localized abscess and peritonitis, CT-directed abscess aspiration may be first indicated with an appendectomy after appropriate antimicrobial therapy.

Discussion Source

Hektor Dunphy, L. (1999). *Management Guidelines for Adult Nurse Practitioners*. Philadelphia: FA Davis. Pp. 290–292.
McQuaid, K. (1999). Alimentary tract. In Tierney, L., McPhee, S., & Papadakis, M. *Current Diagnosis and Treatment* (38th ed.). Norwalk, CT: Appleton & Lange. Pp. 638–647.

QUESTIONS

9. Which of the following is not a risk factor for bladder cancer?

   A. occupational exposure to textile dyes
   B. cigarette smoking
   C. occupational exposure to heavy metals
   D. chronic aspirin use

10. A 68-year-old man presents with suspected bladder cancer. You consider that its most common presenting sign and symptom is:

   A. painful urination
   B. fever and flank pain
   C. hematuria
   D. palpable abdominal mass

11. The patient in Question 10 is diagnosed with superficial bladder cancer without evidence of metastases. As a result, you realize that:

   A. His prognosis for 2-year survival is poor.
   B. A cystectomy is indicated.
   C. Despite successful initial therapy, local recurrence is common.
   D. Systemic chemotherapy is the treatment of choice.

ANSWERS

   9. D
   10. C
   11. C

DISCUSSION

Bladder cancer is the second most common urologic malignancy after prostate cancer. Usually a disease of later in life, the mean age at diagnosis is 65 years, and it is more common in men. Risk factors include cigarette smoking, accountable for the majority of cases, and exposure to industrial chemicals, including paints, dyes, and solvents. Primary prevention of bladder cancer through risk reduction is critically important.

Gross or microscopic hematuria is the most common presenting sign of bladder cancer. Irritative voiding symptoms and frequency without fever may be reported occasionally. Abdominal mass is only palpable with advanced disease.

The majority of those with newly diagnosed bladder cancer have superficial disease, allowing for effective treatment through bladder-sparing surgery and intravesical chemotherapy. Meticulous follow-up is critical because recurrence is often seen, necessitating repeat chemotherapy. Long-term survival is the norm with this noninvasive form of the disease.

Discussion Source

Hektor Dunphy, L. (1999). *Management Guidelines for Adult Nurse Practitioners*. Philadelphia: FA Davis. Pp. 292–295.

QUESTIONS

12. A 43-year-old woman has a 12-hour history of sudden onset of right upper quadrant abdominal pain with radiation to the shoulder, fever, and chills. She has had similar, milder episodes in the past. Examination reveals marked tenderness to right upper quadrant abdominal palpation. Her most likely diagnosis is:

    A. hepatoma
    B. cholecystitis
    C. acute hepatitis
    D. cholelithiasis

13. Which of the following is not seen in the diagnosis of acute cholecystitis?

    A. elevated lactic dehydrogenase (LDH) level
    B. increased alkaline phosphatase level
    C. leukocytosis
    D. elevated aspartate aminotransferase (AST) level

14. Murphy's sign can be best described as abdominal pain elicited by:

   A. right upper quadrant abdominal palpation
   B. deep palpation
   C. asking the patient to cough
   D. percussion

15. Risk factors for cholelithiasis include all of the following except:

   A. oral contraceptive use
   B. rapid weight loss
   C. obesity
   D. high-fiber diet

ANSWERS

12. B
13. A
14. A
15. D

DISCUSSION

Cholelithiasis is the formation of calculi or gallstones. The most common form of stones is cholesterol. About 75% of all of those with cholelithiasis have no symptoms and only become aware of the condition when it is found during evaluation for another health problem. About 10–25% of those initially without symptoms become symptomatic over the next decade. Prophylactic cholecystectomy is not indicated. However, the remainder of patients with cholelithiasis have intermittent right upper quadrant abdominal pain. Cholecystectomy is then indicated. Stone-dissolving medications such as ursodeoxycholic acid are available but take up to 2 years to dissolve stones, and 50% of patients have a return of stones within 5 years.

Cholecystitis is an acute inflammation of the gallbladder, nearly always caused by gallstones. Right upper quadrant or epigastric pain and tenderness is present along with fever and vomiting. Tenderness on palpating right upper quadrant of the abdomen (Murphy's sign) is nearly always present. Leukocytosis typical total WBC count = 12,000 to 15,000, rise in AST and ALP (alkaline phosphatase). ALP is an enzyme found in rapidly dividing or metabolically active tissue such as the liver, bone, intestine, and placenta. Elevated levels can reflect damage or accelerated cellular division in any of these areas. ALP increases in response to any obstruction in the biliary systems, it is a sensitive indicator of intra- or extrahepatic cholestasis.

Gamma glutamyl transferase (GGT), an enzyme involved in the transfer of amino acids across cell membranes, is found primarily in the liver and kidney. In liver disease, its increased level usually parallels changes in ALP, making it a useful marker of hepatic disease in obstructive jaundice, hepatic metastasis to the liver, and intrahepatic cholestasis. In addition, GGT can serve as a backup marker in elevated ALP. For example, if the ALP level is elevated and the GGT level is normal, ALP elevation is likely caused by its bone, and not hepatic, fraction. Acute cholecystis symptoms usually subside with conservative therapy such as low fat, clear liquid diet and analgesics. Cholecystectomy should be considered due to the likelihood of recurrence.

Discussion Sources

Friedman, L. (1999). Liver, biliary tract and pancreas. In Tierney, L., McPhee, S., & Papadakis, M. *Current Diagnosis and Treatment* (38th ed.). Norwalk, CT: Appleton & Lange. Pp. 638–677.
Hektor Dunphy, L. (1999). *Management Guidelines for Adult Nurse Practitioners*. Philadelphia: FA Davis. Pp. 295–299.

QUESTIONS

16. Which of the following is true concerning colorectal cancer?

    A. The majority are found during rectal examination.

    B. Rectal carcinoma is more common than cancers involving the colon.

    C. Early manifestations include abdominal pain and cramping.

    D. Later disease presentation often includes iron deficiency anemia.

17. According to the U.S. Preventive Clinical Services Guidelines, which of the following is the preferred method for annual colorectal cancer screening in a 50-year-old man?

    A. digital rectal examination

    B. fecal occult blood test (FOBT)

    C. flexible sigmoidoscopy

    D. barium enema

18. A patient with colorectal cancer typically presents with:

    A. gross rectal bleeding
    B. weight loss
    C. few symptoms
    D. nausea and vomiting

19. Which of the following does not increase a patient's risk of developing colorectal cancer?

    A. family history of colorectal cancer
    B. familial polyposis
    C. personal history of neoplasm
    D. chronic aspirin therapy

ANSWERS:

16. D
17. B
18. C
19. D

DISCUSSION

Colorectal cancer is second leading cause of cancer death in the United States, with 5% of the population developing the disease. Most are adenocarcinomas, with about 70% found in the colon and 30% in the rectum. Risk factors include a history of inflammatory bowel disease, personal history of neoplasia, age older than 50 years, a family history of colorectal cancer as well as familial polyposis syndrome. In addition, an autosomal dominant condition known as hereditary nonpolyposis colorectal cancer has been recently identified. Although this accounts for about 3% of all colorectal cancers, those with this risk factor tend to develop disease earlier and have as much as a 70% likelihood of colon cancer by age 65 years. A thorough family history is important when assessing an individual's risk of colorectal cancer. In addition, a high-fat, high-meat, low-calcium diet has also been implicated as contributing factor. The use of antioxidants, calcium supplements, and low-dose aspirin may reduce colorectal cancer rates.

    A patient with colorectal cancer is usually asymptomatic until disease is advanced. At that time, vague abdominal complaints coupled with iron deficiency anemia (as a result of chronic low-volume blood loss) may be found. The offending mass is most often beyond the examining digit. As a result, digital rectal examination is an ineffective method of colorectal cancer screening. In an effort to detect colorectal cancer, the U.S. Preventive Services Task Force recommends an annual FOBT. However, this has a high rate of both false-positive and false-negative results. Periodic sigmoidoscopy perhaps every 5 to 10 years is also recommended.

Individuals with increased risk for colorectal cancer have special screening needs. In those who have one first-degree relative with colorectal cancer developed after age 55 years, routine FOBT and sigmoidoscopy testing should begin at age 40 years. Patients with two or more relatives or one first-degree relative with adenomatous polyp before age 60 years should be screened periodically with colonoscopy. With a polyposis or a history of familial nonpolyposis colorectal cancer, expert consultation and period screening with colonoscopy is warranted.

Treatment of colorectal cancer usually includes surgery and adjunctive chemotherapy. Long-term survival depends on a number of factors, including the size and depth of the tumor, presence of positive nodes, and the overall health of a patient.

Discussion Sources

Hektor Dunphy, L. (1999). *Management Guidelines for Adult Nurse Practitioners*. Philadelphia: FA Davis. Pp. 304–306.
McQuaid, K. (1999). Alimentary tract. In Tierney, L., McPhee, S., & Papadakis, M. *Current Diagnosis and Treatment* (38th ed.). Stamford, CT: Appleton & Lange. Pp. 538–637.

QUESTIONS

20. Which of the following is most consistent with the presentation of a patient with diverticulosis?

   A. diarrhea and leukocytosis
   B. constipation and fever
   C. left-sided abdominal cramping
   D. frank blood in the stool with reduced stool caliber

21. Which of the following is most consistent with the presentation of a patient with diverticulitis?

   A. cramping, diarrhea, and leukocytosis
   B. constipation and fever
   C. left-sided abdominal pain
   D. frank blood in the stool with reduced stool caliber

22. One of the preferred antibiotics in the treatment of diverticulitis includes:

    A. metronidazole
    B. clindamycin
    C. azithromycin
    D. cefprozil

23. Prevention of diverticulitis includes:

    A. use of antidiarrheal agents
    B. avoiding gas-producing foods
    C. high-fiber diet
    D. low-dose antibiotic therapy

ANSWERS

20. C
21. A
22. A
23. C

DISCUSSION

Diverticulosis is a condition in which bulging pockets are present in the intestinal wall. However, inflammation is not present, and the patient is usually asymptomatic. When symptoms are present, left-sided abdominal cramping, increased flatus, and a pattern of constipation alternating with diarrhea are often reported.

In diverticulitis, the diverticula are inflamed, causing fever, leukocytosis, diarrhea, and abdominal pain. Conservative management of patients with diverticulitis includes increased fluid intake, rest, and a low-residue diet for the duration of the illness. Antibiotic therapy appears to shorten the course of illness. The organisms most often implicated in diverticulitis are *Bacteroides* spp. and enterococci. Metronidazole is one of the antibiotics of choice because it has excellent activity against anaerobic organisms such as *Bacteroides* spp. A second agent with strong gram-negative activity such as ciprofloxacin, ofloxacin, or trimethoprim sulfa should be added because the infection is often polymicrobial.

Prevention of diverticulosis and diverticulitis includes actions, such as regular aerobic exercise, adequate hydration, and a high-fiber diet, that increase bowel motility.

Discussion Sources

Hektor Dunphy, L. (1999). *Management Guidelines for Adult Nurse Practitioners*. Philadelphia: FA Davis. Pp. 306–309.
Gilbert, D., Moellering, R., Sande, M. (1998). *The Sanford Guide to Antimicrobial Therapy* (28th ed.). Vienna, VA: Antimicrobial Therapy, Inc. P. 14.

QUESTIONS

24. The gastric parietal cells produce:

    A. hydrochloric acid

    B. a protective mucosal layer

    C. prostaglandins

    D. prokinetic hormones

25. Antiprostaglandin drugs cause stomach mucosal injury primarily by:

    A. direct irritative effect

    B. altering the thickness of the protective mucosal layer

    C. decreasing peristalsis

    D. modifying stomach pH level

26. A 24-year-old man presents with a 3-month history of upper abdominal pain. He describes it as an intermittent, centrally located "burning" feeling in his upper abdomen, most often occurring 2 to 3 hours after meals. His presentation is most consistent with the diagnosis of:

    A. gastritis

    B. gastric ulcer

    C. duodenal ulcer

    D. cholecystitis

27. When choosing pharmacologic intervention to prevent recurrence of duodenal ulcer in a middle-aged man, you prescribe:

    A. a proton pump inhibitor

    B. timed antacid use

    C. antimicrobial therapy

    D. a histamine$_2$ receptor antagonist (H_2RA)

28. The H_2RA most likely to cause drug interactions with phenytoin and theophylline is:

    A. cimetidine
    B. famotidine
    C. nizatidine
    D. ranitidine

29. Which of the following is least likely to be found in a patient with gastric ulcer?

    A. history of long-term naproxen use
    B. age younger than 50 years
    C. previous use of H_2RA or antacids
    D. cigarette smoking

30. Nonsteroidal anti-inflammatory (NSAID)-induced peptic ulcer can be best limited by the use of:

    A. antacids
    B. HR_2As
    C. taking the medication with food
    D. misoprostol

31. Cyclooxygenase 1 (COX1) contributes to:

    A. inflammatory response
    B. pain transmission
    C. maintenance of gastric protective mucosal layer
    D. renal arteriole constriction

ANSWERS

24. A
25. B
26. C
27. C
28. A
29. B
30. D
31. C

DISCUSSION

Gastrointestinal irritation and ulcer occurs when there is an imbalance between gastric protective mechanism and irritating factors. Gastric parietal cells secrete hydrochloric acid, mediated by histamine$_2$ receptor sites.

The normal stomach pH is about 2, which kills many swallowed bacteria and viruses. Gastric acid production is about 1 to 2 mEq/hour in the resting, empty stomach and increases to 30 to 50 mEq/hour after a meal. Consequentially, symptoms associated with gastritis and gastric ulcer often become worse with eating because of the increase of irritating stomach acid on top of the lesion. The symptoms may become somewhat lessened because food buffers the acid. In contrast, duodenal ulcer symptoms often become worse as the stomach pH decreases when emptying after a meal.

The stomach is protected by a number of mechanisms, including a mucous coat with a gel layer. This layer provides mechanical protection from shearing as a result of ingestion of rough substances. In addition, bicarbonate is held within the protective layer and helps maintain pH to protect the mucosa from stomach acidity. Endogenous prostaglandins stimulate and thicken the mucus layer as well as enhance bicarbonate secretion and promote cell renewal and blood flow. Endogenous prostaglandins normally decrease with age, placing older adults at increased risk. As part of the stress response, there is an increase in endogenous gastric acid and pepsin production and the potential for gastric mucosa injury and gastritis. Exogenous reasons for damage to the stomach's protective mechanism include the use of standard (non-COX1–sparing) NSAIDs, steroids, smoking, and *Helicobacter pylori* infection.

Peptic ulcer disease is located in areas, such as the duodenum, stomach, esophagus, and small intestine, that are exposed to peptic juices such as acid and pepsin. Peptic ulcer disease usually includes loss of mucosal surface, extending to muscularis mucosae, that is at least 5 mm in diameter, with most being 2 to 5 times this size. Whereas an upper GI series identifies more than 80% of all ulcers larger than 0.5 cm, upper GI endoscopy identifies nearly all of them. Ulcers are capable of brisk bleeding, scarring, and perforation. GI erosion is usually seen in patients with gastritis. These are superficial mucosal lesions, usually less than 5 mm in diameter, that ooze rather than bleed. With healing, there is no scarring (Table 6–1).

Duodenal ulcer is more common than gastric ulcer. The most potent risk factor for this condition is most likely infection with *H. pylori*, a gram-negative, spiral-shaped organism with sheathed flagella found in at least 90% of those with duodenal ulcer. The pathogen is found in about

TABLE 6–1.
ASSESSING A PATIENT WITH PEPTIC ULCER DISEASE

Location and Type of Peptic Ulcer Disease	Risk and Contributing Factors	Presenting Signs and Symptoms	Diagnostic Testing
Duodenal ulcer	*Helicobacter pylori* infection, NSAID use, steroid use (much less common)	Epigastric burning, gnawing pain about 2–3 h PC; relief with foods, antacids Clusters of symptoms with periods of feeling well; awakening at 1 to 2 AM with symptoms common, morning waking pain rare Tender at the epigastrium, left upper quadrant abdomen, slightly hyperactive bowel sounds	*H. pylori* serologic testing Anti-*H. pylori* antibodies present with acute infection and take up to decades to decline If positive and PUD history, assume active infection and treat Cost of treatment less than endoscopy Urea breath test establishes presence of acute infection Consider as follow-up test of care, 1–3 months after treatment with positive serology results Endoscopy with biopsy and urease testing of biopsy or staining looking *for H. pylori* organism

Gastric ulcer	NSAID use potent risk factor Cigarette smoking Male: female ratio equal Peak incidence in fifth and sixth decades of life; nearly all found in those without *H. pylori* infection are caused by NSAID use	Pain often reported with or immediately after meals Nausea, vomiting, weight loss common	Difficulty distinguishing gastric ulcer from stomach cancer through UGI Upper GI endoscopy with biopsy vital Need confirmation of presence of *H. pylori* before treatment, as is present in some of cases
Nonerosive gastritis, chronic type B (antral) gastritis	Most likely caused by *H. pylori* infection	Nausea Burning and pain limited to upper abdomen without reflux symptoms	Upper endoscopy helpful diagnostic test
Erosive gastritis	Usually secondary to alcohol and NSAID use, ASA use, stress *H. pylori* infection usually not a factor	Nausea Burning and pain limited to upper abdomen without reflux symptoms; bleeding common	Upper endoscopy helpful diagnostic test

40–70% of those with gastric ulcer. *H. pylori* has an oral-fecal and oral-oral route of transmission, and rates of infection approach 100% in developing nations with poor water supplies. In developed nations with pure water supplies, at least 75% of the population older than age 50 years old has been infected at some time. Eradication of the organism dramatically alters the risk of relapse. A number of antibiotic combinations are effective (Table 6–2).

H. pylori produces urease, which then breaks down urea into ammonia and CO_2. This allows the organism to control pH in its local environment in the stomach by neutralizing H^+ ions in gastric acid. Therefore, urea breath testing is a helpful diagnostic procedure when attempting to establish the presence of *H. pylori* infection. *H. pylori* serologic titers can be helpful. However, titers may take years to decline after effective treatment. Correlating elevated titers with acute symptoms is helpful and assures the most accurate diagnosis.

In the past, the adage "no stress, no extra acid, no ulcer" was often quoted. Treatment for peptic ulcer disease often included the use of psychotropic medications for relief of stress, hypothesizing that this would reduce the acid production. In reality, only 30–40% of those with duodenal ulcer have higher-than-average acid secretion rates. In addition, coffee drinking and occasional alcohol use are not ulcer risk factors. However, alcohol abuse with cirrhosis remains a risk factor. *H. pylori* is also found in those with asymptomatic gastritis and dyspepsia without ulceration; eradication of the organism does not appear to make a difference in symptoms in patients with these conditions.

Suppression or neutralization of gastric acid is a critical part of peptic ulcer disease therapy. The H_2RAs (-tidine suffix) competitively block the binding of histamine to H_2 receptor site, thus reducing the secretion of gastric acid. Whereas, in prescription doses, these products suppress approximately 90% of hydrochloric acid production, the over-the-counter doses suppress about 80%. These products are generally well tolerated. Cimetidine is the only H_2RA that significantly inhibits CYP 450, thus slowing metabolism of certain drugs. As a result, drug interactions between cimetidine and warfarin, diazepam, phenytoin, quinidine, carbamazepine, theophylline, and imipramine may occur.

Omeprazole (Prilosec) and lansoprazole (Prevacid) are examples of proton pump inhibitors (PPIs). These drugs inhibit gastric acid secretion by inhibiting the final step in acid secretion by altering the activity of the "proton pump" (H = K + -ATPase). As a result, there is a virtual cessation of stomach hydrochloric acid production. PPI use is indicated in the treatment of peptic ulcer disease and gastroesophageal reflux disease (GERD) when an H_2RA is ineffective as well as in refractory erosive esophagitis and Zollinger-Ellison syndrome.

A significant amount of peptic ulcer disease, in particular gastric ulcer and gastritis, is caused by use of NSAIDs. This is partly because of the action of these products against cyclooxygenase. COX1 is an enzyme found in gastric, small and large intestine mucosa, kidneys, platelets, and vascular epithelium. It contributes to the health of these organs through a number of mechanisms, including the maintenance of the protective gastric mucosal layer and proper perfusion of the kidneys. COX2 is an enzyme that produces prostaglandins important to inflammatory cascade and pain transmission. The standard NSAIDs and steroids inhibit the synthesis of COX1 and COX2, thus controlling pain and inflammation but having gastric and renal complications. NSAIDs such as celecoxib (Celebrex) that spare COX1 and are more COX2-selective afford control of the potential for arthritis symptoms but have less risk of gastric and renal problems.

Besides the use of a non-COX1-sparing NSAID, major risk factors for gastric ulcer include age older than 60 years, history of peptic ulcer disease (especially gastric ulcer), and previous use of H_2RA or antacids for GI symptoms. Additional, less-potent risk factors include cigarette smoking, cardiac disease, and alcohol use; taking more than one NSAID; and the concurrent use of NSAIDs and anticoagulants.

H_2RAs likely offer protection against NSAID-induced duodenal ulcer and perhaps gastritis, but not against gastric ulcer. PPIs afford better protection against peptic ulcer disease. A prostaglandin analogue, misoprostol, is the only drug specifically designed for gastric protection with NSAID use and is the preferred drug for this purpose. It may be helpful in preventing renal injury secondary to NSAID use. Arthrotec is a fixed-drug combination of misoprostol and diclofenac (Voltaren) designed for the treatment of osteoarthritis and rheumatoid arthritis (OA and RA).

Discussion Source

Hektor Dunphy, L. (1999). *Management Guidelines for Adult Nurse Practitioners*. Philadelphia: FA Davis. Pp. 337–339.

QUESTIONS

32. An obese 45-year-old man presents complaining of periodic "heartburn." Examination reveals epigastric tenderness without rebound. As first-line therapy, you advise:

    A. avoiding high-fat foods
    B. the use of a prokinetic agent
    C. a daily dose of a PPI (proton pump inhibitor)
    D. increased fluid intake with meals

TABLE 6–2.
TREATMENT OPTIONS IN *HELICOBACTER PYLORI* INFECTION ASSOCIATED WITH PEPTIC ULCER DISEASE

Antimicrobials and Acid-Suppressing Medication	Duration of Therapy	Comments
Bismuth 2 tabs QID; metronidazole 250 mg TID; tetracycline 500 mg QID; omeprazole 20 mg BID	1 week for bismuth, metronidazole, and tetracycline Omeprazole for 4–8 weeks	Less effective if doxycycline substituted for tetracycline; about 95% effective
Bismuth subsalicylate 2 tabs QID, amoxicillin 500 mg TID or tetracycline 500 mg, metronidazole 250 mg QID	Bismuth for 6 weeks, amoxicillin for 2 weeks, metronidazole for 2 weeks. Antisecretory therapy for 4 to 8 weeks	The original treatment recommendation Low rate of adherence because of length of therapy with bismuth subsalicylate If not taken properly, rapid development of metronidazole resistance
Pepto Bismol Metronidazole 250 mg QID Tetracycline 500 mg QID		Prepackaged as Helidac 77–82% effective if taken as directed; if not taken properly, rapid development of metronidazole resistance

Metronidazole 500 mg TID, clarithromycin 500 mg BID, omeprazole 20 mg BID	Metronidazole and clarithromycin for 14 days, omeprazole for 28 days	FDA approved 70–80% effective if taken as directed; if not taken properly, rapid development of metronidazole resistance
Clarithromycin 500 mg BID, ranitidine bismuth citrate (Tritec) 400 mg BID	Clarithromycin for 14 days, ranitidine bismuth citrate for 28 days	FDA approved Well tolerated 84% effective if taken as directed
Amoxicillin 1 g BID, clarithromycin 500 mg BID omeprazole 20 mg BID	Amoxicillin and clarithromycin for 14 days, omeprazole for 4 to 8 weeks	Well tolerated 85–95% effective if taken as directed

Reference: Gilbert, D., Moellering, R., Sande, M. (1998). *The Sanford Guide to Antimicrobial Therapy* (38th ed.). Vienna, VA: Antimicrobial Therapy, Inc.

33. You see a 62-year-old man diagnosed with esophageal columnar epithelial metaplasia. You realize he is at increased risk for:

    A. esophageal stricture
    B. adenocarcinoma
    C. gastroesophageal reflux
    D. *H. pylori* colonization

34. In caring for a patient with symptomatic gastroesophageal reflux, you prescribe cisapride in order to:

    A. enhance motility
    B. raise the stomach's pH level
    C. reduce lower esophageal pressure
    D. help limit *H. pylori* growth

35. Which of the following represents the optimal dosing schedule for sucralfate (Carafate)?

    A. Take each tablet with a snack.
    B. The medication should be taken with a full meal for buffering effect.
    C. The drug must be taken on an empty stomach.
    D. Sucralfate should be taken with other prescribed medications to enhance compliance.

36. Which of the following is most likely to be found in a patient with erosive gastritis?

    A. NSAID use
    B. weight gain
    C. melena
    D. *H. pylori* infection

37. Which of the following is likely to be reported in a patient with severe GERD?

    A. hematemesis
    B. chronic sore throat
    C. diarrhea
    D. melena

38. A 58-year-old man recently began taking an antihypertensive medication and reports that his "heartburn" had become much worse. He is most likely taking:

A. atenolol

B. trandolapril

C. nifedipine

D. losartan

ANSWERS

32. **A**

33. **B**

34. **A**

35. **C**

36. **A**

37. **B**

38. **C**

DISCUSSION

Gastroesophageal reflux disease (GERD) is a common yet troublesome condition. Reflux of stomach contents occurs regularly. Most is asymptomatic with no resulting esophageal injury. GERD is present when there are symptoms or evidence of tissue damage. Presentation of GERD includes dyspepsia, chest pain at rest, and postprandial fullness. In addition, chronic hoarseness, sore throat, nocturnal cough, and wheezing are often reported, on occasion in the absence of more classic GERD symptoms.

Reflux-induced esophageal injury, also known as reflux esophagitis, is present in 40% with GERD. Erosions and ulcerations in squamous epithelium of esophagus are present and are most common in the elderly. Complications of reflux esophagitis include esophageal stricture and columnar epithelial metaplasia, also known as Barrett's esophagus. This is a risk factor for adenocarcinoma of the esophagus. Decreased lower esophageal sphincter tone and the resulting reflux of gastric contents cause GERD. Esophageal mucosal irritation results from exposure to HCl and pepsin.

In GERD, there is often delayed esophageal peristalsis and gastric emptying. Certain medications can cause a decrease in lower esophageal sphincter pressure and worsen GERD; these include estrogen, progesterone, theophylline, calcium channel blockers, and nicotine. Other agents can enhance lower esophageal sphincter pressure and help improve GERD; these include antacids, histamine, and cisapride.

Initial therapy for patients with GERD includes reducing intake of offending medications and of GERD-enhancing foods such alcohol, tomato-based products, chocolate, peppermint, colas, and citrus juices. Behavioral intervention includes avoiding assuming the supine position within 3 hours of a meal, not overeating, and abstaining from high-fat meals. Because abdominal obesity contributes to GERD, weight loss can be helpful.

The use of antacids after meals and at bedtime is often sufficient to control GERD symptoms. Antacids neutralize secreted acids and inactivate pepsin and bile salts. Antacids are most effective when used at 1 and 3 hours after meals and at bedtime (HS). Antacids interact with many other medications and should therefore be used at least 2 hours apart.

If the use of antacids and lifestyle modification are inadequate to control symptoms of GERD, add a histamine-2 receptor antagonist (H_2RA) at full prescription strength BID. If there is no improvement in 4 weeks, the patient should be referred for upper GI endoscopy, if possible, and the diagnosis of esophagitis should be entertained. Additional GERD therapy includes adding cisapride (Propulsid), a prokinetic agent. Cisapride's mechanism of action is as a prokinetic agent that helps increase lower esophageal sphincter tone, thereby assisting in esophageal barrier but promoting gastric emptying. Any medication with a narrow therapeutic range must be carefully evaluated in a patient receiving cisapride because of potential interference related to increased gastric emptying. In addition, cisapride is an inhibitor of CYP450 3A4 and may cause drug interactions with digoxin, theophylline, warfarin, and many of the antiepileptic drugs. Because of these problems, cisapride is only available through a special program. Avoid concurrent use of cisapride with other products inhibiting this enzyme. Since this can result in elevated cisapride plasma concentrations. Excessive plasma cisapride levels can lead to prolonging of the QT interval and the potential for lethal cardiac dysrhythmias; concurrent use of ketoconazole, itraconazole, fluconazole, erythromycin, cimetidine, astemizole (Hismanal), and cisapride should be avoided for this reason.

With moderate to severe esophagitis that does not respond to a prescription dose of H_2RA, discontinue the drug and initiate therapy with a PPI such as omeprazole (Prilosec) or lansoprazole (Prevacid). Consider adding sucralfate 1 g QID on an empty stomach in presence of esophagitis. If there are continued symptoms in 2 to 4 weeks, consider adding cisapride QID 15 minutes after a meal (PC) and HS to enhance motility and strengthen lower esophageal sphincter tone. If this treatment regimen is unsuccessful, expert consultation with a gastroenterologist should be sought. Also consider GI referral if there is concurrent anemia or weight loss.

Sucralfate's mechanism of action is as a mucosal protective agent that acts by forming an adhesive gel that binds to the site of an ulcer. A small amount adheres to normal mucosa. It has no effect on acid formation and inactivates pepsin while stimulating the formation of prostaglandins. Because it can inactivate many other drugs, sucralfate should be taken at least 2 hours before or after any medication. In addition, it should be taken on an empty stomach.

Discussion Source

Hektor Dunphy, L. (1999). *Management Guidelines for Adult Nurse Practitioners*. Philadelphia: FA Davis. Pp. 314–316.

QUESTIONS

39. You are caring for a woman from a developing Asian country. She reports that she had "yellow jaundice" as a young child. Her physical examination is unremarkable. Her laboratory studies are as follows: AST = 22 U/L (0–31); ALT = 25 U/L (0–50); hepatitis A virus (HAV) IgG = positive; HAV IgM = negative. Laboratory testing reveals:

    A. chronic hepatitis A
    B. no evidence of prior or current hepatitis A infection
    C. resolved hepatitis A infection
    D. prodromal hepatitis A

40. The most common source for hepatitis A infection is:

    A. sharing intravenous drug equipment
    B. cooked seafood
    C. contaminated water supplies
    D. sexual contact

41. In addition to the laboratory work given above, results also reveal the following for the patient in Question 40: hepatitis B surface antigen (HbsAg) = positive; hepatitis B surface antibody (HbsAb) = negative. These findings are most consistent with:

    A. no evidence of hepatitis B infection
    B. resolved hepatitis B infection
    C. chronic hepatitis B
    D. evidence of effective hepatitis B immunization

42. An intravenous drug user presents with malaise, nausea, fatigue, and "yellow eyes" for the past week. After ordering diagnostic tests, you confirm the diagnosis of acute hepatitis B. Anticipated laboratory results include:

    A. HBsAB
    B. neutrophilia
    C. lymphopenia
    D. HbsAg

43. Clinical findings in patients with acute viral hepatitis B likely include all of the following except:

    A. rebound tenderness
    B. scleral icterus
    C. a smooth, tender, palpable hepatic border
    D. report of myalgia

44. You examine a woman who has been sexually involved with a man newly diagnosed with acute hepatitis B. You advise her to:

    A. start hepatitis B immunization series
    B. limit the number of sexual partners
    C. be tested for HBsAb
    D. receive hepatitis B immunoglobulin and hepatitis B immunization series

45. Which of the following is true concerning hepatitis C infection?

    A. It usually presents with jaundice, fever, and significant hepatomegaly.
    B. Among health care workers, it is most commonly found in nurses.
    C. More than 50% of those with hepatitis C infection go on to develop chronic liver disease.
    D. Interferon therapy is highly effective.

46. Which of the following is predictive of severity of chronic liver disease in a patient with chronic hepatitis C?

A. female gender, age < 30

B. coinfection with hepatitis B, daily alcohol use

C. acquisition of virus through intravenous drug use, history of hepatitis A infection

D. frequent use of aspirin, nutritional status

47. When answering questions about hepatitis A vaccine, you consider that it:

A. contains live virus

B. should be offered to those who frequently travel to developing countries

C. usually is a required immunization for health care workers

D. is given as a single dose

48. In order to prevent an outbreak of hepatitis D infection, an NP plans to:

A. promote a campaign for clean food supplies

B. immunize the population against hepatitis B

C. offer antiviral prophylaxis against the agent

D. encourage frequent hand washing

49. Which of the following is true concerning hepatitis B vaccine?

A. The vaccine contains live hepatitis B virus.

B. The NP should consider checking post-vaccine HBsAb titers for those at highest risk for infection or with poor immunization response.

C. The vaccine is contraindicated in the presence of HIV infection.

D. Post-vaccine arthralgias are often reported.

50. Hyperbilirubinemia can cause all of the following except:

A. displacement of highly protein-bound drugs

B. scleral icterus

C. cola-colored urine

D. reduction in urobilinogen

51. Monitoring for hepatoma in a patient with chronic hepatitis B or C includes periodic evaluation of:

    A. sedimentation rate
    B. HBsAb
    C. alpha-fetoprotein (AFP)
    D. urobilinogen

52. Which of the following is an expected laboratory result in a patient with acute hepatitis A? (norms: AST = 0–31 U/L; ALT = 0–31 U/L)

    A. AST = 55 U/L; ALT = 50 U/L
    B. AST = 320 U/L; ALT= 190 U/L
    C. AST =320 U/L; ALT = 300 U/L
    D. AST = 440 U/L; ALT = 670 U/L

53. Which of the following is most likely to be reported in a patient taking an HMG CoA reductase inhibitor?

    A. AST = 55 U/L; ALT = 28 U/L
    B. AST = 320 U/L; ALT = 190 U/L
    C. AST =32 U/L; ALT = 120 U/L
    D. AST = 440 U/L; ALT = 670 U/L

ANSWERS

39. C
40. C
41. C
42. D
43. A
44. D
45. C
46. B
47. B
48. B
49. B
50. D
51. C
52. D
53. A

DISCUSSION

A number of infective agents cause viral hepatitis (Tables 6–3 and 6–4). Hepatitis A infection is caused by HAV (hepatitis A virus), a small RNA virus. Transmitted primarily by fecal-contaminated drinking water and food supplies, hepatitis A is typically a self-limiting infection with a very low mortality rate. In developing countries with limited pure water, the majority of the children contract this disease by age 5 years. In North America, adults ages 20 to 39 account for nearly 50% the reported cases.

The hepatitis A vaccine (Table 6–5), which contains dead virus, consists of two injections 6 months apart. Candidates include those who reside or travel to areas where disease is endemic, such as developing nations with impure water supplies. Consideration should be given to offering this vaccine to food handlers, day care and long-term care workers, and military and laboratory personnel. Intravenous drug users may also benefit from the vaccine. However, hepatitis A is rarely transmitted sexually or from needle sharing. Rather, intravenous drug users often live in conditions that facilitate the oral-fecal transmission of the hepatitis A virus.

A small, double-stranded DNA virus that contains the inner-core protein of hepatitis B core antigen and an outer surface of HbsAg causes hepatitis B. The virus is transmitted through exchange of body fluids. Hepatitis B infection can be prevented by limiting exposure to blood and body fluids as well as through immunization. Recombinant hepatitis B vaccine, which does not contain live virus, is well tolerated. About 90–95% of those who receive the vaccine develop HbsAb after three doses, implying protection from the virus. Consider HBsAb testing to confirm the development of HBV protection in those with high risk for infection (e.g., health care workers, intravenous drug uses, sex workers) as well as those at risk for poor immune response (e.g., dialysis patients, immune-suppressed patients).

The presentation of viral hepatitis, regardless of the agent, usually includes malaise, myalgia, fatigue, nausea, and anorexia. Aversion to cigarette smoking is often reported. Occasionally, arthritis-like symptoms and skin rash are also noted. Mild fever is occasionally found. Hepatomegaly with usually mild right upper quadrant abdominal tenderness without rebound is found in about 50%, with splenomegaly in about 15%. Jaundice typically occurs about 1 week after the onset of symptoms. However, jaundice is not found in most cases. The course of the illness is typically 2 to 3 weeks. During this period, a gradual increase in energy, appetite, and well-being is reported.

Laboratory findings common to all forms of viral hepatitis include leukopenia with lymphocytosis. Atypical lymphocytes are often found.

TABLE 6–3.
SEROLOGIC MARKERS OF VIRAL HEPATITIS A TO D

Serologic Marker	Time of Appearance	Comments
Anti-hepatitis A virus IgM (anti-HAV IgM or HAV IgM)	Early in infection Marker of acute hepatitis A infection	Disappears within 3 to 6 months
Anti-hepatitis A virus IgG (anti-HAV, HAB IgG)	Approximately 1 to 2 months after exposure to hepatitis A virus	In absence of anti-HAV IgM, marks immunity to hepatitis A virus through prior infection or vaccine Persists for years
Hepatitis B virus surface antigen (anti-HBsAg)	First marker of infection May be present before increase in level of hepatic enzymes	Indicative of HBV's presence Remains throughout course of acute and chronic hepatitis B Presence HBsAg for 6 months or greater after acute infection indicative of chronic hepatitis B and presence of HBV, a potentially oncogenic virus and risk for hepatocellular carcinoma as well as continued ability to transmit the disease
Hepatitis B surface antibody (anti-HBs or HBsAb)	In HBV infection, presence of HBsAg implied clearance of HBV, recovery from infection, and future immunity With HBV immunization, 90–95% develop HBsAb	In HBV infection, presence of HBsAg implies clearance of HBV and recovery from infection With immunization, HBsAb is usually present in measurable levels A protective antibody, infection with HBV is not possible when HBsAb present Postimmunization testing should be considered in those at risk for impaired immune response (adults > age 30 years, dialysis patients, those with chronic illness) or those at exceptionally high risk for HBV infection (intravenous drug users, sex workers, health care workers)

(continued)

TABLE 6–3. (continued)

Serologic Marker	Time of Appearance	Comments
Anti-HBc (IgM anti-HBc)	Found early in HBV infection when HBsAg present	May be present during period in which HBsAg is cleared and HBsAb response is mounted Persists for 3 to 6 months or longer
HBeAg (hepatitis Be antigen)	Found early in HBV infection when HBsAg present	Found during period of viral replication and greatest risk of infectivity If this marker persists 3 months or more after onset of acute infection, increased likelihood of chronic hepatitis B
HBV DNA	Found during period of HBV viral replication and infectivity	More sensitive marker than HBeAg
Anti-HCV (hepatitis C antibody)	Found about 2–3 months after infection with hepatitis C virus	May persist for lifetime Not a protective antibody marker Is found in those with acute and chronic infection
HCV RNA	Within weeks of infection with hepatitis C virus	Indicates presence of HCV infection If anti-HCV found without HCV RNA, assume past infection
HDAg (hepatitis D antigen)	Within weeks of infection with hepatitis D virus Found in presence of HBsAg	Hepatitis D virus can cause infection only in presence of hepatitis B virus

TABLE 6–4.
RISK FACTORS AND ROUTES OF TRANSMISSION OF VIRAL HEPATITIS

Infectious Agent	Route of Transmission	Risk Factors	Comments
Hepatitis A virus (HAV)	Oral-fecal	Ingestion of impure (fecal-contaminated) water Ingestion of fecal-contaminated food supplies such as raw shellfish grown in contaminated water, fresh fruits and vegetables cleaned with contaminated water or fertilized with human waste	Usually a self-limiting illness with low mortality Acute infection only, no chronic hepatitis or chronic carrier state Prevent infection through food and water safety, immunization, and postexposure immune globulin use
Hepatitis B virus (HBV)	Blood and body fluids	Sexual contact, intravenous drug use with needle sharing, occupational exposure in health care workers	Acute infection is usually symptomatic and mild to life threatening Prevent with universal precautions, clean needle exchange, immunization, safer sex
Hepatitis C virus (HCV)	Blood and body fluids	Intravenous drug use with needle sharing, blood transfusion before 1990, sexual contact, maternal-fetal transmission (rare)	Acute infection is typically asymptomatic Majority of those with infection develop chronic hepatitis with considerable risk of chronic liver disease Prevent with universal precautions, clean needle use, safer sex

Hepatitis D virus (HDV)	Blood and body fluid	Intravenous drug use with needle sharing, sexual contact	A coinfective agent seen only in the presence of acute hepatitis B Prevent with hepatitis B immunization, universal precautions, clean needle programs, safer sex
Hepatitis E virus (HEV)	Oral-fecal	Ingestion of impure (fecal-contaminated) water Ingestion of fecal-contaminated food supplies such as raw shellfish grown in contaminated water, fresh fruits and vegetables cleaned with contaminated water or fertilized with human waste	Common infection in Mexico, India, with occasional reports in the United States Generally a self-limiting illness; however, significant maternal mortality (~10–20%) with hepatitis E infection during pregnancy Prevent infection through food and water safety

TABLE 6–5.
VIRAL HEPATITIS PREVENTION THROUGH THE USE OF VACCINES AND IMMUNE GLOBULIN

Condition	Immunization Available	Groups at Greatest Risk for Infection (Immunization Advisable)	Postexposure Recommendation for Unimmunized Patients
Hepatitis A	Inactivated hepatitis A virus vaccine, 2 immunizations about 6 months apart	Children in day care and day care workers, travelers to endemic areas, intravenous drug users, military members, food handlers, men who have sex with men, consumers of at-risk food (raw shellfish, fecal-contaminated food), health care workers, those with chronic liver disease, large population in face of endemic exposure, those with chronic hepatitis B or C	Immune globulin (IG) 0.02 mL/kg IM up to 2 weeks after exposure (80–90% effective) Administer hepatitis A vaccine series
Hepatitis B	Recombinant DNA vaccine three-dose series at 0, 1, and 6 months. May use accelerated schedule (0,1,4 months or 0,2,4 months) in those >6 months of age with considerable risk, likelihood of poor follow-up	All children and adolescents Those with high-risk sexual exposure (men who have sex with men, heterosexuals with > one partner in a 6-month period, patients with an STD, partner of intravenous drug user, sex partner of patient with chronic HBV), household contacts of patients chronically infected with HBV, pregnant women in any high-risk category, those with chronic hepatitis C	Hepatitis B immune globulin (HBIG) 0.06 mL/kg within 7 days of exposure as well as hepatitis B vaccine on accelerated schedule

Note: There is no currently available immunization against HCV, or no postexposure recommendations. Immunizing against HBV can prevent hepatitis D.

Bilirubin in the urine is usually found in the absence of icterus. Hepatic enzyme elevation is universal (Table 6–6).

The test of liver enzymes is an evaluation of the degree of hepatic inflammation. General rules on the cause of the hepatic inflammation are as follows.

- AST/ALT rise in viral hepatitis (A, B, C, D, E)
  - AST >100 U/L
  - ALT >300 U/L
  - ALT:AST >1
- AST/ALT rise in selected prescription drugs and alcohol abuse
  - AST <300 U/L (typically <150 U/L)
  - ALT <100 U/L
  - AST:ALT >1

Hepatitis C infection is transmitted through the exchange of blood and body fluids. A single-strained RNA virus causes the infection. Although the most frequent cause of blood transfusion–associated hepatitis, only 4% of all cases of hepatitis C can be attributed to this cause. Because of the onset of screening of the blood supply for hepatitis C virus (HCV), the risk of transfusion-associated hepatitis C has decreased from 10% 20 years ago to 0.1% today. More than 50% of cases of HCV infection are caused by intravenous drug use with needle sharing. Transmission through sexual contact is possible, but this risk appears relatively low. Maternal-fetal transmission is also uncommon and is usually limited to women with high circulating HCV levels. Transmission through breast-feeding has not been reported.

The HCV incubation period is about 6 to 7 weeks, and the infection rarely causes a serious acute illness. Diagnosis is made by the presence of anti-HCV, an antibody that persists in the presence of the virus and is not protective. At least 50–80% of those with hepatitis C go on to develop chronic infection and exhibit anti-HCV along with a positive hepatitis C viral load. If anti-HCV persists in the absence of a positive hepatitis C viral load, this suggests that the virus has cleared and active infection is not present.

Because the hepatitis D virus (HDV) is an RNA virus that can only occur concurrently in the presence of HBV, it is only found in those with acute or chronic hepatitis B. A patient with hepatitis B and D acute co-infection has a course of illness similar to a patient with hepatitis B infection only. If a patient with chronic hepatitis B becomes superinfected with HDV, a fulminant or severe chronic hepatitis often results. Prevention of hepatitis B through immunization will also prevent hepatitis D.

Hepatic enzymes are found in circulation because of hepatic growth and repair. AST increases in response to hepatocyte injury, as may occur

TABLE 6–6.
HEPATIC ENZYMES ELEVATIONS AND THEIR SIGNIFICANCE

Enzyme Elevation	Associated Condition	Comments
ALT increases to greater than AST	Hepatitis A, B, C, D, E, and so on Hepatitis associated with drugs or industrial chemicals	A memory jog for recalling reasons for rise is that the "L" in ALT symbolizes "liver infection," the "T" symbolizes "troglitazone" (Rezulin) and other "therapeutic" agents
AST increases to greater than ALT	Alcohol-related hepatic injury (two times the norm), HMG-CoA reductase inhibitor (-statin suffix) use, acetaminophen overdose	A memory jog for recalling reasons for increase is AST symbolizes "Alcohol, -Statin, Tylenol"
AST/ALT elevation one to five times the norm	Alcohol use Skeletal muscle injury secondary to seizure, protracted immobilization	Example: 38-year-old man with a 10-year history of increasingly heavy alcohol use AST = 83 U/L (0–31) ALT = 50 U/L (0–31)
AST/ALT elevation more than five times the norm	Infectious hepatitis	Example: 22-year-old woman who recently returned from a volunteer trip to a developing nation AST = 678 U/L (0–31) ALT= 828 U/L (0–31)

(continued)

in alcohol abuse, the therapeutic use of HMG CoA reductase inhibitors (lipid-lowering drugs with -statin suffix such as lovastatin), and acetaminophen overdose. This enzyme is also found in skeletal muscle, myocardium, brain, and kidney in smaller amounts, so damage to these areas may also cause an AST rise.

AST has a circulatory half-life of approximately 12 to 24 hours; therefore, levels rise in response to hepatic damage and clear quickly after

TABLE 6–6. (continued)

Enzyme Elevation	Associated Condition	Comments
Gamma glutamyl transferase (GGT)	Enzyme involved in the transfer of amino acids across cell membranes Found primarily in the liver and kidney In liver disease, usually parallels changes in alkaline phosphatase Useful marker of hepatic disease in the following conditions, with marked elevation often noted in obstructive jaundice, hepatic metastasis, intrahepatic cholestasis In response to binge drinking, GGT leaks out of cells in greater amounts than do other hepatic enzymes; GGT elevation is marked, sustained in high alcohol intake Will elevate modestly with lower ETOH consumption	Example: 40-year-old woman with cholecystitis AST = 45 U/L (0–31) ALT= 55 U/L (0–31) Alkaline phosphatase = 175 U/L (0–125) GGT = 245 U/L (0–45) Example of patient with alcohol abuse: 38-year-old man with a 10 year history heavy alcohol use with recent binge AST = 83 U/L (0–31) ALT =50 U/L (0–31) GGT = 150 U/L (0–45)

damage ceases. AST elevation is generally found in only about 10% of problem drinkers. However, if AST is elevated with normal ALT and mild macrocytosis (MCV > 100 fL, seen in about 30–60% of men who drink five or more drinks per day and in women at a threshold of three or more drinks per day), long-standing alcohol abuse is the likely cause.

Alanine aminotransferase (ALT; formerly known as SGPT) is more specific to the liver, having limited concentration in other organs. This enzyme has a longer half-life than AST at 37 to 57 hours. Therefore, elevation persists longer after hepatic damage has ceased. This enzyme's greatest elevation is likely seen in hepatitis caused by infection or inflammation. This enzyme is unlikely to increase in the presence of alcohol abuse. When evaluating a patient with suspected substance abuse causing hepatic dysfunction, the NP must note both the degree of AST or ALT elevation as well as the AST-to-ALT ratio.

An increase in bilirubin level is typically found in patients with viral hepatitis. Clinical jaundice is found when total bilirubin exceeds 2.5 mg. Bilirubin is the degradation product of heme, with 85–90% arising from hemoglobin and a smaller percentage from myoglobin. About 4 mg/kg per day of bilirubin is produced in healthy individuals, and because the rate of excretion usually matches rate of production, the levels stay low and stable. Reticuloendothelial cells take in haptoglobin, a protein that binds with hemoglobin from aged RBCs. The reticuloendothelial cells remove the iron from hemoglobin for recycling. The remaining substances are then degraded to bilirubin in its unconjugated, or indirect, form. This form is not water soluble.

When unconjugated bilirubin is released into circulation, it binds to albumin and is transported to the liver. When unconjugated bilirubin arrives at the liver, hepatocytes detach bilirubin from the albumin. It is now in a water-soluble form, also know as conjugated, or direct, bilirubin. Conjugated bilirubin loosely attaches to albumin and is easily detached in the kidney. The passing of small amounts of conjugated bilirubin through the kidney gives urine its characteristic yellow color.

Conjugated bilirubin not excreted by the kidney is reabsorbed by the small intestine and converted to urobilinogen by bacterial action in the gut. This can be reabsorbed into circulation, and excess amounts can appear in the urine. Small amounts of urobilinogen may also be found in fecal-contaminated urine because this substance is normally found in the large intestine.

When there is an excess of urinary excretion of bilirubin, as found in patients with viral hepatitis, urine develops a characteristic brown color, often described by a patient as looking like "cola." Also, bilirubin in excess may push drugs with high propensity for protein (albumin) binding, thus increasing free drug and possibly causing drug toxicity.

Treatment of acute viral hepatitis is largely supportive. Steroids, antiviral agents, and interferon are used on occasion, often with equivocal outcomes. Given the seriousness of hepatitis B and C sequelae, considerable research is under way to develop effective, well-tolerated therapies.

Chronic hepatitis B and C are potent risk factors for hematoma or primary hepatocellular carcinoma. Periodic monitoring for Alpha-fetoprotein (AFP) is indicated, looking for an increase in the level that indicates hepatic tumor growth.

Discussion Sources

Friedman, L. (1999). Liver, biliary tract and pancreas. In Tierney, L., McPhee, S., & Papadakis, M. *Current Diagnosis and Treatment* (38th ed.). Stamford, CT: Appleton & Lange. Pp. 638–677.

Hektor Dunphy, L. (1999). *Management Guidelines for Adult Nurse Practitioners*. Philadelphia: FA Davis. Pp. 332–335.

QUESTIONS

54. Which of the following is an expected finding in a patient with chronic renal failure?

    A. hypokalemia

    B. hypotension

    C. constipation

    D. anemia

55. The use of which of the following medications can precipitate acute renal failure in a patient with renal artery stenosis?

    A. steroids

    B. angiotensin$_2$- receptor antagonists

    C. beta adrenergic blockers

    D. cephalosporins

56. A 78-year-old man presents with fatigue and difficulty with bladder emptying. Examination reveals a distended bladder but is otherwise unremarkable. BUN = 88 mg/dL; Cr = 2.8 mg/dL. The most likely diagnosis is:

    A. prerenal azotemia

    B. acute glomerulonephritis

    C. tubular necrosis

    D. postrenal azotemia

57. A 68-year-old woman with congestive heart failure presents with tachycardia, S_3 heart sounds, and basilar crackles bilaterally. Blood pressure (BP) = 90/68 mm Hg; BUN = 58 mg/dL, Cr = 2.4 mg/dL. The most likely diagnosis is:

    A. prerenal azotemia

    B. acute glomerulonephritis

    C. tubular necrosis

    D. postrenal azotemia

58. Which of the following is found early in the development of chronic renal failure?

    A. proteinuria
    B. elevated creatinine level
    C. uremia
    D. hyperkalemia

59. Angiotensin-converting enzyme (ACE) inhibitors can limit the progress of some forms of renal disease by:

    A. increasing intraglomerular pressure
    B. lowering efferent arteriolar resistance
    C. enhancing afferent arteriolar tone
    D. increasing urinary protein excretion

60. Objective findings in patients with glomerulonephritis include all of the following except:

    A. edema
    B. urinary RBC casts
    C. proteinuria
    D. hypotension

ANSWERS

54. D
55. B
56. D
57. A
58. A
59. B
60. D

DISCUSSION

Renal failure can occur either acutely or chronically. In acute renal failure, a precipitating event or cause is often easily identifiable. With prerenal azotemia, the most common cause of acute renal failure, the kidneys are hypoperfused, often leading to acute tubular necrosis, the cause of 85% of all acute renal failure. Reasons for this include decreased circulating volume as seen in patients with dehydration and acute blood loss, decreased cardiac output as seen in patients with congestive heart failure, or excessive sequestering of fluid as seen in patients with burns. Postrenal azotemia, caused by obstruction to urine flow, accounts for about 5% of all renal failure. Intrinsic renal failure is found when there is disease within the kidney at the levels of the renal tubules, glomerularis, interstitium, or vessels. Etiologies include glomerulonephritis and acute interstitial nephritis. Laboratory findings in these more common forms of acute renal failure vary (Table 6–7).

Typical findings in renal failure include increased serum creatinine and urea nitrogen levels. Creatinine is the end product of creatine metabolism, which arises from skeletal muscle. Its measurement is a surrogate marker of kidney function because creatinine excretion by the healthy kidney is very efficient. As the kidney fails, creatinine increases. BUN is derived from the breakdown of protein from dietary or other sources. BUN level typically increases (uremia) more rapidly than creatinine in response to decreased renal perfusion and can increase from the prerenal, renal, and postrenal causes of kidney failure. In particular, elevated BUN level with a normal creatinine level may be found in patients with healthy kidneys but with severe dehydration. In addition, GI bleeding usually causes a marked increase in BUN level as the gut digests and absorbs proteins found in the blood.

TABLE 6–7.
ETIOLOGY OF AND FINDINGS IN PATIENTS WITH ACUTE RENAL FAILURE

Disease Causing Acute Renal Failure	Typical Etiology	Laboratory Findings
Acute glomerulonephritis	Post–streptococcal infection, autoimmune diseases	BUN: Cr ratio ≥ 20:1 Urinalysis: renal casts, RBCs
Acute interstitial nephritis	Allergic reaction, drug reaction	BUN: Cr ratio ≤ 20:1 Urinalysis: WBC casts, eosinophils
Acute tubular necrosis	Hypotension, nephrotoxins	BUN: Cr ratio ≤ 20:1 Urinalysis: granular casts, renal tubular cells

Anemia is typically seen in patients with chronic renal failure. Erythropoietin, a glycoprotein growth factor produced primarily by the kidneys, influences the undifferentiated stem cell to form the RBC precursor. With end-stage renal disease (ESRD), there is reduced erythropoietin response because of limited supply. That is, as the kidney fails, erythropoietin production declines. In addition, as is common in chronic illness, RBC life-span is shortened. These factors result in a normocytic, normochromic anemia in the presence of a low reticulocyte count. This can be treated by the use of recombinant erythropoietin and transfusion.

Discussion Sources

Hektor Dunphy, L. (1999). *Management Guidelines for Adult Nurse Practitioners*. Philadelphia: FA Davis. Pp. 340–344.
Fitzgerald, M. (1999). Hematologic disorders. In Youngkin E., Sawin, K., Kissinger, J., & Israel, D. *Pharmacotherapatics: A Primary Care Clinical Guide*. Stamford, CT: Appleton & Lange. Pp. 605–620.
Watnick, S., Morrison, G. (1999), Kidney. In Tierney, L., McPhee, S., & Papadakis, M. *Current Diagnosis and Treatment* (38th ed.) Norwalk, CT: Appleton & Lange. Pp. 863–894.

QUESTIONS

61. A 36-year-old afebrile woman without health problems presents with dysuria and frequency of urination. Her urinalysis findings include results positive for nitrites and leukocyte esterase. You evaluate these results and consider that she likely has a:

    A. purulent vulvovaginitis

    B. gram-negative urinary tract infection (UTI)

    C. cystitis caused by *S. saprophyticus*

    D. urethral syndrome

62. The most likely causative organism in community-acquired UTI is:

    A. *Klebsiella* spp.

    B. *mirabilis*

    C. *E. coli*

    D. *S. saprophyticus*

63. Preferred therapy for an uncomplicated UTI in an otherwise healthy woman includes:

    A. trimethoprim-sulfamethoxazole

    B. amoxicillin

    C. azithromycin

    D. cephalexin

64. The notation of alkaline urine in a patient with a UTI may point to infection caused by:

  A. *Klebsiella* spp.
  B. *P. mirabilis*
  C. *E. coli*
  D. *S. saprophyticus*

65. Which of the following is most accurate information when caring for a 40-year-old man with cystitis?

  A. This is a common condition in men of this age.
  B. A gram-positive organism is the likely causative pathogen.
  C. A urologic evaluation should be considered.
  D. Pyuria is rarely found.

66. Which of the following is the best advice on the post-UTI treatment urine culture?

  A. recommended with each UTI
  B. should be considered in all patients approximately 1 month after UTI
  C. indicated about 1 week after completion of antibiotic therapy in patients with pyelonephritis
  D. may have false-positive results if obtained immediately after antibiotic therapy

67. Activities to prevent UTIs in women include all of the following except:

  A. increased fluid intake
  B. drinking cranberry juice
  C. voiding after vaginal intercourse
  D. twice-a-week erythromycin therapy

68. A 44-year-old woman presents with pyelonephritis. The report of her urinalysis is least likely to include:

  A. WBC casts
  B. positive nitrites
  C. 3+ protein
  D. rare RBCs

69. An example of a first-line therapeutic agent for the treatment of pyelonephritis is:

    A. ampicillin
    B. sulfisoxazole
    C. levofloxacin
    D. nitrofurantoin

70. Length of antimicrobial therapy for uncomplicated pyelonephritis is typically:

    A. 5–7 days
    B. 1–2 weeks
    C. 2–3 weeks
    D. 3–4 weeks

ANSWERS

61. B
62. C
63. A
64. B
65. C
66. C
67. D
68. C
69. C
70. A

DISCUSSION

Urinary tract infections (UTIs) can involve mucosal tissue (in cystitis) or soft tissue (in pyelonephritis and prostatitis). Acute uncomplicated cystitis typically presents in an otherwise-healthy adult woman who complains of dysuria and frequency of urination but without fever and constitutional symptoms. The physical examination may reveal suprapubic tenderness but may also be normal. The infection is limited to the bladder.

TABLE 6–8.
COMMON URINALYSIS DIPSTICK FINDINGS IN PATIENTS WITH URINARY TRACT INFECTIONS

Finding	Significance	Comments
Leukocyte esterase	Positive results indicate presence of neutrophils > 5 white blood cells/high powered field, an indicator of UTI	Results not valid in neutropenic patients Decreased sensitivity with increased urinary glucose concentration, high urinary specific gravity, and presence of antibiotic in urine
Nitrites	Positive nitrite is an indicator of gram-negative organism, such as *E. coli* or *P. mirabilis*, in the urine	Indicates bacterial reduction of dietary nitrates to nitrites Absent in gram-positive UTIs such as caused by *S. saprophyticus* infection Best done on well-concentrated urine such as first AM void Urine should be held in bladder for at least ½ hour for nitrite to nitrate conversion to take place.
Protein	Common in febrile response or represent presence of protein-containing substance such as WBCs, bacteria, mucus	Not greater than 100 mg/dL (2+), frequently trace to 30 mg/dL (1+); consider presence of glomerulonephritis or nephropathy with higher levels
pH	If alkaline urine is found in presence of UTI symptoms and positive results for leukocyte esterase, likely that *Proteus* spp. or *Pseudomonas* spp. is the causative organism	These organisms split urea into CO_2 and ammonia, causing an increase in the urine's normally acidic pH

TABLE 6–9.
SANFORD GUIDE RECOMMENDATIONS FOR TREATMENT OF COMMUNITY-ACQUIRED URINARY TRACT INFECTIONS

Type of Infection	Usual Pathogens	Primary Regimen	Alternative Regimen
Acute, uncomplicated UTI (cystitis, ureteritis) in women who are not pregnant	E. coli, S. saprophyticus, enterococci	All recommended for 3 days Trimethoprim-sulfamethoxazole double strength BID, ciprofloxacin 250 mg BID, norfloxacin 400 mg BID, lomefloxacin 400 mg QID, enoxacin 200 mg BID	Oral cephalosporin, nitrofurantoin, fosfomycin
Recurrent UTIs (three or more years)	E. coli, S. saprophyticus, enterococci, other pathogens possible	Eradicate organisms then trimethoprim-sulfamethoxazole DS QID long term	Single dose of trimethoprim sulfa DS two tablets at onset of symptoms One trimethoprim sulfa DS tablet after coitus
Acute uncomplicated pyelonephritis suitable for outpatient therapy	E. coli, enterococci	All therapies for 14 days Ciprofloxacin 500 mg BID, norfloxacin 400 mg BID, levofloxacin 250 mg QID, lomefloxacin 400 mg QID, enoxacin 400 mg BID	Amoxicillin with clavulanate, oral cephalosporin

Most community-acquired infections are caused by enteric gram-negative rods from the Enterobacteriaceae group such as *E. coli* and *Proteus mirabilis*, as well as the less commonly encountered *Klebsiella pneumoniae*. These organisms are capable of reducing dietary nitrates to nitrites. This, coupled with the inflammatory changes seen in UTIs, leads to the typical urinalysis dipstick's revealing the presence of leukocyte esterase, nitrites, and small amounts of protein (Table 6–8).

Usually cystitis is easily eradicated with 3-day antibiotic therapy (Table 6–9). However, even uncomplicated cystitis in men may be a harbinger of structural urinary tract abnormality and should trigger a longer course of therapy and urologic evaluation.

Patients with acute pyelonephritis report symptoms of cystitis along with fever and flank pain, often with vomiting. Physical examination findings include costovertebral tenderness and the general appearance of an acutely ill patient. Typically, this infection of the renal parenchyma and renal pelvis is caused by an ascending cystitis. Because pyelonephritis is a complicated UTI, therapy includes 1–2 weeks treatment with a fluoroquinolone (see Table 6–9). A urine culture about 1 week after completion of antibiotic therapy is important to confirm resolution of infection. Further diagnostic testing is not required unless there is evidence of other conditions such as nephrolithiasis.

Prevention of UTIs includes high fluid intake (2 to 3 L per day) and voiding at regular intervals. For women, voiding after vaginal intercourse may also be helpful. Drinking 12 oz of cranberry juice daily may help limit bacteria from adhering to bladder mucosa and limit UTI recurrence. In addition, cranberry juice has bacteriostatic activity.

Discussion Sources

Gilbert, D., Moellering, R., Sande, M. (1998) The *Sanford Guide to Antimicrobial Therapy* (28th ed.). Vienna, VA: Antimicrobial Therapy, Inc. Pp. 15–17.

Hektor Dunphy, L. (1999). *Management Guidelines for Adult Nurse Practitioners*. Philadelphia: FA Davis. Pp. 346–349.

Presiti, J., Stoller, M., Carroll, P. (1999) Urology. In Tierney, L., McPhee, S., & Papadakis, M. *Current Diagnosis and Treatment* (38th ed.). Norwalk, CT: Appleton & Lange. Pp. 894–931.

Youngkin, E., Israel, D. (1999). Herbal therapies for common health problems. In Youngkin E., Sawin, K., Kissinger, J., Israel, D. *Pharmacotherapeutics: A Primary Care Clinical Guide*. Stamford, CT: Appleton & Lange. Pp. 127–150.

7 CHAPTER

Male
Genitourinary
Disorders

QUESTIONS

1. Which of the following is not consistent with the description of benign prostatic hyperplasia (BPH)?

   A. obliterated median sulcus
   B. size larger than 2.5 cm x 3 cm
   C. sensation of incomplete emptying
   D. boggy gland

2. In choosing an antihypertensive agent for a 68-year-old man with symptomatic BPH, the NP considers prescribing:

   A. hydrochlorothiazide
   B. doxazosin
   C. lisinopril
   D. atenolol

3. When assessing a 78-year-old man with suspected BPH, the NP considers that:

   A. Prostate size does not correlate well with severity of symptoms.
   B. It affects about 50% of men of this age.
   C. He is at increased risk for prostate cancer.
   D. Limiting fluids is a helpful method of relieving severe symptoms.

4. Which of the following medications can cause urinary retention in a man with BPH?

   A. amitriptyline
   B. trimethoprim sulfa
   C. enalapril
   D. atenolol

5. A 78-year-old man presents with fatigue and difficulty with bladder emptying. Examination reveals a distended bladder but is otherwise unremarkable. Blood urea nitrogen (BUN) = 88 mg/dL; creatinine (Cr) = 2.8 mg/dL. The most likely diagnosis is:

   A. prerenal azotemia
   B. acute glomerulonephritis
   C. tubular necrosis
   D. postrenal azotemia

ANSWERS

1. D
2. B
3. A
4. A
5. D

DISCUSSION

Benign prostatic hyperplasia is a common disorder in older men, with a prevalence of approximately 50% by age 60 years and 90% by age 85 years. This benign enlargement of the prostate can lead to bladder outlet obstruction. There is both an enlargement in prostatic connective tissue as well as an increase in the number of epithelial and smooth muscle cells. The cause of BPH is not fully understood but may be in response to androgenic hormones.

BPH can lead to bladder outlet obstruction from urethral narrowing. As a result, men with BPH develop symptoms of increased frequency of urination, decreased force of urinary stream, nocturia, and the sensation of incomplete emptying. Postrenal azotemia, caused by obstruction to urine flow, accounts for about 5% of all renal failure.

Patient education about BPH should include information on measures to avoid making symptoms worse. Drugs with anticholinergic effect, such as tricyclic antidepressants and first-generation antihistamines, can cause urinary retention in men with BPH. In addition, urinary frequency may become worse with ingestion of certain bladder irritants such as caffeine and artificial sweeteners. Although men with BPH may be tempted to limit fluid intake, this may yield a more concentrated and perhaps irritating urine, possibly leading to increased symptoms.

Discussion Sources

Hektor Dunphy, L (1999). *Management Guidelines for Adult Nurse Practitioners*. Philadelphia: FA Davis. Pp. 352–357.
Presti, J., Stoller, M., Carrol, P. (1999). Urology. Tierny, L. McPhee, S., & Papadakis, M. *Current Medical Diagnosis and Treatment* (38th ed.). Stamford, CT: Appleton and Lange. Pp. 894–931.

QUESTIONS

6. You examine a 32-year-old man with chancroid and anticipate finding the following:

    A. a vesicular-form lesion

    B. painful ulcer

    C. painless craterlike lesion

    D. plaquelike

7. The causative organism of chancroid is:

    A. ureaplasma

    B. *Chlamydia trachomatis*

    C. *Mycoplasma homili*

    D. *Hemophilus ducreyi*

8. Treatment options for chancroid include all of the following except:

    A. azithromycin

    B. ciprofloxacin

    C. ceftriaxone

    D. amoxicillin

9. When ordering laboratory tests to confirm chancroid, the NP considers that:

    A. Concomitant infection with herpes simplex is often found.

    B. A disease-specific serum test is available.

    C. A WBC count with differential is indicated.

    D. Dark-field examination is needed.

ANSWERS

6. C
7. D
8. D
9. A

DISCUSSION

The gram-negative bacillus *H. ducreyi* causes chancroid. The organism is most often contracted sexually. However, transmission to health care providers through direct contact with chancroid lesions has been documented. The chancroid lesion is typically found at the site of inoculation with a vesicular to pustular-form lesion that forms a painful, soft ulcer with a necrotic base. Multiple lesions, acquired through autoinoculation, are usually found. A dense, matted lymphadenopathy can be found on the ipsilateral side of the lesion. The affected nodes may spontaneously rupture. Treatment options include azithromycin, ciprofloxacin, and ceftriaxone (Table 7–1).

As with all sexually transmitted diseases (STDs), a critical part of care is discussion of prevention strategies, including condom use and limiting the number of sexual partners. Offer and encourage testing for other STDs, including HIV. Concomitant infection with syphilis, herpes simplex, and HIV is often found.

Discussion Sources

Hektor Dunphy, L (1999). *Management Guidelines for Adult Nurse Practitioners*. Philadelphia: FA Davis. Pp. 357–358.
Chambers, H. (1999). Infectious disease: Bacterial and chlamydia. Tierny, L. McPhee, S., & Papadakis, M. *Current Medical Diagnosis and Treatment* (38th ed.). Stamford CT: Appleton and Lange. Pp. 1291–1331.

QUESTIONS

10. The most common causative organism of lymphogranuloma venereum is:

    A. ureaplasma

    B. *C. trachomatis*

    C. *N. gonorrhoeae*

    D. *H. ducreyi*

TABLE 7–1.
GUIDELINES FOR TREATMENT OF GENITOURINARY INFECTION

Conditions	Causative Organism	Clinical Presentation	Treatment Options
Chancroid	*H. ducreyi*	Painful genital ulcer	Azithromycin 1 g PO; or ceftriaxone 250 mg IM; or ciprofloxacin 500 mg PO BID for 3 days; or erythromycin 500 mg PO QID for 7 days
Herpes simplex	Herpes simplex virus 1 or 2	Painful ulcerated lesions, lymphadenopathy	For initial infection: Acyclovir 400 mg PO TID for 7-10 days; or acyclovir 200 mg 5ID for 7-10 days; or famciclovir 250 mg PO TID for 7-10 days; or valacyclovir 1 g PO BID for 7-10 days For episodic recurrent infection: Acyclovir 400 mg PO TID for 5 days; or famciclovir 250 mg PO BID for 5 days; or valacyclovir 1 g PO QD for 5 days; or valacyclovir 500 mg PO BID for 5 days For suppression of recurrent infection: Acyclovir 400 mg PO BID; or famciclovir 250 mg PO BID; or valacyclovir 1 g PO QID; or valacyclovir 500 mg PO for extended period of time

Lymphogranuloma venereum	Invasive serovar L1, L2, L3 of *C. trachomatis*	Vesicular or ulcerative lesion on the external genitalia with inguinal lymphadenitis or buboes	Doxycycline 100 mg PO BID for 21 days or erythromycin 500 mg QID for 21 days
Nongonococcal urethritis	*C. trachomatis*	Irritative voiding symptoms, occasional mucopurulent discharge	Azithromycin 1 g PO as a single dose; or doxycycline 100 mg po BID for 7 days; or erythromycin 500 mg PO QID for 7 days; or ofloxacin 300 mg BID for 7 days
Gonococcal urethritis	*N. gonorrhoeae*	Irritative voiding symptoms, occasional purulent discharge	Single-dose therapy for uncomplicated infection: Cefixime 400 mg, ceftriaxone 125 mg IM, or ciprofloxacin 500 mg, or ofloxacin 400 mg Concurrently treat with azithromycin 1 g as a single dose or doxycycline 100 mg BID for 7 days because of risk of concurrent nongonococcal urethritis
Epididymitis	*N. gonorrhoeae, C. trachomatis*	Irritative voiding symptoms; fever; and an acutely painful, enlarged epididymis	Ceftriaxone 125 mg IM as a single dose plus doxycycline 100 mg BID for 10 days With penicillin or cephalosporin allergy: Ofloxacin 300 mg PO BID for 10 days
Genital warts (condyloma acuminata)	Human papilloma virus	Verruca-form lesions or may be subclinical or unrecognized	For treatment of visible lesions: Podofilox, imiquimod, trichloroacetic acid, cryotherapy, interferon, or surgery

(continued)

TABLE 7-1. (continued)

Conditions	Causative Organism	Clinical Presentation	Treatment Options
Acute prostatitis in men < 35 years or with STD risk	*N. gonorrhoeae, C. trachomatis*	Irritative voiding symptoms; suprapubic and perineal pain; fever; tender, boggy prostate	Ofloxacin 400 mg × 1 dose then 300 mg BID for at least 7 days
Acute prostatitis in men >35 years	Coliform organisms	Irritative voiding symptoms; suprapubic and perineal pain; fever; tender, boggy prostate	Ciprofloxacin 500 mg PO BID trimethoprim sulfamethoxazole DS PO BID for 10–14 days
Chronic bacterial prostatitis	Enterobacteriaceae, enterococci, *P. aeruginosa*	Low back pain, afebrile, pain with defecation tender, boggy prostate	Ciprofloxacin 500 mg BID × 4 wks, ofloxacin 300 mg BID × 6 wks Trimethoprim sulfamethoxazole DS BID × 1–3 months

Reference: Center for Disease Control and Prevention. (1998). *1998 Guidelines for Treatment of Sexually Transmitted Disease.* Available at http://www.cdc.gov.epo/mmwr/preview/mmwrhtml/00050909.htm Sanford Guide (1999) pp. 19.

11. Physical examination findings in lymphogranuloma venereum include:

   A. verruca-form lesions
   B. inguinal lymphadenitis
   C. firm, painless ulcer
   D. plaquelike lesions

12. Treatment options for lymphogranuloma venereum include:

   A. tetracycline
   B. penicillin
   C. ceftriaxone
   D. dapsone

ANSWERS

10. **B**
11. **B**
12. **A**

DISCUSSION

Lymphogranuloma venereum is an STD caused by *C. trachomatis* types L1 to L3. The clinical presentation, usually occurring approximately 1 to 4 weeks after contact with an infected host, consists of a vesicular or ulcerative lesion on the external genitalia with inguinal lymphadenitis or buboes. These may fuse and then drain, forming multiple sinus tracts with resultant scarring. Treatment options include tetracycline, doxycycline, erythromycin, or trimethoprim sulfisoxazole (see Table 7–1).

As with all STDs, a critical part of care is discussion of prevention strategies, including condom use and limiting the number of sexual partners. Offer and encourage testing for other STDs, including HIV.

Discussion Source

Chambers, H. (1999). Infectious disease: Bacterial and chlamydia. In Tierny, L. McPhee, S., & Papadakis, M. *Current Medical Diagnosis and Treatment* (38th ed.). Stamford, CT: Appleton and Lange. Pp. 1291–1331.

QUESTIONS

13. The presentation of acute epididymitis includes:
    A. Prehn's sign
    B. low back pain
    C. absent cremasteric reflex
    D. diffuse abdominal pain

14. The most likely causative pathogens in a 26-year-old man with acute epididymitis include:
    A. *E. coli*
    B. Enterobacteriaceae
    C. *Chlamydia trachomatis*
    D. *Pseudomonas* spp.

15. Which of the following is a reasonable treatment option for a 30-year-old man with acute epididymitis?
    A. ofloxacin
    B. amoxicillin
    C. metronidazole
    D. clindamycin

ANSWERS

13. A
14. C
15. A

DISCUSSION

Acute epididymitis is an infectious disease caused by a variety of pathogens. In men younger than age 40 years, it is usually caused by *C. trachomatis* or *N. gonorrhoeae*, with the organism acquired through sexual contact. In older men, acute epididymitis is often seen secondary to prostatitis and is typically caused by a gram-negative organism. This condition presents with irritative voiding symptoms; fever; and an acutely painful, enlarged epididymis. Pain may radiate up the spermatic cord to the ipsilateral lower abdomen. Prehn's sign, a reduction in pain when the scrotum is elevated above the symphysis pubis, is typically noted. Urethritis, scrotal swelling, and penile discharge are often found.

Treatment options differ according to age and risk factors. In younger men with low risk for epididymitis as a complication of urinary tract infection (UTI), particularly with risk for STD, antimicrobials effective against gonorrhea and chlamydia such as ceftriaxone and azithromycin or ofloxacin should be used. In men at risk for epididymitis as a UTI complication, the choice of an antimicrobial agent should be directed by urine culture. A fluoroquinolone such as ciprofloxacin will likely be effective.

As with all STDs, a critical part of care is discussion of prevention strategies, including condom use and limiting the number of sexual partners. Offer and encourage testing for other STDs, including HIV.

Discussion Source

Hektor Dunphy, L (1999). *Management Guidelines for Adult Nurse Practitioners*. Philadelphia: FA Davis. Pp. 359–360.

QUESTIONS

16. Gram stain of the urethral discharge of a 37-year-old man with dysuria reveals gram-negative cocci. This most likely represents:

    A. *C. trachomatis*
    B. ureaplasma
    C. *N. gonorrhoeae*
    D. *E. coli*

17. Treatment options for uncomplicated gonococcal proctitis include:

    A. ceftriaxone 125 mg IM as a single dose
    B. erythromycin 500 mg BID for 7 days
    C. norfloxacin 400 mg BID for 3 days
    D. azithromycin 1 g as a single dose

18. Which of the following is recommended by the Centers for Disease Control and Prevention (CDC) as single-dose therapy for uncomplicated gonorrhea?

    A. cefixime
    B. metronidazole
    C. azithromycin
    D. amoxicillin

19. In gonococcal infection, which of the following is true?

    A. Risk of transmission from an infected woman to a male sexual partner is about 20%.

    B. Most men have symptomatic infection.

    C. The incubation period is about 2 to 3 weeks.

    D. The organism rarely produces beta-lactamase.

ANSWERS

16. C

17. A

18. A

19. A

DISCUSSION

Gonorrhea, caused by the gram-negative diplococci *N. gonorrhoeae*, is one of the most common STDs. It has a short incubation period of 1 to 5 days and is likely to cause infection in approximately 20% of men who have sexual contact with an infected woman and approximately 80% of women who have sexual contact with an infected man.

In men, presentation typically includes dysuria with a milky, occasionally blood-tinged, penile discharge. However, the majority of men are asymptomatic. With anal-insertive sex, rectal infection leading to proctitis is often seen. Because the organism frequently produces beta-lactamase, the choice of a therapeutic agent should include agents with beta-lactamase stability and include select fluoroquinolones, ceftriaxone, and cefixime (see Table 7–1).

As with all STDs, a critical part of care is discussion of prevention strategies, including condom use and limiting the number of sexual partners. Offer and encourage testing for other STDs, including HIV.

Discussion Source

Hektor Dunphy, L (1999). *Management Guidelines for Adult Nurse Practitioners*. Philadelphia: FA Davis. Pp. 362–364.

QUESTIONS

20. When choosing an antimicrobial agent for the treatment of chronic bacterial prostatitis, the NP considers that:

A. Gram-positive organisms are the most likely cause of infection.
B. Cephalosporins are first-line choice of therapy.
C. Choosing an antibiotic with gram-negative coverage is critical.
D. Length of antimicrobial therapy is typically 10 days.

21. All of the following are likely to be reported by patients with acute bacterial prostatitis except:

A. perineal pain
B. irritative voiding symptoms
C. penile discharge
D. fever

22. During acute bacterial prostatitis, the digital rectal examination usually reveals a gland described as:

A. boggy
B. smooth
C. irregular
D. cystic

23. Symptoms in chronic bacterial prostatitis often include:

A. fever
B. gastrointestinal upset
C. low back pain
D. penile discharge

24. The most common causative organisms in chronic bacterial prostatitis include:

A. gram-negative rods
B. gram-positive cocci
C. gram-negative cocci
D. gram-positive coccobacilli

25. Which of the following is the best choice of therapy in chronic bacterial prostatitis?

   A. trimethoprim sulfamethoxazole for 2 weeks
   B. amoxicillin for 4 weeks
   C. ciprofloxacin for 4 weeks
   D. gentamicin for 8 weeks

ANSWERS

20. C
21. C
22. A
23. C
24. A
25. C

DISCUSSION

Gram-negative rods such as *E. coli* and *Pseudomonas* spp. usually cause acute bacterial prostatitis in older men. In younger men or men at risk for STDs, gonorrhea or chlamydia are most often implicated. Less often, gram-positive organisms such as enterococci are implicated. Irritative voiding symptoms are typically reported as well as suprapubic and perineal pain. Objective findings include fever; a tender, boggy prostate; leukocytosis; and a urine culture positive for the causative organism. Treatment options for acute bacterial prostatitis are similar to those of acute pyelonephritis: that is, an antimicrobial agent with activity against gram-negative organisms and excellent tissue penetration. These include select fluoroquinolones and trimethoprim sulfamethoxazole. Length of therapy is usually 7–14 days.

In patients with chronic bacterial prostatitis, irritative voiding symptoms, low back and perineal pain, as well as a history of urinary tract infection are typically reported. Objective findings include a tender, boggy prostate. Urinalysis results are usually normal. Obtaining urinalysis and culture after prostatic message will typically yield leukocytes and the causative organism. Two to twelve weeks of antimicrobial therapy is usually required (see Table 7–1).

Discussion Sources

Hektor Dunphy, L (1999). *Management Guidelines for Adult Nurse Practitioners*. Philadelphia: FA Davis. Pp. 372–375.
Presti, J., Stoller, M., Carrol, P. (1999). Urology. In Tierny, L. McPhee, S., & Papadakis, M. *Current Medical Diagnosis and Treatment* (38th ed.). Stamford, CT: Appleton and Lange. Pp. 894–931.

QUESTIONS

26. You perform a rectal examination on a 72-year-old man and find a lesion suspicious for prostate cancer. The findings are described as a(n):
    A. rubbery, enlarged prostatic lobe
    B. discrete hard nodule
    C. tender, boggy gland
    D. asymmetric gland

27. Which of the following prostate-specific antigen (PSA) results is most consistent with prostate cancer?
    A. a single elevated PSA result in a man recovering from prostatitis
    B. a doubling of PSA value in serial annual tests in the presence of a normal prostatic digital rectal examination
    C. elevated, unchanged serial PSA level in a man with BPH
    D. a markedly abnormal PSA result immediately postcystoscopy

28. Risk factors for prostate cancer include all of the following except:
    A. African ancestry
    B. history of genital trauma
    C. family history of prostate cancer
    D. high-fat diet

ANSWERS

26. **B**
27. **B**
28. **B**

DISCUSSION

Prostate cancer is the most common cancer in men in the United States. Although clinically detectable prostate cancer is a cause of considerable mortality and morbidity, the majority is likely occult and limited to the prostate with little risk of metastasis. Prostate cancer has been found on autopsy in two-thirds of men age 80 to 89 years. The average American man has a 40% lifetime risk of latent prostate cancer, an approximate 10% risk of clinically significant disease, and an approximate 3% risk of dying of prostate cancer. Risk factors include advancing age, high-fat diet, family history of prostate cancer, and African ancestry. Vasectomy has been suggested as a prostate cancer risk factor.

Most men with prostate cancer are asymptomatic unless the disease is advanced. The prostate examination may reveal a discrete lesion or induration. Measurement of PSA, a glycoprotein produced in benign and malignant prostate cells, is used to screen for prostate cancer. Although nearly two-thirds of men with PSA level of more than 10 ng/mL (normal PSA: < 4 ng/mL) will have prostate cancer, about 25% of those with values between 4 and 10 ng/mL will have disease. Correlating an abnormal prostate examination finding with an abnormal PSA level increases the likelihood of a diagnosis of prostate cancer. PSA level is typically elevated during prostatitis or prostatic instrumentation such as cystoscopy. Levels may remain chronically elevated in patients with BPH. Serial increases even in the presence of a normal prostate examination should be further evaluated. Prostate cancer screening should begin at age 50 years in men with no risk factors and at age 40 years in those with one or more risk factors.

Pathology and disease staging guide prostate cancer treatment options. Watchful waiting is often a reasonable option for older men with local disease.

Discussion Sources

Hektor Dunphy, L (1999). *Management Guidelines for Adult Nurse Practitioners*. Philadelphia: FA Davis. Pp. 369–371.
Presti, J., Stoller, M., Carrol, p. (1999). Urology. Tierny, L. McPhee, S., & Papadakis, M. *Current Medical Diagnosis and Treatment* (38th ed.). Pp. 894–931.

QUESTIONS

29. A 19-year-old man presents with sudden onset of left-sided scrotal pain and unilateral loss of the cremasteric reflex. This most likely represents:

   A. acute epididymitis

   B. testicular torsion

    C. testicular neoplasia

    D. incarcerated hernia

30. In assessing men with testicular torsion, the NP is most likely to note:

    A. relief of pain with scrotal elevation

    B. white blood cells reported in urinalysis

    C. a swollen, tender testicle

    D. increased testicular blood flow by color-flow Doppler ultrasound

31. Anticipated organ survival exceeds 85% with testicular decompression within how many hours of torsion?

    A. 1

    B. 6

    C. 16

    D. 24

32. In order to prevent a recurrence of testicular torsion, which of the following is recommended?

    A. use of a scrotal support

    B. avoidance of testicular trauma

    C. orchiopexy

    D. limiting the number of sexual partners

ANSWERS

29. B

30. C

31. B

32. C

DISCUSSION

Testicular torsion is a urologic emergency caused by a twisting of the testis and spermatic cord around a vertical axis. This results in arterial and venous compression, testicular swelling, and testicular death. Findings include severe unilateral scrotal pain and swelling, the affected testicle held high in the scrotum, absent cremasteric reflex, and lack of relief of pain with scrotal elevation. Radionuclide testicular scan and color-flow Doppler ultrasound may demonstrate reduction of blood flow.

Prompt referral to a urologic surgeon to detort the organ and restore testicular blood flow is indicated. If accomplished within 6 hours, testicular survival surpasses 85%. A bilateral orchiopexy, a procedure in which both testes are brought down and tacked lower in the scrotum, is usually performed in order to avoid subsequent torsion.

Discussion Sources

Hektor Dunphy, L (1999). *Management Guidelines for Adult Nurse Practitioners*. Philadelphia: FA Davis. Pp. 337–338.
Presti, J., Stoller, M., Carrol, P. (1999). Urology. In Tierny, L, McPhee, S., & Papadakis, M. *Current Medical Diagnosis and Treatment* (38th ed.). Stamford, CT: Appleton and Lange. Pp. 894–931.

QUESTIONS

33. A 42-year-old man has a nontender "bag of worms" mass within the left scrotum that disappears when he is in the supine position. This most consistent with:

    A. testicular neoplasm
    B. varicocele
    C. inguinal hernia
    D. epididymitis

34. Which of the following is a common finding in a man with varicocele?

    A. low sperm count with abnormal forms
    B. increased rate of testicular cancer
    C. recurrent scrotal pain
    D. BPH

ANSWERS

33. B
34. A

DISCUSSION

A varicocele is an abnormally dilated spermatic vein within the scrotum. Typically described as a "bag of worms" lesion and most often found in the left scrotum, the varicocele is present while standing and disappears in the supine position. A decreased sperm count with an increase in abnormal forms is noted in about two-thirds of men with varicocele. Surgery is curative. A scrotal support may be helpful for relief of discomfort associated with varicocele.

Discussion Source

Hektor Dunphy, L. (1999). *Management Guidelines for Adult Nurse Practitioners*. Philadelphia: FA Davis. Pp. 379–380.

QUESTIONS

35. How long after contact does the onset of clinical manifestations of syphilis typically occur?

   A. < 1 week
   B. 1–3 weeks
   C. 2–4 weeks
   D. 4–6 weeks

36. Which of the following is not representative of the presentation of primary syphilis?

   A. painless ulcer
   B. palpable inguinal nodes
   C. flulike symptoms
   D. spontaneously healing lesion

37. Which of the following is not representative of the presentation of secondary syphilis?

   A. generalized rash
   B. chancre
   C. arthralgia
   D. aortic regurgitation

38. Which of the following is found in tertiary syphilis?

   A. arthralgia
   B. lymphadenopathy
   C. macropapular lesions involving the palms and soles
   D. gumma

39. Syphilis is most contagious during which of the following?

    A. before onset of signs and symptoms
    B. primary stage
    C. secondary stage
    D. tertiary stage

40. First-line treatment options for syphilis include:

    A. penicillin
    B. ciprofloxacin
    C. erythromycin
    D. ceftriaxone

ANSWERS

35. C
36. C
37. B
38. D
39. C
40. A

DISCUSSION

Caused by the spirochete *Treponema pallidum,* syphilis is a complex, multiorgan disease. Sexual contact is the usual route of transmission. The initial lesion forms about 2 to 4 weeks after contact; contagion is greatest during the secondary stage. Treatment is guided by the stage of disease and clinical manifestation (Table 7–2).

As with all STDs, a critical part of care is discussion of prevention strategies, including condom use and limiting the number of sexual partners. Offer and encourage testing for other STDs, including HIV.

Discussion Sources

Hektor Dunphy, L. (1999). *Management Guidelines for Adult Nurse Practitioners.* Philadelphia: FA Davis. Pp. 375–377.

Center for Disease Control and Prevention. (1998). 1998 Guidelines for Treatment of Sexually Transmitted Disease. Available at http://www.cdc.gov.epo/mmwr/preview/mmwrhtml/00050909.htm

TABLE 7-2.
STAGES OF SYPHILIS, CLINICAL MANIFESTATIONS, AND TREATMENT CONSIDERATIONS

Stage of Syphilis	Clinical Manifestations	Treatment Options
Primary syphilis	Painless genital ulcer with a clean base and indurated margins, localized lymphadenopathy	Benzathine penicillin G 2.4 million U IM In penicillin allergy: Doxycycline 100 mg PO BID for 2 weeks or tetracycline 500 mg PO QID for 2 weeks
Secondary syphilis	Diffuse maculopapular rash involving palms and soles, generalized lymphadenopathy, low-grade fever, malaise, arthralgias and myalgia, headache	Benzathine penicillin G 2.4 million U IM In penicillin allergy: Doxycycline 100 mg PO BID for 2 weeks or tetracycline 500 mg PO QID for 2 weeks
Late syphilis (tertiary syphilis)	Gumma (granulomatous lesions involving skin, mucous membranes, bone), aortic insufficiency, aortic aneurysm, Argyle Robertson pupil, seizures	Benzathine penicillin G 2.4 million U IM weekly for 3 weeks In penicillin allergy: Doxycycline 100 mg PO BID for 4 weeks or tetracycline 500 mg PO QID for 4 weeks

Reference: Center for Disease Control and Prevention. (1998). *1998 Guidelines for Treatment of Sexually Transmitted Disease.* Available at http://www.cdc.gov.epo/mmwr/preview/mmwrhtml/00050909.htm

QUESTIONS

41. Sequelae of genital condyloma acuminata may include:

    A. anal carcinoma
    B. low sperm count
    C. paraphimosis
    D. Reiter's syndrome

42. Which of the following best describes the lesions associated with condyloma acuminata?

    A. verruca form
    B. plaquelike
    C. vesicular form
    D. bullous

43. Treatment options for patients with condyloma acuminata include:

    A. podofilox
    B. penicillin
    C. acyclovir
    D. metronidazole

ANSWERS

41. A
42. A
43. A

DISCUSSION

Condyloma acuminata are verruca-form lesions seen in genital warts. It is an STD. The causative agent is human papilloma virus (HPV), with infection with multiple HPV types usually seen with genital infection. Anal, penile, and cervical carcinoma can be consequences of HPV infection. However, not all HPV types are correlated with malignancy. About 50% have a spontaneous regression of warts without intervention. Treatment options include podofilox, imiquimod, trichloroacetic acid, or cryotherapy; the patient, saving the cost and inconvenience of office visits may administer podofilox and imiquimod cream. Interferon therapy or surgery is typically reserved for complicated, recalcitrant lesions (see Table 7–1).

As with all STDs, a critical part of care is discussion of prevention strategies, including condom use and limiting the number of sexual partners. Offer and encourage testing for other STDs, including HIV.

8
CHAPTER

Musculoskeletal
Disorders

QUESTIONS

1. The most common cause of bursitis is:

   A. inactivity
   B. joint overuse
   C. fibromyalgia
   D. gonoccocal infection

2. First-line bursitis treatment options likely include:

   A. steroid bursal injection
   B. heat to area
   C. weight-bearing exercises
   D. nonsteroidal anti-inflammatory drugs (NSAIDs)

3. Patients with olecranon bursitis typically present with:

   A. swelling and redness over the affected area
   B. limited elbow range of motion (ROM)
   C. nerve impingement
   D. destruction of the joint space

4. Patients with subscapular bursitis typically present with:

   A. limited shoulder ROM
   B. heat over the affected area
   C. localized tenderness under the superomedian angle of the scapula
   D. cervical nerve root irritation

5. Patients with gluteus medius or deep trochanteric bursitis typically present with:

   A. increased pain by resisted hip abduction
   B. limited hip ROM
   C. sciatic nerve pain
   D. heat over the affected area

6. Likely sequelae of intrabursal steroid injection include:

A. irreversible skin atrophy
B. infection
C. inflammatory reaction
D. soreness at the site of injection

7. First-line prepatellar bursitis therapy should include:

A. bursal aspiration
B. intrabursal steroid injection
C. acetaminophen
D. knee splinting

ANSWERS

1. **B**
2. **D**
3. **A**
4. **C**
5. **A**
6. **D**
7. **A**

DISCUSSION

Bursitis, inflammation of the fluid-filled sacs that act as a cushion between tendons and bones, most commonly affects the subdeltoid, olecranon, ischial, trochanter, and prepatellar bursae. Unlike arthritis, bursitis typically has an abrupt onset with focal tenderness and swelling. The joint ROM is usually full but may be limited by pain (Table 8–1).

Risk factors for bursitis include joint overuse, trauma, infection or arthritis conditions such as rheumatoid or osteoarthritis. Because recurrence is common, prevention of further joint overuse and trauma should be emphasized.

With prepatellar bursitis, bursal aspiration should be considered as a first-line therapy because it affords significant pain relief as well as allows the bursa to reapproximate. In other sites, first-line bursitis therapy includes minimizing or eliminating the offending activity, applying ice to

TABLE 8–1.
CLINICAL PRESENTATION OF BURSITIS

Location of Bursitis	Clinical Presentation	Comments
Prepatellar (knee)	Knee swelling and pain in front of the knee, normal ROM	Risk factors include frequent kneeling (housemaid's knee)
Olecranon (elbow)	Pain and swelling behind the elbow; swelling in same area, often described as a ball or sac hanging from the elbow	Risk factors include prolonged pressure or trauma to the elbow (draftsman's elbow)
Trochanter (hip)	Gait disturbance, local trochanter tenderness, pain on hip rotation, and resisted hip abduction with normal hip ROM	Risk factors include back disease, leg length discrepancy, and leg problems that lead to altered gait; osteoarthritis is seldom implicated
Subscapular (shoulder)	Local tenderness under the superomedian angle of the scapula over the adjacent rib, normal shoulder ROM, no nerve root impingement	Risk factors include repeated back and forth motion; common in assembly workers
Pre-Achilles (heel)	Pain and localized swelling behind the heel, minimal pain with dorsiflexion, normal ankle ROM	Usually not disabling and does not contribute to tendon rupture; often confused with Achilles tendonitis
Retrocalcaneal (heel)	Pain behind ankle made worse by walking; patient often runs fingers along both sides of Achilles tendon	Risk factors include wearing high-heeled shoes as well as repetitive ankle motion such as stair climbing, running, jogging, walking

the affected area for 15 minutes at least 4 times per day, and the use of NSAIDs. If these conservative measures have not worked after approximately 4 to 8 weeks, intrabursal steroid injection should be given. Before injection, patients should be informed of the risks of this procedure, including the most common problem, soreness at the injection site. Infection, tissue atrophy, and inflammatory reaction are rarely encountered.

Discussion Source

Anderson, B. (1999). Office orthopedics for primary care. *Diagnosis and Treatment* (2nd ed.). Philadelphia: W. B. Saunders Company.

QUESTIONS

8. Patients with lateral epicondylitis typically present with:

    A. electric-like pain with tapping over the median nerve
    B. hand numbness
    C. pain that is at its worst with elbow flexion
    D. decreased grip strength

9. Risk factors for lateral epicondylitis include all of the following except:

    A. repetitive lifting
    B. playing tennis
    C. hammering
    D. gout

10. First-line therapy for treatment of lateral epicondylitis includes:

    A. long arm cast
    B. short arm cast with thumb spica
    C. wrist splint with metal stays
    D. shoulder sling

11. Patients with median epicondylitis typically present with:

    A. forearm numbness
    B. reduction of ROM
    C. pain on elbow flexion
    D. decreased grip strength

12. Risk factors for median epicondylitis include playing:

   A. tennis
   B. golf
   C. baseball
   D. volleyball

ANSWERS

   8. D
   9. D
   10. C
   11. D
   12. B

DISCUSSION

The painful condition that arises as a result of injury to the extensor tendon at the lateral epicondyle is often called *tennis elbow* or *lateral epicondylitis*. Patients usually give a history of an aggravating activity followed by forearm weakness and point to tenderness over the inner aspect of the humerus (Table 8–2). Median epicondylitis is often called *golfer's elbow*.

Conservative therapy in the first 3 to 4 weeks should include avoidance of the precipitating activity, application of a forearm splint, and NSAIDs use. If symptoms persist, a short arm cast may be used to further limit arm movement. Local steroid injection may be helpful if symptoms persist beyond 6 to 8 weeks or are particularly severe. The use of a tennis elbow band may help prevent recurrence.

Discussion Source

Anderson, B. (1999). *Office orthopedics for primary care. Diagnosis and Treatment* (2nd ed.). Philadelphia: W. B. Saunders Company.

QUESTIONS

13. Risk factors for gout include:

   A. thiazide diuretic use
   B. female gender

TABLE 8–2.
CLINICAL PRESENTATION OF EPICONDYLITIS

Condition	Presentation	Comments
Median epicondylitis	Patient complains of pain over median epicondyle or inner aspect of lower humerus; local epicondylar tenderness, elbow pain, forearm weakness, pain aggravated by resisting writing flexion and radial deviation, decreased grip strength, full ROM	Often called "golfers elbow"; results from repetitive activity such as lifting, using tools, sports involving a tight grip; patients should avoid recurrence by using palm-up lifting or a tennis elbow band
Lateral epicondylitis	Patient complains of pain over the lateral epicondyle or outer aspect of the lower humerus; local epicondylar tenderness, elbow pain, forearm weakness, pain aggravated by resisting writing flexion and radial deviation, decreased grip strength, full ROM	Often called "tennis elbow"; results from repetitive activity such as lifting, using tools, sports involving a tight grip; patients should avoid recurrence by stretching exercises, minimizing length of time spent with light grip

Reference: Hektor Dunphy, L. (1999). *Management Guidelines for Adult Nurse Practitioners*. Philadelphia: FA Davis. Pp. 401–402.

    C. rheumatoid arthritis

    D. joint trauma

14. The clinical presentation of gout includes:

    A. slow onset of discomfort over a number of days

    B. greatest swelling and pain along the median border of the joint

    C. improvement of symptoms with joint rest

    D. fever

15. The most helpful diagnostic test to perform during acute gouty arthritis is:

A. erythrocyte sedimentation rate (ESR)
B. serum uric acid
C. analysis of joint aspirate
D. joint radiograph

16. First-line therapy for the treating patients with acute gouty arthritis includes:

A. aspirin
B. naproxen sodium
C. allopurinol
D. probenecid

17. Which of the following patients with acute gouty arthritis is the best candidate for local corticosteroid injection?

A. a 66-year-old patient with a gastric ulcer
B. a 44-year-old patient taking a thiazide diuretic
C. a 68-year-old patient with type 2 diabetes mellitus
D. a 32-year-old patient who is a binge drinker

ANSWERS

13. A
14. B
15. C
16. B
17. A

DISCUSSION

Primary gout is an acute monoarticular arthritis caused by a disorder in uric acid excretion allowing an accumulation of urates in joints, bones, and subcutaneous tissues. It is most often seen in men. Risk factors include excessive alcohol use, obesity, presence of diabetes mellitus, and thiazide diuretic use. Less often, it is caused by excessive uric acid production and seen with hemolytic anemia, leukemia, or psoriasis; this type is known as secondary gout. This acutely painful condition typically affects the metacarpophalangeal joint of the great toe. The onset is sudden and is accompanied by significant distress. Patients report the inability to move the joint, walk, or even tolerate the weight of a bed sheet on the affected joint because of pain. The entire great toe is usually reddened and enlarged, and the greatest amount of swelling is noted along the median border of the joint; this usually is also the point of greatest discomfort. Although the presentation of gout can mimic an acutely infected joint, it is important to remember that gout is 100 times more common than septic arthritis.

The diagnosis of acute gouty arthritis is usually straightforward, particularly in repeat episodes. With the first episode, uric acid levels may be obtained. However, levels may be reduced during the acute phase. Analysis of joint aspirate for urate crystals is diagnostic; ESR is usually high, but this is neither sensitive nor specific for gout. Radiographs are not needed unless there is a concurrent history of trauma and risk of fracture.

The treatment of acute gouty arthritis should include minimizing or removing contributing factors such as alcohol or thiazide diuretic use. A loading dose of a NSAID, such as naproxen 750 mg or indomethacin 50 mg followed by lower doses, can be helpful. Colchicine 0.6 mg every hour up to 7.2 mg or when gastrointestinal symptoms occur can be used. Because its use can precipitate gout, aspirin is contraindicated. Local injection with corticosteroids can provide significant relief and offers a treatment alternative to NSAIDs, particularly in the face of warfarin use, renal failure, or peptic ulcer disease.

After the acute flare-up has subsided, a 24-hour urine collection for uric acid will help assess if the patient overproduces or undersecretes uric acid. Long-term care to avoid future attacks will be directed by this, with undersecretors benefiting from probenecid and overproducers by allopurinol.

Discussion Sources

Anderson, B. (1999). *Office orthopedics for primary care. Diagnosis and Treatment* (2nd ed.). Philadelphia: W. B. Saunders Company.
Hektor Dunphy, L. (1999). *Management Guidelines for Adult Nurse Practitioners*. Philadelphia: FA Davis. Pp. 389–391.

QUESTIONS

18. Which of the following joints is most likely to be affected by osteoarthritis?

   A. wrists
   B. elbows
   C. metacarpophalangeal
   D. distal interphalangeal

19. Deformity of the proximal interphalangeal joints found in an elderly patient with osteoarthritis is known as:

    A. Heberden nodes
    B. Bouchard nodes
    C. valgus halgas
    D. Dupytrene's contracture

20. Which of the following best describes the presentation of a patient with osteoarthritis?

    A. worst symptoms in weight-bearing joints later in the day
    B. symmetric early morning stiffness
    C. sausage-shaped digits with associated skin lesions
    D. back pain with rest and anterior uveitis

21. As part of the evaluation of patients with osteoarthritis, the NP anticipates finding:

    A. anemia of chronic disease
    B. elevated C-reactive protein level
    C. narrowing of the joint space on radiograph
    D. elevated antinuclear antibody titer

22. First-line pharmacologic intervention for osteoarthritis should be:

    A. acetaminophen
    B. piroxicam
    C. methylprednisolone
    D. intra-articular corticosteroid injection

23. In caring for a patient with osteoarthritis of the knee, you advise that:

    A. Straight-leg raising should be avoided.
    B. Heat should be applied to painful joints after exercise.
    C. Quadriceps strengthening exercises should be performed.
    D. Exercise should be avoided.

24. Glucosamine and chondroitin are nutritional supplements that may help in the treatment of:

    A. rheumatoid arthritis
    B. osteoarthritis
    C. prevention of upper respiratory infections
    D. insomnia

ANSWERS

18. D
19. B
20. A
21. C
22. A
23. C
24. B

DISCUSSION

Osteoarthritis (OA) is the most common joint disease in the United States, affecting more than 20 million people. It is a degenerative disease without systemic manifestations or inflammation. The most problematic joint involvement is the hip and knee. Worst symptoms are reported with use of the joints, and there is minimum morning stiffness (in contrast to rheumatoid arthritis). Risk factors for osteoarthritis include a positive OA family history and contact sport participation. Obesity is also a risk factor, especially with hip and knee involvement.

In osteoarthritis, the articular cartilage becomes rough and wears away. Bone spurs may form, and the synovial membrane thickens. Consequently, the joint space narrows.

The clinical presentation in patients with osteoarthritis includes an insidious onset of symptoms, including use-related joint pain that is relieved by rest, and joint stiffness that occurs with rest but resolves with less than 15 minutes of activity. Physical examination reveals smooth, cool joints and coarse crepitus. Particularly when the knee is affected, joint effusion is common and may be minimal to severe with up to 20 mL of fluid. Patients cannot reach full knee flexion in the effused joint. The knee often locks or pops, suggesting a degenerative meniscal tear.

Radiologic findings in patients with osteoarthritis include narrowing of the joint space and increased density of subchondral bone. Bony cysts and osteophytes are often present. However, only about 50% with radiologic findings have symptoms. Because osteoarthritis is typically a noninflammatory disease, ESR and C-reactive protein, both markers of inflammation, are typically normal. Unlike in patients with rheumatoid arthritis and systemic lupus erythematosus, antinuclear antibodies are absent from the serum.

Therapeutic goals for those with osteoarthritis include preventing further articular cartilage destruction, minimizing pain, and enhancing mobility. Therapies for symptom control include lifestyle modification such as weight loss and minimum weight-bearing exercise such as swimming or water-based activities as well as exercise to maintain joint flexibility and enhance strength in the surrounding muscles (Table 8–3). Application of heat to minimize pain and stiffness in the morning before activity can be helpful, but applying ice to the joint after activity can minimize discomfort. Acetaminophen and NSAIDs have long been used as arthritis drug treatments. These medications are helpful in controlling pain. Although NSAIDs also have potential anti-inflammatory activity, this is seldom needed in osteoarthritis therapy. Long-acting opioids may be required if symptom control can not be achieved.

Glucosamine, an amino acid, is usually used as first-line treatment for osteoarthritis in many European nations and is available as an over-the-counter nutritional supplement in the United States. It appears to help rebuild damaged joint cartilage and results in reduction in pain, increased joint flexion, and articular function. Glucosamine must be used consistently for a minimum of 2 weeks and likely as long as 3 months before therapeutic effect is seen. Although no drug interactions or hepatoxicity have been noted with its use, glucosamine should be used with caution because there is a risk of bronchospasm. Chondroitin is often used in con-

TABLE 8–3.
EXERCISE REGIMENS IN OSTEOARTHRITIS

Joint Condition	Exercise Regimen	Comments
Osteoarthritis in the knee	Straight-leg raises without weights, advance to using weights as tolerated; quadriceps sets; no or limited weight-bearing aerobic activity	Avoid squatting, kneeling, and high-impact exercise
Osteoarthritis of the hip	Straight-leg raises without weights, advance to using weights as tolerated; stretching exercises of adductor, rotator, and gluteus muscles; isometric exercises of the iliopsoas and gluteus muscles; no or limited weight-bearing aerobic activity	Avoid high-impact exercise

junction with glucosamine because the two appear to have synergistic activity. Chondroitin's mechanism of action is not well understood. It is derived from bovine tracheal cartilage. Although chondroitin is generally well tolerated, it should be used with caution because of potential anticoagulant effect.

Intra-articular corticosteroid joint injection may help when more conservative therapy has failed. In particular with osteoarthritis in the knee, corticosteroid injection can help when joint effusion is present. Hip injection is a technically challenging procedure that can be done with fluoroscopic guidance.

Joint replacement should be considered when pain is intractable, when function is severely compromised, or when more than 80% of the articular cartilage is worn away. Duration of prosthetic joint function is typically 10 to 15 years. As a result, the ideal candidate for joint replacement is older than age 60 years and is able to tolerate a surgical procedure that lasts for several hours followed by an aggressive postoperative course of rehabilitation. A patellar restraining brace, walker, or wheelchair may be needed for patients with advanced osteoarthritis of the knee and hip that cannot be surgically repaired.

Discussion Sources

Anderson, B. (1999). Office orthopedics for primary care. *Diagnosis and Treatment* (2nd ed.). Philadelphia: W. B. Saunders Company.
Hektor Dunphy, L. (1999). *Management Guidelines for Adult Nurse* Practitioners. Philadelphia: FA Davis. Pp. 392–394.

QUESTIONS

25. In order to confirm the results of a McMurray test, you ask the patient to:

    A. squat
    B. walk
    C. flex the knee
    D. rotate the ankle

26. Which of the following best describes the presentation of a patient with complete median meniscus tear?

    A. joint effusion
    B. heat over the knee
    C. inability to kneel
    D. loss of smooth joint movement

27. In order to help prevent meniscal tear, you advise:

    A. limiting participation in sports
    B. quadriceps strengthening exercises
    C. using a knee brace
    D. applying ice to the knee before exercise

28. Initial treatment for meniscus tear includes all of the following except:

    A. NSAIDs
    B. applying ice
    C. elevation
    D. joint aspiration

ANSWERS

25. A
26. C
27. B
28. D

DISCUSSION

A meniscal tear is a disruption of the fibrocartilage pad located between the femoral condyles and the tibial plateaus. Because the purpose of the fibrocartilage pad is shock absorption and smooth joint mobility, patients with larger tears often report that the knee locks, pops, or gives out. Effusion is also common, with the patient reporting a sensation of knee tightness and stiffness. With certain positions, there is often sudden-onset, sharp, localized pain, usually on the median aspect of the knee. Over time, premature osteoarthritis is seen as the normal joint space is compromised.

Meniscal tears are often classified in a number of manners, including complex or partial; traumatic or degenerative; lateral, posterior, horizontal or vertical; radial, parrot beak, or bucket handle. Patients with partial, horizontal, and anterior tears may have relatively normal examination findings because the knee's mechanics are relatively unchanged even though these patients continue to have knee locking and pain with certain positions. The McMurray test, a palpable popping on the joint line, is highly specific but poorly sensitive for meniscal tear; the Apley grinding test gives similar results. Squatting or kneeling is nearly impossible for patients with a large, complete, or bucket-handle meniscal tear. Joint effusion is typical with ROM being limited by discomfort.

Knee radiographs, which can reveal osteoarthritic changes and possible foreign bodies, are reasonable as initial diagnostic tests. Initial treatment includes rest, elevation, and ice application as well as analgesia. Because joint effusion is nearly always present but is relatively mild, aspiration should be considered only if no improvement after 2 to 4 weeks of conservative therapy. Crutch walking should be encouraged, and a patellar stabilizer may be needed when significant knee instability is present. Straight-leg raising exercises help strengthen the quadriceps and stabilize the joint.

Magnetic resonance imaging (MRI) can identify the type and extent of the tear and should be considered if milder symptoms do not resolve within 2 to 4 weeks or earlier with severe symptoms. Arthroscopy, which provides the most accurate diagnosis with the possibility of concurrent treatment through debridement, should be considered at 4 to 6 weeks if there is no improvement and earlier if joint locking, giving out, and effusion are particularly problematic.

Discussion Sources

Anderson, B. (1999). Office orthopedics for primary care. *Diagnosis and Treatment* (2nd ed.). Philadelphia: W. B. Saunders Company.
Hektor Dunphy, L. (1999). *Management Guidelines for Adult Nurse Practitioners*. Philadelphia: FA Davis. Pp. 391–392.

QUESTIONS

29. Phalen's sign is described as:

   A. reproduction of symptoms with forced flexion of the wrists
   B. abnormal tingling when the median nerve is tapped
   C. pain on internal rotation
   D. palmar atrophy

30. Tinel's sign is best described as:

   A. reproduction of symptoms with forced flexion of the wrists
   B. abnormal tingling when the median nerve is tapped
   C. pain on internal rotation
   D. palmar atrophy

31. Risk factors for carpal tunnel syndrome (CTS) include all of the following except:

    A. pregnancy
    B. hypothyroidism
    C. repetitive motion
    D. multiple sclerosis

32. Which of the following is least likely to be reported by patients with CTS?

    A. worst symptoms during the day
    B. burning sensation in the affected hand
    C. tingling pain that radiates to the forearm
    D. nocturnal numbness

33. Initial therapy for patients with CTS includes:

    A. intra-articular injection
    B. joint splinting
    C. systemic corticosteroids
    D. referral for surgery

34. Primary prevention of CTS includes:

    A. screening for thyroid dysfunction
    B. treatment of osteoarthritis
    C. stretching and toning exercises
    D. wrist splinting

ANSWERS

29. A
30. B
31. D
32. A
33. B
34. C

DISCUSSION

Carpal tunnel syndrome is a painful syndrome caused by compression of the median nerve between the carpal ligament and other structures within the carpal tunnel. This leads to an entrapment neuropathy, causing symptoms in the distribution of the median nerve.

The most common risk is repetitive motion; the condition is common with protracted computer keyboard use as well as in workers such as cake decorators and soldiers who must continually grasp a small object. Primary prevention of CTS includes limiting time spent in these activities, ensuring proper work breaks, and encouraging toning and stretching exercises.

Patients with CTS usually report a burning, aching, or tingling pain radiating to the forearm and occasionally to the shoulder, neck, and chest. Symptoms are often worst at night. A classic finding is the report of acroparesthesia, awakening at night with numbness and burning pain in the fingers. Diagnostic tests for patients suspected of having CTS include electromyogram (EMG) and nerve conduction studies that can confirm the median neuropathy.

Treatment of patients with CTS includes limiting the activity that caused the condition, elevating the affected extremity, and splinting the hand and forearm. Pain relief with NSAIDs or acetaminophen can be helpful. Steroid injection into the carpal tunnel at 6-week intervals may reduce swelling and symptoms but should only be attempted by a skilled practitioner. Surgery to release the transverse carpal ligament gives symptom relief in the majority of patients who do not respond to conservative therapy. However, about 10% will not respond because of nerve damage or new pressure within the carpal tunnel resulting from recurrent compression caused by scar formation. Vitamin B6 therapy has been reported to be helpful in minimizing CTS symptoms.

Carpal tunnel syndrome is often noted transiently at the end of pregnancy and in patients with untreated hypothyroidism. Pregnancy-induced CTS usually resolves quickly after the woman gives birth, and thyroxine supplements quickly help CTS caused by hypothyroidism. In the interim, splinting and analgesia can be helpful.

Discussion Sources

Anderson, B. (1999). Office orthopedics for primary care. *Diagnosis and Treatment* (2nd ed.). Philadelphia: W. B. Saunders Company.
Hektor Dunphy, L. (1999). *Management Guidelines for Adult Nurse Practitioners*. Philadelphia: FA Davis. Pp. 386–388.

QUESTIONS

35. Most episodes of low back pain are caused by:
    A. an acute precipitating event
    B. disk herniation
    C. muscle or ligamentous strain
    D. nerve impingement

36. With straight-leg raising test, the NP is evaluating tension on which of the following nerve roots?
    A. L1 and L2
    B. L3 and L4
    C. L5 and S1
    D. S2 and S3

37. During acute lumbosacral strain, which of the following is the best advice to give about exercising?
    A. You should not exercise until you are free of pain.
    B. Back-strengthening exercises may cause mild muscle soreness.
    C. Electric-like pain is to be expected.
    D. Conditioning exercises should be started immediately.

38. Early neurological changes in patients with sciatica include:
    A. loss of deep tendon reflexes
    B. poor two-point discrimination
    C. reduced muscle strength
    D. foot drop

39. When evaluating a patient with low back pain, the loss of bowel and bladder control most likely indicates:
    A. cauda equina syndrome
    B. muscular spasm
    C. vertebral fracture
    D. sciatic nerve entrapment

40. Loss of posterior tibial reflex may indicate a lesion at:
    A. L3
    B. L4
    C. L5
    D. S1

41. Loss of Achilles tendon reflex most likely indicates a lesion at:

   A. L1-L2
   B. L3-L4
   C. L5-S1
   D. S2-S3

42. Which test is demonstrated when the examiner applies pressure at the sciatic notch and produces radiating leg pain?

   A. Spurling
   B. McMurray
   C. Lachman
   D. Newman

43. The preferred diagnostic test in a patient with acute lumbar radiculopathy is a(n):

   A. lumbosacral radiograph series
   B. ESR
   C. MRI
   D. bone scan

ANSWERS

35. C
36. C
37. B
38. B
39. A
40. C
41. C
42. A
43. C

DISCUSSION

Low back pain is at least an occasional problem for nearly all adults, with a lifetime prevalence of 60–90%. In about 90% of patients with low back pain, symptoms are short lived and resolve within 1 month without specific therapy. However, a small number have recurrent or chronic low back pain and significant disability.

Lumbosacral strain or disk herniation and its resulting lumbar radiculopathy and sciatica can cause musculoskeletal low back pain. Most often, contributing factors include muscle or ligamentous strain, degenerative joint disease (DJD), or a combination of these factors. Lumbosacral strain is the most common reason for a patient to present to primary care with acute low back pain. In the typical presentation, the patient complains of stiffness, spasm, and reduced ROM. The erector spinae muscle is most often implicated. Sitting usually aggravates the pain, but there may be some relief if the patient lies supine on a firm surface. A precipitating event is reported only by a small number because lumbosacral strain is usually the culmination of a number of events, including repeated used of improperly stretched muscles in patients with overall poor conditioning. In addition, poor posture, scoliosis, and spinal stenosis can be predisposing factors. The physical examination usually reveals a straightening of the lumbosacral curve, paraspinal muscle tenderness, and spasm worst at the level of L3 to L4, as well as decreased lumbosacral flexion and lateral bending. The neurological examination findings are typically within normal limits unless radiculopathy is present.

Diagnostics in lumbosacral strain vary according to the length and severity of symptoms. Radiographs can be of help if spondylolisthesis, scoliosis, or DJD is suspected. However, in the absence of these, little will likely be revealed. Therefore, lumbosacral radiographs should not be routinely obtained. CT scanning or MRI should be considered if radiculopathy is present because these studies could reveal contributing factors such as spinal stenosis and disk herniation.

Lumbosacral disk herniation usually occurs after years of episodes of back pain caused by repeated damage to the annular fibers of the disk and is less common than lumbosacral strain as a cause of low back pain. Lumbar disk herniation often leads to sciatica, neurological changes, and significant distress. Because the intravertebral disks contain less water and are more fibrous, the risk of disk rupture decreases after age 50 years.

The cause of sciatica is usually pressure on lumbosacral nerve roots from a herniated disk, spinal stenosis, or compression fracture. On occasion, sciatica can be caused by external pressure on the sciatic nerve, such as is often found in people who carry a wallet in a rear pants pocket and develop symptoms after prolonged sitting. Patients with sciatica complain of shooting pain that starts over the hip and radiates to the foot, often accompanied by leg numbness and weakness. The degree of pain can vary according to the degree of nerve involvement; it ranges from mildly bothersome and occasionally reported, to more itchy than painful, and to incapacitating pain.

In patients who have herniated disks, the degree of neurological involvement ranges from more minor symptoms of numbness to loss of extremity function. Deep tendon reflexes may be absent. With cauda equina involvement, there is compression of the lower portion of the nerve root inferior to the spinal cord usually secondary to disk herniation. This leads to rectal or perineal pain and disturbance in bowel and bladder function. Signs of lumbosacral strain are present, and the straight-leg-raising maneuver yields reproduction of pain.

Management of patients with low back pain differs according to presentation. In the majority with acute low back pain and intact neurological examination, a short course of 2 to 4 days of bed rest may be helpful; longer periods of immobilization may contribute to deconditioning and are potentially harmful. Application of cold packs for 20 minutes 3 to 4 times a day can help with pain control, and heat applications may help before gentle stretching exercise. NSAIDs or acetaminophen should be prescribed for pain control. Muscle relaxers have demonstrated to be of little help. Treatment should also include initiation of aerobic and toning exercises and teaching the patient to minimize back stress through appropriate use of body mechanics.

Prompt referral to specialty care is needed when there is limb, bowel, or bladder dysfunction. Surgery is usually only considered if severe symptoms persist beyond 3 months. In addition, early referral is indicated in select conditions that are particularly worrisome (Table 8–4).

Discussion Sources

Hektor Dunphy, L. (1999). *Management Guidelines for Adult Nurse Practitioners*. Philadelphia: FA Davis. Pp. 44–47.
Uphold, C., & Graham, V. (1998). *Clinical Guidelines in Family Practice* (3rd ed.). Gainesville, FL: Barmarrae Books. Pp 776–783.

QUESTIONS

44. A 22-year-old man presents with new onset of pain and swelling in his feet and ankles as well as conjunctivitis, oral lesions, and dysuria. The most important test to obtain is:

   A. antinuclear antibody (ANA)
   B. ESR
   C. rubella titers
   D. urethral cultures

**TABLE 8–4.
POTENTIALLY SERIOUS CONDITIONS RELATED TO LOW
BACK PAIN**

Possible Fracture	Possible Tumor or Infection	Cauda Equina Syndrome
History of recent trauma, particularly a fall from significant height or motor vehicle accident	Age younger than 20 years or older than 50 years; constitutional symptoms such as unexplained weight loss, fever; recent bacterial infection, intravenous drug use, immunosuppression	Bladder dysfunction, perineal sensory loss, or anal laxity
In patient with or at risk for osteoporosis, minor trauma or strenuous lifting	Increased pain with rest	Neurological deficit in lower extremities
	History of cancer	Lower extremity motor weakness
		Saddle anesthesia

Reference: Agency for Health Care Policy and Research Guideline on Acute Low Back Problems in Adults. Available at http://text.nlm.nih.gov/ftrs/gateway

45. Treatment for Reiter's syndrome in a sexually active man usually includes:

   A. antimicrobial therapy
   B. corticosteroid therapy
   C. antirheumatic medications
   D. immunosuppresive drugs

ANSWERS

44. D
45. A

DISCUSSION

Reiter's syndrome, a reactive arthritis, causes generalized inflammatory condition. The classic tetrad of the disease consists of urethritis, conjunctivitis, mucocutaneous lesions, and arthritis. The knees and ankles are most often involved, and sacroiliitis is less common. Uveitis may also be seen. This condition is typically seen a number of days to weeks after an episode of acute bacterial diarrhea caused by *Shigella* spp., *Salmonella* spp., *Campylobacter* spp., or a sexually transmitted infection such as *Chlamydia trachomatis* or *Ureaplasma urealyticum*. When seen with infectious diarrhea, the disease is found equally in both genders. When seen with urethritis, there is a male predominance of 9:1. Cultures of joint aspirates in Reiter's syndrome typically have negative results.

Treatment includes the use of anti-inflammatory drugs such as NSAIDs. When Reiter's syndrome occurs with urethritis, tetracycline use is associated with a shorter duration of symptoms. Early antimicrobial treatment of urethritis appears to limit a patient's risk of developing Reiter's syndrome. No change in symptoms is usually seen with antibiotic use if infectious diarrhea was the precipitating event.

Discussion Sources

Hellman, D., & Stone, J. (1999). Arthritis and musculoskeletal disorders. In Tierney, L., McPhee, S., & Papadakis, M. *Current Diagnosis and Treatment* (38th ed.). Norwalk, CT: Appleton & Lange. Pp. 786–837.

QUESTIONS

46. During a preparticipation sports examination, you hear a grade 2/6 early to midsystolic ejection murmur heard best at the second intercostal space of the left sternal boarder in an asymptomatic young adult. This most likely represents:

   A. an innocent flow murmur
   B. mitral valve incompetency
   C. aortic regurgitation
   D. mitral valve prolapse (MVP)

47. You are examining an 18-year-old man who is seeking a sports clearance physical examination. You note a midsystolic murmur that gets louder when he stands. This may represent:

   A. aortic stenosis
   B. hypertrophic obstructive cardiomyopathy
   C. a physiologic murmur
   D. Still's murmur

48. A Still's murmur:

    A. is an indication to selectively restrict sports participation
    B. has a buzzing quality
    C. is usually seen in patients who experience dizziness when exercising
    D. a sign of cardiac structural abnormality

49. A 22-year-old woman with MVP wants to know if she can start a walking program. You respond that:

    A. She should have an exercise tolerance test.
    B. An echocardiogram should be obtained.
    C. She may proceed in the absence of activity intolerance symptoms.
    D. Running should be avoided.

50. You hear a fixed split S_2 heart sound in a 28-year-old man who wants to start an exercise program and consider that it is:

    A. a normal finding in a younger adult
    B. occasionally found uncorrected atrial septal defect
    C. the result of valvular sclerosis
    D. often found in patients with left bundle branch block

51. A 19-year-old man presents with stage 1 hypertension. Which of the following is correct concerning sports participation?

    A. Full activity should be encouraged.
    B. Weight lifting is contraindicated.
    C. An exercise tolerance test is advisable.
    D. A beta adrenergic antagonist should be prescribed.

52. A 25-year-old woman presents with sinus arrhythmia. Which of the following is correct concerning sports participation?

    A. Full activity should be encouraged.
    B. Weight lifting is contraindicated.
    C. An exercise tolerance test is advisable.
    D. A calcium channel antagonist should be prescribed.

ANSWERS

46. A
47. B
48. B
49. C
50. B
51. A
52. A

DISCUSSION

Cardiovascular evaluation is an important component of the sports participation evaluation. Reducing the risk of exercised-induced sudden cardiac death and the progression or deterioration of cardiovascular function caused by exercise are the primary goals of preparticipation evaluation. During the health history, NPs should ask about the major symptoms of heart disease, altered cardiac output, and poor myocardial perfusion. This includes asking about chest pain, heart failure symptoms, palpitations, syncope, or activity intolerance. When examining children, inquire about poor growth and development.

Hypertension is a relatively common problem. Because of the cardiovascular benefit of exercise, activity restriction is usually not advisable unless severely elevated hypertension or target organ damage is present. Certain antihypertensive agents may influence exercise tolerance. In general, the use of angiotensin-converting enzyme (ACE) inhibitors, angiotensin receptor blockers, calcium channel antagonists, and alpha adrenergic blockers has little to no impact on exercise tolerance. However, use of a beta adrenergic antagonist may reduce the ability to exercise because of its ability to blunt normal increase in heart rate in response to exercise. Diuretic use should be avoided because of increased risk of dehydration and hypokalemia.

Cardiac rhythm disturbances are common and are usually benign. In particular, the presence of sinus arrhythmia in a younger adult is a normal finding and is not an indication for curtailing activity. Dysrhythmias associated with ischemic heart disease and certain supraventricular and ventricular rhythms may preclude sports participation.

A cardiac murmur may be benign, in that the examiner simply hears the blood flowing through the heart but no cardiac structural abnormality exists. However, certain cardiac structural problems, such as valvular and myocardial disorders, can contribute to the development of a murmur (Table 8–5).

TABLE 8–5.
FINDINGS AND IMPACT OF CARDIAC CONDITION ON SPORTS PARTICIPATION

Cardiac Condition	Important Examination Findings	Additional Findings	Impact on Sports Participation
Hypertension	Elevated blood pressure	With target organ damage: S_3, S_4 heart sounds, PMI displacement, hypertensive retinopathy	With all but markedly elevated blood pressure or evidence of target organ damage, full participation should be encouraged because of the cardiovascular benefit of exercise
Physiologic, innocent or functional murmur	Gr 1–3/6 early to midsystolic murmur, heard best at LSB but usually audible over precordium	No radiation beyond precordium; softens or disappears with standing, increases in intensity with activity, fever, anemia; S_1, S_2 intact, normal PMI	Full participation; patient should be asymptomatic, with no report of chest pain, CHF symptoms, palpitations, syncope, and activity intolerance
Aortic stenosis	Gr 1–4/6 harsh systolic murmur, usually crescendo-decrescendo pattern, heard best at second RICS, apex	Radiates to carotids, may have diminished S_2, slow filling carotid pulse, narrow pulse pressure, loud S_4; softens with standing; the greater the degree of stenosis, the later the peak of the murmur	Impact on participation varies with degree of stenosis; mild = full participation; moderate = selected participation; severe = no participation; in younger adults, usually congenital bicuspid valve; in older adults, usually calcific, rheumatic in nature; dizziness, syncope, ominous signs pointing to severely decreased cardiac output

Mitral stenosis	Gr 1–3/4 low-pitched late diastolic murmur heard best at the apex, localized; short crescendo-decrescendo rumble, like a bowling ball rolling down an alley or distant thunder	Often with opening snap, accentuated S₁ in the mitral area; enhanced by left lateral decubitus position, squat, cough, immediately after Valsalva maneuver	Impact on participation varies with degree of stenosis; mild = full participation; moderate = selected participation; mild with atrial fibrillation = selected participation; severe = no participation; nearly all rheumatic in origin; protracted latency period, then gradual decreased in exercise tolerance leading to rapid downhill course because of low cardiac output; atrial fibrillation common
Mitral regurgitation	Gr 1–4/6 high-pitched blowing systolic murmur, often extending beyond S₂; sounds like long "haaa" or "hooo"; heard best at RLSB	Radiates to axilla, often with laterally displaced PMI; decreased with standing, Valsalva maneuver; increased by squat, hand grip	Impact on participation varies with ventricular size and function; MR with normal left ventricle size and function = full participation; MR with mild LV enlargement but normal function at rest = selected participation; MR with LV enlargement or any LV dysfunction at rest = no participation; origin: rheumatic, ischemic heart disease, endocarditis, often with other valve abnormalities (AS, MS, AR)

(continued)

TABLE 8–5. (continued)

Cardiac Condition	Important Examination Findings	Additional Findings	Impact on Sports Participation
Aortic regurgitation	Gr 1–3/4 high-pitched blowing diastolic murmur heard best at third LICS	May be enhanced by forced expiration, leaning forward; usually with S_3, wide pulse pressure, sustained thrusting apical impulse	Impact on participation varies with ventricular size, function, and dysrhythmias; AR with normal or mildly increased LV size and function = full participation; AR with moderate LV enlargement, premature ventricular contractions at rest and with exercise = selected participation; mild to moderate AR with symptoms, severe AR, AR with progressive LVH = no participation; more common in men, usually caused by rheumatic heart disease but occasionally because of tertiary syphilis
MVP	Gr 1–3/6 late systolic crescendo murmur with honking quality heard best at apex; murmur follows midsystolic click	With Valsalva maneuver or standing, click moves forward into earlier systole, resulting in a longer-sounding murmur; with hand grasp, squat, click moves back further into systole, resulting in a shorter murmur	Impact in participation varies with ventricular function and dysrhythmia; MVP without = full participation; MVP with mild to moderate regurgitation, dysrhythmias such as repetitive supraventricular tachycardia, complex ventricular dysrhythmias = selected participation; often seen with minor thoracic deformities such as pectus excavatum, strait back, and shallow AP diameter

Hypertrophic cardiomyopathy	Harsh midsystolic crescendo-decrescendo murmur heard best at the lower left sternal border or at the apex	Murmur may increase with standing, squatting, or Valsalva maneuver; triple apical impulse, loud S_4, bisferious carotid pulse	Dyspnea, chest pain, postexertional syncope often reported; sports participation should be determined on an individual basis based on degree of ventricular function and symptoms
Still's murmur (AKA vibratory innocent murmur)	Gr 1–3/6 early systolic ejection, musical or vibratory, short, often buzzing, heard best midway between apex and LLSB	Softens or disappears when sitting, standing, or with Valsalva maneuver; usual onset is at ages 2 to 6 years; may persist through adolescence; benign condition	Benign finding; no limitation on sports participation
Atrial septal defect (without surgical intervention)	Gr 1–3/6 systolic ejection murmur heard best at the ULSB with widely split fixed S_2; may be accompanied by a mid-diastolic murmur heard at the fourth ICS; LSB common, caused by increased flow across tricuspid valve	Twice as common in females; child may be entirely well or present with CHF; often missed in the first few months of life or even entire childhood; watch for the child with easy fatigability	With correction, full sports participation is typical; without correction, sports participation should be determined on an individual basis based on degree of pulmonary hypertension, right-to-left shunt, and symptoms

(continued)

TABLE 8–5. (continued)

Cardiac Condition	Important Examination Findings	Additional Findings	Impact on Sports Participation
Ventricular septal defect (without surgical intervention)	Gr 2–5/6 regurgitant systolic murmur heard best at LLSB; occasionally holosystolic, usually localized	Usually without cyanosis; with small- to moderate-sized left-to-right shunt without pulmonary hypertension likely to have minimal symptoms; larger shunts may result in CHF with onset in infancy	With correction, full sports participation is typical; without correction, sports participation should be determined on an individual basis based on degree of pulmonary hypertension, right-to-left shunt, and symptoms

References: Constant, J. (1999). *Essentials of Bedside Cardiology*. Philadelphia: Lippincott, Williams & Wilkins.
Van Camp, S. (1999). Cardiology. In Sarafan, M., McKeag, D., & Van Camp, S. *Manual of Sports Medicine*. Philadelphia: Lippincott-Raven. Pp. 226–243.
Willms, J., Schneidermans, H., & Algranti, P. (1994). The heart and great vessels. In *Physical Diagnosis: Bedside Evaluation of Diagnosis and Function*. Baltimore: Williams & Wilkins. Pp. 283–346.

Normal heart valves allow one-way, unimpeded forward blood flow through the heart. The entire stroke output is able to pass freely during one phase of the cardiac cycle (diastole with the atrioventricular valves, systole with the others), and there is no backward flow of blood. When a heart valve fails to open to its normal size, it is stenotic. When it fails to close appropriately, the valve is incompetent, causing regurgitation of blood to the previous chamber or vessel. Both of these events place patients at significant risk for embolic disease.

Physiologic murmurs, also known as functional or innocent flow murmurs, are present in the absence of cardiac pathology. There is no obstruction to flow, and there is a normal gradient across the valve. This type of murmur may be heard in up to 80% of thin adults or children if the cardiac examination is performed in a soundproof booth and is best heard at the left sternal border. It occurs in early to midsystole, leaving the two heart sounds intact. In addition, patients with a benign systolic ejection murmur deny having cardiac symptoms and have otherwise normal cardiac examination results, including an appropriately located PMI and full pulses. Because no cardiac pathology is present in patients with a physiologic murmur, full activity should be encouraged.

Aortic stenosis is the inability of the aortic valves to open to optimum size. The aortic valve normally opens to 3 cm^2; aortic stenosis usually does not cause significant symptoms until the valvular orifice is limited to 0.8 cm^2. In children and younger adults, aortic stenosis is occasionally found, usually caused by a congenital bicuspid (rather than tricuspid) valve or with a three-cusp valve with leaflet fusion. This defect is most often found in males and is commonly accompanied by a long-standing history of becoming excessively short of breath with increased activity such as running. The physical examination results are usually normal except for the murmur. The ability to participate in sports or other vigorous activity is dictated by the degree of aortic stenosis and patient symptoms (see Table 8–5).

In older adults, calcification aortic stenosis leading to the inability of the valve to open to its normal size is usually the problem. In middle-aged adults without congenital aortic stenosis, the disease is usually sequelae of rheumatic fever representing about 30% of valvular dysfunction seen in patients with rheumatic heart disease. As with those who have congenital aortic stenosis, the ability to participate in sports or an exercise program is dictated by the degree of valvular dysfunction, ventricular enlargement, and patient symptoms.

The murmur of mitral regurgitation arises from mitral valve incompetency, or the inability of the mitral valve to close properly. This allows a retrograde flow from a high-pressure area (left ventricle) to an area of lower pressure (left atrium). Mitral regurgitation is most often caused by the degeneration of the mitral valve most commonly by rheumatic fever, endocarditis, calcific annulus, rheumatic heart disease, ruptured chordae, or papillary muscle dysfunction. In mitral regurgitation from rheumatic heart disease, some mitral stenosis is usually present. After a patient is symptomatic, the disease progresses, without intervention, in a downhill course of chronic heart failure over the next 10 years. Sports or other vigorous activity participation is dictated by the degree of mitral regurgitation and ventricular chamber enlargement.

Mitral valve prolapse is likely the most common valvular heart problem, perhaps present in 10% of the general population. The majority of patients with MVP have a benign condition in which one of the valve leaflets is unusually long and buckles or prolapses into the left atrium, usually occurring in midsytole. At that time, a click occurs followed by a short murmur caused by regurgitation of blood into the atrium. Cardiac output is usually not compromised, and the event goes unnoticed by patients. However, an examiner may detect this on examination. Echocardiography fails to reveal any abnormality, with simply the valve buckling followed by a small-volume mitral regurgitation noted. If there are no cardiac complaints and the rest of the cardiac examination, including electrocardiogram, is within normal limits, no further evaluation is needed. One way of describing this variation from the norm is to inform patients that one leaflet of the mitral valve is a bit longer than usual. However, the "holder" (valve orifice) is of average size. This variation causes the valve to buckle a bit, just as your foot would if forced into a shoe that is one or two sizes too small. Therefore, the heart makes an extra set of sounds (click and murmur) but is not diseased or damaged. MVP is often found in people with minor thoracic deformities such as pectus excavatum, a dish-shaped concave area at T1, and scoliosis. The second and much smaller group with MVP has systolic displacement of one or more of the mitral leaflets into the left atrium alone with valve thickening and redundancy, usually accompanied by mild to moderate mitral regurgitation. This group typically has additional health problems such as Marfan syndrome or other connective tissue disease. Because structural cardiac abnormality is present in this group, there is a risk of bacterial endocarditis.

Barring other health problems, patients with MVP usually have normal cardiac output and tolerate a program of aerobic exercise well. A program of regular aerobic activity should be encouraged in order to promote health and well-being. Because the mitral valve prolapses more, thus increasing the murmur, when circulating volume is low, maintaining a high level of fluid intake should be encouraged in patients with MVP. Treatment with beta adrenergic agonists (beta blockers) is indicated only when symptomatic recurrent tachycardia or palpitations are an issue. Although this degree of distress (i.e., chest pain, dyspnea) may depend in part on the degree of mitral regurgitation, some studies have failed to reveal any difference in the rates of chest pain in patients with or without MVP. The potentially biggest threat is the rupture of chordae, usually seen only in those with connective tissue diseases (especially Marfan syndrome).

Hypertrophic obstructive cardiomyopathy (HOCM) is a disease of the cardiac muscle. The ventricular septum is thick and asymmetric, leading to potential outflow tract block. Patients with HOCM often exhibit symptoms of cardiac outflow tract blockage with activity because the hypertrophic ventricular walls better approximate with the increased force of myocardial contraction associated with exercise. Unfortunately, the presentation of HOCM may be sudden cardiac death. Idiopathic hypertrophic subaortic stenosis (IHSS) is a type of cardiomyopathy. A strong family history is often present in those who have this autosomal dominant disorder. The typical patient is a young adult with a history of dyspnea with activity, but patients may also be asymptomatic.

In those with congenital heart disease such as atrial or ventricular septal defect, recommendations for sports participation vary according to patient presentation and surgical intervention. Most often, if the defect has been surgically repaired with little residual dysfunction, full sports participation is allowed. If uncorrected or if there is significant alteration in cardiac function despite repair, the degree of participation should be assessed on an individual basis.

Discussion Source

Van Camp, S. (1999). Cardiology. In Sarafan, M., McKeag, D., & Van Camp, S. *Manual of Sports Medicine.* Philadelphia: Lippincott-Raven. Pp. 226–243.

QUESTIONS

53. All of the following are common sites of fracture in patients with osteoporosis except:

A. proximal femur
B. distal forearm
C. vertebrae
D. clavicle

54. Osteoporosis is more common in individuals:

    A. with type 2 diabetes mellitus
    B. taking chronic corticosteroid therapy
    C. who are obese
    D. of African ancestry

55. Osteoporosis screening tests include all of the following except:

    A. quantitative ultrasound measurement
    B. dual-energy radiograph absorptiometry
    C. qualitative computed tomography
    D. wrist, spine, and hip radiographs

56. Osteoporosis prevention measures include all of the following except:

    A. calcium supplementation
    B. hormone replacement therapy (HRT)
    C. vitamin B_6 supplementation
    D. exercise program

57. Early disease presentation in osteoporosis may include:

    A. greater than 1-inch loss in terminal adult height
    B. hip fracture
    C. kyphosis
    D. back pain

58. In counseling a postmenopausal woman, you advise her that HRT users may experience:

    A. an increase in breast cancer rates with long-term use
    B. reduction in high-density lipoprotein cholesterol
    C. a 10% increase in bone mass
    D. no change in the occurrence of osteoporosis

59. When counseling a patient taking alendronate, you advise that the medication should be taken with:

    A. a bedtime snack
    B. a meal
    C. other medications
    D. a large glass of water

ANSWERS

53. D
54. B
55. D
56. C
57. D
58. A
59. D

DISCUSSION

Osteoporosis is a disorder of bone thinning in which bone absorption exceeds its formation to the degree that bone density is insufficient to meet skeletal needs. In addition, osteoporosis is defined as bone density more than 2.5 standard deviations below the average bone mass for women who are younger than age 35 years. For every reduction of bone mass by 1 standard deviation, the relative risk of fracture rises by 1.5- to threefold.

Estrogen deficiency is a potent risk factor, and osteoporosis is most common in postmenopausal women; by age 80 years, the average woman has lost more than 30% of her premenopausal bone density. Men appear to be at significantly less risk; this is partly because of inherently greater bone density. Body habitus and ethnicity can influence the risk of osteoporosis; it is most common in petite women of Asian and European ancestry who usually have lower bone density in adulthood. Obesity appears to minimize osteoporosis risk caused by highly endogenous estrogen production by fatty tissue. Additional risks for osteoporosis include disorders such as thyroidtoxicosis, Cushing disease, and rheumatoid arthritis as well as inactivity and prolonged therapy with anticonvulsants, heparin, and corticosteroids.

In patients with osteoporosis, hip, wrist, and spinal fractures most commonly occur, but all bones are at risk. Early disease usually does not have symptoms, but backache may be reported. Although hip fracture is often the first clinical manifestation of osteoporosis, it usually indicates advanced disease.

In patients with osteoporosis, bone loss takes place over the baseline bone density. A small amount of loss may be of great significance against poor bone density but of little consequence with greater density. Therefore, primary prevention of osteoporosis includes ensuring the development of maximum adult bone density. Because maximum bone density is achieved in the early adult years, encouraging adequate calcium intake and weight-bearing exercise throughout the teen and adult years is important. The calcium intake goal should be the equivalent of 1000 mg/day for men and premenopausal women, increased to 1200 to 1500 mg/day or more in postmenopausal women. Vitamin D 600 to 900 IU daily is also recommended. Food sources should be the main source of nutrition; supplements may be used if dietary intake is inadequate.

A number of tests are available to evaluate osteoporosis risk or detect progress of the disease. Dual-energy x-ray absorptiometry (DEXA) is considered one of the more reliable measures. Qualitative computed tomography is precise but uses more radiation than DEXA. Quantitative ultrasound is relatively inexpensive and can be performed with portable equipment. Plain radiographic films should not be used for screening or evaluation of osteoporosis because disease detection is not possible until 40–50% of bone mass is lost.

When taken with calcium supplements, postmenopausal HRT can help reduce the risk of postmenopausal fracture by as much as 50% by minimizing further bone loss. Raloxifene, an example of a selective estrogen receptor modulator (SERM) indicated for preventing osteoporosis, preserves rather than builds bone. Because it does not attach to estrogen receptor sites in the breast or uterus, a SERM may be an alternative to HRT. Alendronate (Fosamax), a bisphosphate that inhibits the resorptive activity of osteoclasts, can help modestly increase bone mass as well as significantly reduce fracture risk. In order to minimize the risk of drug-induced esophagitis, patients taking alendronate should be cautioned to take the medication in the morning with a full glass of water. At least 30 minutes must elapse before food, other liquids, or medications are ingested. In addition, patients should remain upright for at least 1 hour. Calcitonin is most helpful in building vertebral bone. Because it also has analgesic properties, calcitonin can help in the treatment of vertebral fracture pain and can help minimize the risk of future fracture. With all therapies, calcium supplements should be continued.

Discussion Sources

Hektor Dunphy, L. (1999). *Management Guidelines for Adult Nurse Practitioners*. Philadelphia: FA Davis. Pp. 395–398.
Uphold, C., & Graham, V. (1998). *Clinical Guidelines in Family Practice* (3rd ed.). Gainesville, FL: Barmarrae Books. Pp. 776–783.

QUESTIONS

60. The most common site of sprain is the:

    A. wrist

    B. shoulder

    C. ankle

    D. knee

61. A grade II ankle sprain is best described as:

    A. minor swelling and minimal joint instability

    B. moderate joint instability without swelling or ecchymosis

    C. moderate swelling, mild to moderate ecchymosis, moderate joint instability

    D. complete ankle instability, significant swelling, moderate to severe ecchymosis

62. Patients with a grade III ankle sprain should be advised that full recovery will likely take a:

    A. few days

    B. 2 to 3 weeks

    C. 4 to 6 weeks

    D. a number of months

63. Which of the following is usually not part of treatment of a sprain?

    A. immobilization

    B. applying ice to the area

    C. joint rest

    D. local corticosteroid injection

ANSWERS

60. C

61. C

62. D

63. D

DISCUSSION

A sprain is a partial or complete injury of a ligament either within the ligament body or at its site of attachment to the bone. Inversion injuries of the ankle cause about 85% of all sprains. This is the most common injury that involves jumping or running. Sprains can also involve the wrist, elbow, and knee. Wearing appropriate footwear, improved conditioning, and preexercise warm-up exercises as well as taping can be helpful in avoiding sprains.

Sprains are often graded according to presentation and proposed underlying degree of ligamentous injury (Table 8–6). The ankle anterior

TABLE 8–6.
GRADING, PRESENTATION, AND INTERVENTION OF
LIGAMENTOUS SPRAINS

Grade of Injury	Pathology and Presentation	Intervention
Grade I	Partial tear No instability	RICE (rest, ice, compression, elevation) Immobilizer Limit weight bearing Analgesia Length of disability is usually limited to a few days
Grade II	Partial ligamentous tear Moderate joint instability Moderate swelling Mild to moderate ecchymosis	RICE Immobilizer Limit weight bearing Analgesia Length of disability is usually several weeks to a few months
Grade III	Complete ligamentous tear Complete ankle instability Significant swelling Moderate to severe ecchymosis	Orthopedic referral RICE Immobilizer Limit weight bearing Analgesia Length of disability may be many months

draw test is used to assess for excessive laxity of the tibiotarsal joint. Excessive anterior motion is usually seen with a grade III sprain.

Immobilization is important to help appropriate healing and minimize sequelae. Grade II and III injuries are occasionally associated with joint laxity and a risk of future sprain.

Discussion Sources

Hellman, D., & Stone, J. (1999). Arthritis and musculoskeletal disorders. In Tierney, L., McPhee, S., & Papadakis, M. *Current Diagnosis and Treatment* (38th ed.). Norwalk, CT: Appleton & Lange. Pp. 786–837.

Hektor Dunphy, L. (1999). *Management Guidelines for Adult Nurse Practitioners*. Philadelphia: FA Davis. Pp. 398–401.

QUESTIONS

64. The diagnosis of tendonitis is usually made by:

    A. clinical presentation

    B. plain radiographic films

    C. MRI

    D. arthritis profile

65. Complications of Achilles tendonitis include:

    A. tendon rupture

    B. neurological sequelae

    C. stress fracture

    D. bursitis

66. Which of the following is often found with rotator cuff tendonitis?

    A. osteoarthritis

    B. tendon rupture

    C. bursitis

    D. joint effusion

67. First-line therapy for biceps tendonitis usually includes:

    A. applying ice to the area

    B. local steroid injection

    C. orthopedic referral

    D. nerve block

ANSWERS

64. A

65. A

66. C

67. A

DISCUSSION

The most common sites for tendonitis are the rotator cuff, elbow, biceps (shoulder), wrist, and heel. In the majority, a microscopic tear causes tendon inflammation; the resulting swelling and inflammation in the tendon are a result of overuse. The clinical presentation usually includes report of reduced ROM caused by joint stiffness and discomfort as well as a dull, aching pain over the affected tendon, especially with joint use. This pain can become sharp and acute when the tendon is squeezed. With rotator cuff involvement, abduction and elevation of the shoulder joint worsens symptoms.

The diagnosis of tendonitis is usually straightforward, with no special studies required. If it occurs with a history of recent trauma, plain radiographic films of the affected area may reveal calcium deposits on the tendon. Because bursitis and tendonitis often occur concurrently, assessment may reveal both conditions.

Treatment of tendonitis includes discontinuing the contributing activity. Applying ice to the region is helpful. When the hand or wrist is affected, splinting and NSAIDs are reasonable first-line therapies. Achilles tendonitis may require treatment with a posterior splint to immobilize the heel as well as heel cord stretching and orthotics after the acute phase to prevent recurrence. There is a 10% risk of tendon rupture with recurrent Achilles tendonitis; the risk can exceed 12% with biceps tendonitis. With rotator cuff involvement, the likelihood of concurrent bursitis is high; treatment includes limiting overhead movement as well as intrabursal corticosteroid injection.

Discussion Sources

Anderson, B. (1999). Office orthopedics for primary care. *Diagnosis and Treatment* (2nd ed.). Philadelphia: W. B. Saunders Company.
Hektor Dunphy, L. (1999). *Management Guidelines for Adult Nurse Practitioners*. Philadelphia: FA Davis. Pp. 383–384.

9
CHAPTER

Peripheral
Vascular
Disease

QUESTIONS

1. Who is most likely to have new-onset primary Raynaud's phenomenon?

   A. a 68-year-old man
   B. a 65-year-old woman
   C. a 25-year-old man
   D. an 18-year-old woman

2. All of the following are associated with secondary Raynaud's phenomenon except:

   A. hypertension
   B. scleroderma
   C. repeated use of vibrating tools
   D. use of beta-adrenergic antagonists

3. Lifestyle modification for patients with Raynaud's phenomenon includes:

   A. discontinuing cigarette smoking
   B. increasing fluid intake
   C. avoiding placing hands in warm water
   D. discontinuing aspirin use

4. Medications that may be helpful in treating patients with Raynaud's phenomenon include:

   A. nonsteroidal anti-inflammatory drugs (NSAIDs)
   B. angiotension-converting enzyme (ACE) inhibitors
   C. beta-adrenergic antagonists
   D. diuretics

5. Which of the following is the most common presentation in a patient with Raynaud's phenomenon?

   A. digital ulceration
   B. gangrene of the tip of the second fingers bilaterally

C. a period of intense itchiness after blanching

D. unilateral symptoms

ANSWERS

1. D
2. A
3. A
4. B
5. C

DISCUSSION

Raynaud's phenomenon is characterized by paroxysmal digital vasocon-striction resulting in bilateral symmetric pallor or cyanosis. The hands are nearly always involved; foot involvement is rare. A period of rubor follows this initial response. Primary Raynaud's phenomenon, also known as Raynaud's disease, is idiopathic in origin in most patients and is most often found in women. It usually appears between the ages of 15 and 45 years. Vasoconstriction triggers include exposure to cold relieved by warmth and, less commonly, emotional upset. Symptoms tend to be progressive with vasospasm becoming more frequent and prolonged.

There are no specific studies to help diagnosis primary Raynaud's dis-ease. The diagnosis is made if recurrent episodes occur for a period of more than 3 years without notation of associated disease or secondary cause.

Secondary Raynaud's phenomenon is seen in the presence of an un-derlying condition such as atherosclerosis, collagen vascular disease, and select autoimmune disease such as scleroderma. In addition, the use of vibrating tools, repeated sharp digit movement such as piano playing or typing, frostbite, tobacco, ergotamine, or beta blockers can be contribut-ing factors. The presentation of secondary Raynaud's phenomenon is the same as the idiopathic condition; the degree and length of vasospasm may be more severe. On rare occasions, distal digital ulceration may be seen.

Whatever the cause, Raynaud's phenomenon intervention is primarily aimed at preventing vasospasm by avoiding cold and other known trig-gers. At the onset of an episode, submerging the hands in warm water may be helpful in limiting the length and severity of vasospasm. Because wound healing may be delayed and infection more common, the hands should be protected from even minor injury. Keeping the skin well lubricated can help avoid small fissures. Because tobacco use exacerbates vasospasm, it should be discontinued. Biofeedback can be helpful because the patient can be taught to envision warming the digits, thus reducing symptoms. Oral and topical nitrates, dihydropyridine calcium channel blockers such as nifedipine, and ACE inhibitors such as captopril can be used for their vasodilator effect when lifestyle modification is inadequate. In patients with secondary Raynaud's phenomenon, treatment of the associated condition is important and may help minimize episodes.

Discussion Sources

Hektor Dunphy, L. (1999). *Management Guidelines for Adult Nurse Practitioners*. Philadelphia: FA Davis. Pp. 407–409
Toyoshima, H., Toth, P., & Garber, M. (1999). Rheumatology: Raynaud's phenomenon. *Virtual Hospital: University of Iowa Family Practice Handbook*. Available at http://www.vh.org/Providers/ClinRef/FPHandbook/Chapter06/08–6.html

QUESTIONS

6. Which of the following does not directly contribute to the development of varicose veins?
   A. leg crossing
   B. pregnancy
   C. heredity
   D. Raynaud's disease

7. When advising a woman with varicose veins about the use of support stockings, you consider that the preferred type is:
   A. able to be purchased in the hosiery section of a department store
   B. lightweight and available over the counter
   C. a medium- to heavyweight prescription product
   D. used with a panty girdle

8. In patients with varicose veins, which vessel is most often affected?
   A. femoral vein
   B. posterior tibial vein
   C. peroneal vein

D. saphenous vein

9. Which of the following is most accurate in the assessment of a patient with varicose veins?

   A. The degree of venous tortuosity is well correlated with the amount of leg pain reported.
   B. As the number of affected veins increases, so does the degree of patient discomfort.
   C. Symptoms are sometimes reported with minimally affected vessels.
   D. Lower extremity edema is usually only seen with severe disease.

10. Spider varicosities are:

   A. usually symptomatic
   B. a potential site for thrombophlebitis
   C. responsive to laser obliteration
   D. caused by sun exposure

ANSWERS

   6. D
   7. C
   8. D
   9. C
   10. C

DISCUSSION

Seen in 15% of the adult population, varicose veins are most often found in the lower extremities. Tortuous, dilated, superficial veins are characteristic. An inherited venous defect of either a valvular incompetence or a weakness in the walls of the vessel likely plays a significant role. In addition, situations that cause high venous pressure such as leg crossing, wearing of constricting garments, prolonged standing, heavy lifting, and pregnancy contribute to their development. Women are affected twice as often as men.

The vessel most often affected is the great saphenous vein and its tributaries. Often asymptomatic, varicose veins may also be associated with leg aching but usually not severe pain. The degree of discomfort poorly correlates with the number and appearance of the affected veins. Mild edema in the ankle area, particularly at the end of the day and in warm weather, is common. When palpated, the vein compresses easily and without pain. No specific diagnostic tests are needed with typical presentation.

In uncomplicated varicose veins, lifestyle modification usually helps minimize the symptoms and disease progress. Attaining and maintaining normal weight helps to reduce intravenous pressure and discourage the development and progress of varicose veins. Periodic leg elevation is helpful in minimizing edema and encouraging venous return. The use of medium- to heavyweight elastic support hose such as Jobst stockings should be encouraged. Support hose purchased in a department or drug store do not supply enough compression. Wearing possibly constricting garments such as panty girdles and garters should be avoided. Surgery may be needed for symptomatic varicose veins that do not respond to conservative therapy. Sclerotherapy involves injecting a sclerosing agent into the affected vein, followed by a period of compression, resulting in vessel obliteration.

Possible complications of varicose veins include superficial thrombophlebitis. Over time, varicose veins tend to progressively dilate. This can lead to secondary changes in the lower extremities, including chronic edema, skin hyperpigmentation, and the development of chronic venous insufficiency.

Spider varicosities are visible surface vessels usually seen with varicose veins. These vessels do not usually cause symptoms and pose no thromboembolic risk. Laser obliteration is helpful in reducing the appearance of spider varicosities and is considered a cosmetic procedure.

Discussion Sources

Hektor Dunphy, L. (1999). *Management Guidelines for Adult Nurse Practitioners*. Philadelphia: FA Davis. Pp. 405–406.
Tierney, L., & Messina, L. (1999). Blood vessels and lymphatics. In Tierney, L., McPhee, S., & Papadakis, M. *Current Diagnosis and Treatment* (38th ed.). Norwalk, CT: Appleton & Lange. Pp. 453–484.

QUESTIONS

11. Which of the following is a not a contributing factor to development of thrombophlebitis?

    A. venous status
    B. injury to vascular intima

    C. malignancy-associated hypercoagulation states

    D. isometric exercise

12. Presentation of superficial thrombophlebitis includes:

    A. Homan's sign

    B. diminished dorsalis pedis pulse

    C. dilated vessel

    D. dependent pallor

13. Treatment of superficial thrombophlebitis in a low-risk, stable patient includes use of:

    A. compression stockings

    B. dicoumarol

    C. warfarin

    D. heparin

14. In providing care for a patient with superficial thrombophlebitis, the NP considers that:

    A. It is a benign, self-limiting disease.

    B. Evaluation should include duplex ultrasound.

    C. A chest radiograph should be obtained.

    D. Limited activity enhances recovery.

15. Which of the following is the most likely to be found in deep vein thrombophlebitis (DVT)?

    A. unilateral leg edema

    B. leg pain

    C. warmth over the affected area

    D. fever

16. The NP considers that Homan's sign is present is approximately what percentage of patients with DVT?

    A. 25

    B. 33

    C. 50

    D. 75

17. Diagnostic evaluation of a clinically stable patient with suspected DVT is usually:

    A. impedance plethysmography

    B. 125-I fibrinogen scan

    C. contrast venography

D. duplex ultrasonography

18. Which of the following is the preferred medication used to reverse the anticoagulant effects of unfractionated heparin?

    A. vitamin K
    B. protamine sulfate
    C. platelet transfusion
    D. plasma components

19. Which of the following is the preferred medication used to reverse the anticoagulant effects of warfarin?

    A. vitamin K
    B. protamine sulfate
    C. platelet transfusion
    D. plasma components

20. Warfarin's onset of anticoagulation effect usually occurs how soon after the onset of therapy?

    A. immediately
    B. 1 to 2 days
    C. 3 to 5 days
    D. 5 to 7 days

21. When compared with unfractionated heparin, characteristics of low-molecular-weight heparin include all of the following except:

    A. more antiplatelet effect
    B. decreased need for monitoring of anticoagulant effect
    C. longer half-life
    D. superior bioavailability

22. Which of the following is least likely to be found in patients with pulmonary embolus (PE)?

    A. pleuritic chest pain
    B. tachypnea
    C. DVT signs and symptoms
    D. hemoptysis

23. The most commonly used method of preventing venous thromboembolism in higher-risk surgical patients is:

    A. antiplatelet therapy
    B. low-dose heparin
    C. vena cava filter

D. warfarin

24. When taken with warfarin, which of the following causes a possible increased anticoagulant effect?

   A. cisapride
   B. carbamazepine
   C. oral contraceptives
   D. sucralfate

25. When taken with warfarin, which of the following causes a possibly decreased anticoagulant effect?

   A. cholestyramine
   B. allopurinol
   C. cephalosporins
   D. chloral hydrate

26. What is the INR range recommended for warfarin therapy during DVT treatment?

   A. 1.5 to 2
   B. 2 to 3
   C. 2.5 to 3.5
   D. 3 to 4

ANSWERS

11. **D**
12. **C**
13. **A**
14. **B**
15. **A**
16. **B**
17. **D**
18. **B**
19. **A**
20. **C**
21. **A**
22. **C**
23. **B**
24. **A**

25. A
26. B

DISCUSSION

Virchow's triad of stasis, injury to the vascular intima, and abnormal co-agulation leading to clot usually contributes to the development of vessel inflammation and the resulting thrombophlebitis. The lower extremities are most often affected.

Thrombophlebitis can occur in superficial or deep veins. Risk factors for superficial thrombophlebitis include local trauma, prolonged travel or rest, presence of varicose veins, and history of prior episodes as well as pregnancy and use of estrogen-containing hormonal contraceptives. Characteristics of superficial thrombophlebitis include a localized, tender, inflamed, dilated, thrombosed vessel, often in the popliteal fossa. Homan's sign is absent. Having the patient stand for 2 minutes before examination enhances the findings because less severe cases may be missed on supine examination.

Superficial thrombophlebitis is often considered a benign condition. However, extension into a deep vein is typically present in 45% of patients with the condition. In particular, superficial thrombophlebitis in hospitalized patient is more likely to be associated with DVT and PE. Duplex ultrasound should be performed to help rule out concurrent DVT. Because superficial thrombophlebitis is often accompanied by DVT in a different location or extremity, the study should not be limited to the affected area. Serial studies may be needed if initial examination findings are negative but symptoms persist. Impedance plethysmography is a noninvasive test that helps detect disturbances in normal physiologic flow state through the venous system. Although a venogram is the most sensitive and specific test, its use has been limited because these less invasive tests have become available. A chest radiograph and V/Q scan should be obtained if shortness of breath or friction rub is present and the diagnosis of PE considered. Coagulation studies should be obtained, particularly if there is a history of episodes.

After it is confirmed that the thrombophlebitis is indeed superficial, intervention is dictated by DVT risk factors and patient history. In the absence of risk factors and history of similar episodes, warm packs, compression hose, and NSAIDs can treat superficial thrombophlebitis. Ambulation should be encouraged because rest may encourage stasis and enhance coagulation. In the face of prior episodes, a history of DVT, decreased mobility, hypercoagulability, or extensive saphenous vein involvement, subcutaneous low-molecular-weight heparin therapy should be initiated with consideration for long-term warfarin use. The inflammation associated with superficial thrombophlebitis usually subsides over 2 weeks, with a firm cord remaining for a much longer period.

Acute DVT usually involves the veins of the lower extremities and pelvis. Pulmonary embolism (PE), a potentially fatal condition, is largely a DVT sequelae. Long-term sequelae of DVT include chronic venous insufficiency and venous ulceration.

Because the triad of venous stasis, vessel wall injury, and altered state is the primary mechanism of DVT (as it is with superficial thrombophlebitis), risk factors include prolonged rest, recent trauma, recent surgery (especially hip replacement), pregnancy, and recent childbirth. The hypercoagulation state associated with many malignancies presents considerable risk. The use of estrogen-containing oral contraceptives can increase the risk of DVT particularly in cigarette smokers. Disorders of coagulation such as factor V Leiden, protein C and S deficiencies, and antithrombin III deficiencies have been recognized as a cause of DVT in younger, otherwise healthy adults.

Because the presentation of DVT varies, making the diagnosis by clinical presentation alone is problematic (Table 9–1). The minority of patients with suspected DVT have the diagnosis supported unless Virchow's triad of venous stasis, vessel wall injury, and coagulation abnormalities is present.

In order to establish the diagnosis and develop an appropriate plan of intervention, a thorough diagnostic evaluation is needed in patients suspected of having DVT. Contrast venography is considered the diagnostic standard. However, because of cost and the invasive nature of the test as well as the risk of contrast allergy, noninvasive tests are used more commonly. Both duplex ultrasound and impedance plethysmography (IPG) are helpful for diagnosing venous thrombosis; duplex studies that have increased sensitivity and specificity over IPG are the preferred tests for evaluating ambulatory patients with DVT. Both may have difficulty assessing calf vein thrombosis. False-positive IPG results may occur with the increased lower extremity pressure seen in those with congestive heart failure. The 125-I fibrinogen scan can be helpful in detecting active clot formation and ongoing calf thrombi. However, cost and difficulty with length of examination limit its usefulness.

Therapy for patients with DVT should be aimed at minimizing the risk of PE and extension of peripheral thrombus. Anticoagulation therapy, aimed at allowing natural fibrinolysis action and clot resolution to take place, is usually prescribed for 3 to 6 months after the first DVT episode.

Because rapid anticoagulation is needed in DVT therapy, heparin is usually the initial treatment (Table 9–2). A naturally occurring acidic carbohydrate, heparin potentiates antithromboplastin III (a naturally occur-

TABLE 9–1.
CLINICAL PRESENTATION OF PATIENTS WITH
DEEP VEIN THROMBOPHLEBITIS

Finding	Comments
Edema	Usually unilateral; most specific finding
Leg pain	Usually described as a tugging pain, heaviness, ache; present in ~50%; degree of pain does not correlate well with extent of thrombus
Homan's sign	Pain on dorsiflexion of the foot; present in about 33% with DVT and up to 50% without DVT
PE signs and symptoms	Present in ~10%
Warm over area of thrombosis	Relatively rare
Venous distention and prominence of subcutaneous veins	Relatively uncommon
Fever	If present, typically mild
Tenderness	Found in about 75%; may also be found in many conditions other than DVT; degree of tenderness does not correlate well with extent of thrombus

Reference: Adapted from Schrieber, D. (1999). *Deep Vein Thrombosis and Thrombophlebitis*. Available at http://www.emedicin.come/EMERG/topic122.htm

ring antithrombotic agent) and inhibits the activity of a number of coagulating factors. Its effect on thrombus formation is immediate in contrast to warfarin (Coumadin), which usually requires 3 to 5 days of use before therapeutic effect is seen.

Heparin is available in the standard unfractionated form (UFH) with an average molecular weight of 15,000 daltons (d), as well as a low-molecular-weight form (LMWH) with a molecular weight 4000 to 6500 d; an example is the product enoxaparin (Lovenox). LMWH selectively enhances factor Xa and accelerates antithrombin III activity; because of limited bleeding risk, PTT monitoring is not required during its use. LMWH has certain additional advantages, including superior bioavailability, a longer half-life that allows for twice-a-day dosing, ease of calculating dose, and limited antiplatelet effect (see Table 9–2). However, LMWH is more expensive than UFH. Patients with an isolated calf vein DVT who are clinically stable with few risks for further embolic process and the ability to access careful provider follow-up can be considered for initial outpatient treatment with self-administered injections of LMWH twice a day. In the absence of this, inpatient admission and heparin anticoagulation are indicated.

Long-term warfarin therapy usually follows an initial heparin course. As a result of vitamin K antagonism, warfarin acts against coagulation factors II, VII, IX, and X. Warfarin is highly (99%) protein bound, primarily to albumin, and has a narrow therapeutic range. In order to avoid problems with warfarin therapy, patients must be well informed of the drug-to-drug and drug-to-food interactions (Table 9–3). Because cigarette smoking likely increases thrombotic risk while reducing warfarin's efficacy, developing a smoking cessation plan is important.

Prothrombin time (PT) is used as the measure of warfarin's efficacy and is reported as an international normalized ratio (INR). INR prolongation is seen in about 48 to 72 hours after the first warfarin dose (Table 9–4).

Because it can cause an initial hypercoagulation state during the first days of use, warfarin therapy should be started only after the patient is fully anticoagulated with heparin; heparin should then be discontinued only after the prothrombin time is prolonged as reflected by an increase in INR. Daily testing is generally done until the desired INR is reached; then weekly to monthly testing continues throughout therapy (Table 9–5).

Approximately 2–10% of patients taking warfarin develop hemorrhage. This complication, however, is rarely seen in those with INR of 2.0 to 3.0. In the presence of significant bleeding in patients taking warfarin, the drug should be discontinued and vitamin K should be given promptly. However, vitamin K has little effect on hemostasis for 24 hours afterward. If more prompt action is needed, such as in the case of hemorrhage or bleeding into an enclosed space, fresh frozen plasma must be given. If anticoagulation therapy is continued after the bleeding crisis, response to warfarin may fluctuate, necessitating close monitoring.

With a mortality rate as high as 20–40%, PE is a feared complication of DVT. However, the diagnosis is often missed because presentation is nonspecific. PE presentation usually includes dyspnea, pleuritic chest pain, and accentuation of the pulmonic component of S_2 heart sound; tachypnea (RR > 16 breaths per minute) is nearly a universal finding. DVT signs and symptoms may be noted, but their absence should not

TABLE 9–2.
CLINICAL ISSUES IN HEPARIN THERAPY

Clinical Condition	Heparin Type, Dose, and Frequency	Comment
Prophylaxis for deep venous thrombus formation in select clinical conditions • Higher-risk surgical patients, such as orthopedics • Acute myocardial infarction • Ischemic stroke with lower extremity paralysis • Patients with congestive heart failure or pneumonia • Pregnant women with previous thrombotic disease or with antiphospholipid antibody	Low-dose UFH therapy • Usually 5000u SC every 8–12 hours	• PTT monitoring usually not indicated • Major complications include bruising at site of injection

Indication	Treatment	Comments
• DVT • PE • Unstable angina • Those receiving thrombolytic therapy • Perioperative management of patients taking warfarin	• High-dose UFH therapy • Intravenous or subcutaneous administration to maintain a therapeutic PTT between 1.5–2.5 • Dose variable, usually titrate in response to PTT • Check PTT every 6 h • Usual heparin dose • UFH 40–120 U/kg or approximately 10,000/70 kg followed by infusion at 20 U/kg/h • If PTT < 1.5, give heparin 5000 U bolus and increase infusion rate by 10% • If PTT > 2.5 but not extremely high, decrease infusion rate by 10% • For markedly high PTT (> 100 s), hold heparin infusion for 1 h, then decrease infusion rate by 10%	• Can cause hemorrhagic complications • For significant bleeding complications, protamine sulfate 15 mg can reverse heparin's anticoagulant effect • Possibly triggers immune thrombotic thrombocytopenia 1–2 weeks after beginning of therapy; sequelae includes widespread thrombosis refractory to treatment
• Outpatient anticoagulation of patient with superficial thrombophlebitis who has a history of DVT, venous thrombus risk factors, or involvement of the saphenous vein above the knee	• LMWH at 1 mg/kg SC every 12 h	• LMWH has limited antiplatelet effect and does not require monitoring of anticoagulant effect • Use with hot packs and compression hose • Careful clinical evaluation and serial duplex examinations are needed to ensure safe care
• DVT in clinically stable patient with few risks for further embolic phenomena	• LMWH at 1 mg/kg/d SC in divided dose every 12 hours	• The ability to access careful provider follow-up is essential to safe and effective care

TABLE 9–3.
DRUG AND FOOD INTERACTIONS OF WARFARIN

Increased Anticoagulant Effect	Decreased Anticoagulant Effect	Variable Effects
Acetaminophen (inconsistent effect)	Barbiturates	Phenytoin
Acute alcohol use	Carbamazepine	• Both increased
Allopurinol	Chronic alcohol abuse	and decreased
Amiodarone	Cholestyramine	effect noted, as
Cisapride	Griseofulvin	well as increase
Cephalosporins	Oral contraceptives	in phenytoin
Chloral hydrate	Rifampin	level
Disopyramide	Spironolactone	
Disulfiram	Sucralfate	
Erythromycin		
Ethacrynic acid		
Fluoroquinolones		
Gemfibrozil		
H_2 blockers		
Fluconazole, ketoconazole, miconazole (oral or parenteral)		
Metronidazole		
Narcotics		
NSAIDs		
Penicillins		
Propranolol		
Quinidine		
SSRIs		
Sulfonylureas		
Tetracycline		
Trimethoprim-sulfamethoxazole		
Valproate		
Vitamins A, C, E		

Reference: Adapted from Rizack, M. (1998). *Handbook of Adverse Drug Interactions*. New Rochelle, NY: The Medical Letter.

eliminate the consideration of a PE diagnosis. Hemoptysis, cyanosis, and change in level of consciousness are rarely encountered yet often considered to be part of the presentation.

In treating patients with PE, thrombolytic therapy may be used followed by heparin followed by warfarin therapy for a minimum of 3 to 6

TABLE 9–4.
WARFARIN: INITIATION OF THERAPY AND
LONG-TERM MANAGEMENT

General principles
- The overlapping period of heparin and warfarin is 4 to 5 days because of warfarin's delayed onset of action and the hypercoagulable state that occurs when heparin use is discontinued
- Discontinue heparin after INR is within desired range for 2 days
- The initial warfarin dose should be the anticipated daily dose; a loading dose is not recommended; 2 to 4 days is usually safer than giving a large, loading dose (50–75 mg)
- Warfarin's half-life is 20 to 60 hours, with approximately 48 hours needed before maximum of effect of a dose

INR Goal = 2 to 3	Action	Comments
At desired range	Repeat INR at interval determined by duration of therapeutic INR and underlying condition	Repeat INR in: • 4–6 weeks with stable condition and long-term therapeutic INR • At least weekly when underlying condition can impact coagulation state (malignancy, clotting disorder, use of medications that can influence warfarin effect)
INR < 2	• Increase weekly dose by 5–20% • Repeat INR 2–3 times per week until within desired range	Check for: • Adherence to recommended therapy • Use of medications or foods that may interfere with warfarin effect
INR 3–3.5	• Decrease weekly dose by 5–15% • Repeat INR 2–3 times per week until within desired range	Check for: • Adherence to recommended therapy • Use of medications or foods that may enhance warfarin effect

(continued)

TABLE 9–4. (continued)

INR Goal = 2 to 3	Action	Comments
INR 3.6–4	• Consider withholding 1 dose, decrease weekly dose by 10–15% • Repeat INR 2–3 times per week until within desired range	Check for: • Adherence to recommended therapy • Use of medications or foods that may enhance warfarin effect
INR > 4 without complications and no indication for rapid reversal of anticoagulation effect	• Consider withholding 1 dose, decrease weekly dose by 10–20% • Repeat INR 2–3 times per week until within desired ranges	Check for: • Adherence to recommended therapy • Use of medications or foods that may enhance warfarin effect
INR > 4 and need for rapid reversal of anticoagulant effect	Vitamin K 3 mg SC or slow IV	Check INR at 6 and 24 hours May repeat dose

INR Goal = 2.5 to 3.5	Action	Comments
At desired range	• Repeat INR at interval determined by duration of therapeutic INR and underlying condition • Repeat INR 2–3 times per week until within desired range	Repeat INR in: • 4–6 weeks with stable condition and long-term therapeutic INR • At least weekly when underlying condition can impact coagulation state; malignancy, clotting disorder, use of medications that can influence warfarin effect
INR < 2	• Increase weekly dose by 10–20% • Repeat INR 2–3 times per week until within desired range	Check for: • Adherence to recommended therapy • Use of medications or foods that may interfere with warfarin effect

(continued)

TABLE 9-4. (continued)		
INR Goal = 2.5 to 3.5	**Action**	**Comments**
INR 2–2.4	• Increase weekly dose by 5–15% • Repeat INR 2–3 times per week until within desired range	Check for: • Adherence to recommended therapy • Use of medications or foods that may interfere with warfarin effect
INR 3.5–4.6	• Decrease weekly dose by 5–5% • Repeat INR 2–3 times per week until within desired range	Check for: • Adherence to recommended therapy • Use of medications or foods that may enhance warfarin effect
INR 4.7–5.2	• Consider withholding one dose, decrease weekly dose by 10–20% • Repeat INR 2–3 times per week until within desired range	Check for: • Adherence to recommended therapy • Use of medications or foods that may enhance warfarin effect
INR > 5.2 without complications and no indication for rapid reversal of anticoagulation effect	• Consider withholding 1–2 doses, decrease weekly dose by 10–20% • Repeat INR 2–3 times per week until within desired range	Check for: • Adherence to recommended therapy • Use of medications or foods that may enhance warfarin effect
INR > 5.2 and need for rapid reversal of anticoagulant effect	• Vitamin K 3 mg SC or slow IV	Check INR at 6 and 24 h May repeat dose

Reference: Adapted from Horton, J., & Bushwick, B. (1999). Warfarin therapy: Evolving strategies in anticoagulation. *American Family Physician.* 59 (3) 635–647.

TABLE 9–5.
INDICATIONS FOR AND LENGTH OF
WARFARIN TREATMENT

Condition	INR	Duration of Therapy
Acute venous thrombosis		
• First episode	• 2–3	• 3–6 months
• High risk of recurrence	• 2–3	• Indefinite
• In presence of antiphospholipid antibody	• 3–4	• Lifelong
Prevention of systemic emboli		
• Tissue heart valves	• 2–3	• 3 months
• Valvular heart disease after thrombotic event	• 2–3	• Indefinite
• Mechanical heart valve	• 2.5–3.5	• Indefinite
• Acute myocardial infarction	• 2–3	• As deemed by clinical presentation
Atrial fibrillation		
• Chronic or intermittent	• 2–3	• Lifelong
• Cardioversion	• 2–3	• 3 weeks before and 4 weeks after conversion to sinus rhythm

Reference: Adapted from Horton, J., & Bushwick, B. (1999). Warfarin therapy: Evolving strategies in anticoagulation. *American Family Physician.* 59 (3) 635–647.

months. If the patient is not a candidate for long-term anticoagulation therapy, a vena cava filter is often used to minimize the risk of future PE. Follow-up is recommended as needed to monitor INR and the underlying clinical condition.

Discussion Sources

Feied, C., & Seim, S. (1999). *Superficial Thrombophlebitis.* Available at http://www.emedicine.com/ emerg/topic582.htm

Hektor Dunphy, L. (1999). *Management Guidelines for Adult Nurse Practitioners.* Philadelphia: FA Davis. Pp. 411–413.

Horton, J., & Bushwick, B. (1999). Warfarin therapy: Evolving strategies in anticoagulation. *American Family Physician.* 59 (3) 635–647.

Rizck, M. (1998). *Handbook of Adverse Drug Interactions.* New Rochelle, NY: The Medical Letter.

Schrieber, D. (1999). *Deep Vein Thrombosis and Thrombophlebitis.* Available http://www.emedicine.com/EMERG/topic122.htm

Tierney, L., & Messina, L. (1999). Blood vessels and lymphatics. In Tierney, L., McPhee, S., & Papadakis, M. *Current Diagnosis and Treatment* (38th ed.). Norwalk, CT: Appleton & Lange. Pp. 453–484.

QUESTIONS

27. Which of the following is the most potent peripheral vascular disease (PVD) risk factor?

   A. hypertension
   B. older age
   C. cigarette smoking
   D. leg injury

28. Clinical presentation of advanced vascular disease includes all of the following except:

   A. resting pain
   B. absent posterior tibialis pulse
   C. blanching of the foot with elevation
   D. spider varicosities

29. Drug therapy for patients with arterial vascular disease includes:

   A. aspirin
   B. nitrates
   C. pentoxifylline
   D. propranolol

30. Typically, the earliest sign of venous insufficiency is:

   A. edema
   B. altered pigmentation
   C. skin atrophy
   D. shiny skin

31. Which of the following is the most appropriate topical antimicrobial therapy for patients with venous stasis ulcer treatment?

   A. mupirocin
   B. bacitracin
   C. metronidazole
   D. polymixin

ANSWERS

27. C
28. D
29. C
30. A
31. C

DISCUSSION

Peripheral vascular disease, a common condition found in up to 10% of older adults, is a term used to describe a group of conditions in which there is a reduction of blood flow to the extremities. Risk factors include diabetes mellitus, hypertension, and hyperlipidemia; tobacco use is the most potent risk factor. In the absence of these risk factors, PVD is rare except in advanced age.

In those with PVD, the venous, arterial, or lymphatic systems may be affected. Disease caused by atherosclerosis in the distal aorta or iliac, femoral, or popliteal arteries is the greatest clinical problem. Presentation varies according to the area of vessel disease and dysfunction (Table 9–6). Atherosclerotic and calcific lesions usually cause occlusive disease of the aorta and its branches. Disease is often asymmetric because the distribution of obstructive lesions usually occurs in segments rather than continuous.

The diagnosis of arterial PVD is largely made by clinical presentation. Ankle-to-brachial index measurement, Doppler ultrasonography, and transcutaneous oximetry can help confirm the diagnosis and monitor disease progress.

Because patients with arterial PVD usually have other health problems, prevention and intervention measures, such as aggressive risk factor reduction, including cessation of tobacco use, blood pressure, glucose and lipid control, helps improve overall well-being. In addition, the presence of concomitant disease such as cardiovascular or cerebrovascular disease may limit ability to exercise. Exercise such as walking helps develop collateral circulation and minimize symptoms and therefore should be encouraged. Meticulous skin care is needed, and periodic podiatric care is recommended.

Pharmacotherapy for those with arterial PVD includes the use of pentoxifylline (Trental), a medication thought to reduce blood viscosity and improve blood flow by altering the ability of red blood cells to pass through diseased vessels. Its use does not alter the course of the disease

TABLE 9–6.
CLINICAL PRESENTATION OF PERIPHERAL VASCULAR DISEASE

Patient Presentation	Clinical Significance
Burn or ache with walking	Usually indicates femoropopliteal arterial disease
Pain in calf, hip, or buttock with activity; relieved by rest	Classic report in intermittent claudication
Foot pain at rest	Blood flow to extremity ≤ 10% of normal
Numbness, coldness, pain in extremity	More common than claudication report in older adults
Absent posterior tibialis pulse	Always present in healthy adults; dorsalis pedis pulse absent in about 5% of healthy adults
Nail thickening	As numbness is often also a problem, meticulous nail hygiene while minimizing injury is needed; onychomycosis is often seen in PVD
Sexual dysfunction	Most common in presence of smoking, hyperlipidemia, diabetes mellitus; PVD contributes to its development but is likely one of a number of influencing factors
Absent dorsalis pedis and tibial pulses	Proximal pulses may remain palpable
Blanching of the foot with elevation, poor capillary return, dependent rubor	≤ 10% of normal blood flow to extremity
Ache in anterior tibial muscles, foot; and metatarsal arch with activity	Most common with long-standing poorly controlled diabetes mellitus; can be confused with peripheral neuropathy

but rather reduces symptoms. Outcomes with pentoxifylline use are variable; patients without diabetes mellitus and milder symptoms appear to gain the most benefit. Clopidogrel (Plavix) has been used in PVD therapy; it prevents fibrinogen binding and may reduce the risk of thrombus formation. Although vasodilators and anticoagulants appear to be of no help, low-dose aspirin therapy is likely indicated, in part because of the increased risk of heart disease with the condition.

Surgical evaluation should be part of the care of patients with PVD. Angioplasty and grafting procedures can help improve blood flow and minimize symptoms and complications.

Chronic venous insufficiency is a common sequelae of DVT and leg trauma, although the absence of this history is noted in about 25% of patients. There is decreased venous return because of vessel damage, and lower extremity edema is usually the earliest sign. Symptoms usually include leg aching and itchiness. Over time, edema becomes progressively worse; this results in the development of thin, shiny, atrophic skin, often with brown pigmentation. Subcutaneous tissue thickens and becomes fibrous.

The stage is set for stasis ulceration. Inflamed, red, pruritic patches usually precede the formation of an irregular ulceration with a clean base. Yellow eschar, which is occasionally found, requires debridement. After the ulcer base is clean, metronidazole gel should be applied to reduce bacterial growth and odor. An occlusive hydroactive dressing such as Duoderm followed by an Unna zinc paste boot is applied and changed weekly. If healing does not ensue within a few weeks, refer for surgical evaluation for possible skin grafts.

Discussion Sources

Hektor Dunphy, L. (1999). *Management Guidelines for Adult Nurse Practitioners*. Philadelphia: FA Davis. Pp. 404–414.

Kennedy-Malone, L., Fletcher, K., & Plank, L. (2000). *Management Guidelines for Gerontologic Nurse Practitioners*. Philadelphia: F.A. Davis. Pp. 230–237.

Tierney, L., & Messina, L. (1999). Blood vessels and lymphatics. In Tierney, L., McPhee, S., & Papadakis, M. *Current Diagnosis and Treatment* (38th ed.). Norwalk, CT: Appleton & Lange. Pp. 453–484.

10
CHAPTER

Endocrine
Disorders

QUESTIONS

1. Which of the following characteristics applies to type 1 diabetes mellitus?

   A. Significant hyperglycemia and ketoacidosis result from lack of insulin.
   B. It is commonly diagnosed on routine examination or workup for other health problem.
   C. Initial response to oral agents is usually favorable.
   D. Insulin resistance is a significant part of the disease.

2. Which of the following characteristics apply to type 2 diabetes mellitus?

   A. Major risk factors are heredity and obesity.
   B. Pear-shaped body type is commonly found.
   C. Exogenous insulin is needed for control of disease.
   D. Exercise increases insulin resistance.

3. You consider using Ultralente insulin because of its:

   A. extended duration of action
   B. rapid onset of action
   C. ability to prevent diabetic end-organ damage
   D. ability to preserve pancreatic function

4. Humalog's (lispro) onset of action is:
   A. <15 minutes
   B. approximately 1 hour
   C. 1–2 hours
   D. 3–4 hours

5. A 56-year-old obese man of Scandinavian ancestry presents for care with type 2 diabetes mellitus with FPG = 280 mg/dL and HgbA$_{1c}$ = 10%. He is currently not taking medications and works as a landscaper. Which of the following is the most appropriate choice of therapeutic agent for this patient?

   A. metformin
   B. glyburide
   C. Ultralente insulin
   D. NPH insulin

6. Metformin's (Glucophage's) mechanism of action is as a(n):

   A. insulin-production enhancer
   B. product virtually identical in action to the sulfonylureas
   C. drug that increases insulin action in the peripheral tissues and reduces hepatic glucose production
   D. facilitator of renal glucose excretion

7. According to the American Diabetes Association (ADA) Clinical Practice Guidelines, criteria for testing for type 2 diabetes mellitus in asymptomatic, undiagnosed individuals older than age 45 years should be conducted every _____years.

   A. 1
   B. 3
   C. 5
   D. 10

8. According to the ADA Clinical Practice Guidelines, criteria for testing for type 2 diabetes mellitus in asymptomatic, undiagnosed individuals younger than age 45 years should be considered when there is:

   A. a family history of obesity
   B. a personal history of high-density lipoprotein (HDL) < 35 mg/dL
   C. activity intolerance reported by the patient
   D. poor response to efforts to maintain normal body mass index (BMI)

9. Criteria for the diagnosis of type 2 diabetes mellitus include:

   A. classic symptoms regardless of fasting plasma glucose measurement
   B. plasma glucose ≥ 126 mg/dL as a random measurement
   C. 2-hour glucose measurement ≥ 156 mg/dL after a 75-g anhydrous glucose load dissolved in water
   D. plasma glucose ≥ 126 mg/dL after an 8-hour fast on more than one occasion

10. Recommendations for glucose control according to the ADA include:

    A. fasting glucose between 80–120 mg/dL
    B. bedtime glucose measurement between 110–150 mg/dL
    C. HgbA$_{1c}$ 7–8%
    D. consistent measurements between 80–140 mg/dL

11. Which of the following should be the goal measurement when treating a person with diabetes mellitus and hypertension?

    A. blood pressure (BP) < 130 mm Hg systolic; < 85 mm Hg diastolic
    B. low-density lipoprotein cholesterol (LDL-C) <130 mg/dL in the presence of coronary heart disease (CHD)
    C. triglycerides 200–300 mg/dL
    D. HDL < 35mg/dL

12. In caring for a patient with diabetes mellitus, microalbuminuria measurement should be obtained:

    A. annually if urine protein is present
    B. periodically in relationship to glycemia control
    C. yearly if urinalysis is negative for protein
    D. with each office visit related to diabetes mellitus

13. The mechanism of action of sulfonylureas is as:

    A. enhancer of insulin receptor site activity
    B. product that enhances insulin release
    C. facilitator of renal glucose excretion
    D. agent that can reduce hepatic glucose production

14. When caring for a patient with diabetes mellitus and hypertension, the NP considers prescribing:

   A. atenolol
   B. hydrochlorothiazide
   C. fosinopril
   D. nifedipine

ANSWERS

   1. A
   2. A
   3. A
   4. A
   5. A
   6. C
   7. B
   8. B
   9. D
   10. A
   11. A
   12. C
   13. B
   14. C

DISCUSSION

Type 1 diabetes mellitus is a disease of insulin deficiency. The onset of this disease is usually in the person less than age 30 years with symptomatic presentation often as the classic "polys"—polydipsia, polyphagia, and polyuria. If associated with ketoacidosis, type 1 diabetes mellitus presentation can be dramatic with severe dehydration, abdominal pain, vomiting, and decreased level of consciousness. In any event, prompt intervention with appropriate insulin therapy is indicated.

Patients with type 2 diabetes mellitus are most often asymptomatic at onset. As a result, the ADA recommends periodic fasting plasma glucose

(FPG) screening in those with risk factors for type 2 diabetes mellitus. These risk factors include:

- First-degree relative with type 2 diabetes mellitus
- Being overweight
- HDL < 35 mg/dL
- Triglycerides > 250 mg/dL
- Member of a high-risk ethnic group (African ancestry, Asian, Native American, Latino)
- High BP (HBP)
- Gestational diabetes mellitus or (GDM) giving birth to a baby weighing more than 9 lb
- Previous glucose intolerance
- Older than age 45 years

According to the ADA recommendations, if the initial FPG is within normal limits, it should be repeated every 3 years or more frequently as the provider determines as directed by risk factors. For those younger than age 45 years, periodic FPG screening should be determined by the presence of risk factors. When a threshold of FPG of greater than 126 mg/dL after an 8-hour fast is used, this testing is 98% specific and 40–88% sensitive for type 2 diabetes mellitus. Typically, wide-scale screening done using these guidelines yields a 6% true positive rate. Additional ADA diagnostic criteria for type 2 diabetes mellitus include a casual (random) plasma glucose level greater than 200 mg/dL with classic diabetic symptoms or oral glucose tolerance greater than 200 mg/dL at 2 hours. At this time, the ADA does not recommend the use of $HgbA_{1c}$ as a tool for diagnosing diabetes mellitus.

Sulfonylureas have been used for many years for the treatment of type 2 DM. These drugs help to control diabetes mellitus by stimulating of insulin release from functioning beta cells and, to a lesser degree, help enhance insulin sensitivity. However, type 2 DM is a progressive disease, with about 5–20% patients per year failing therapy on sulfonylurea alone. As a result, multiple treatment modalities should be considered. (See Table 10–1.)

Metformin, a biguanide, increases muscle and adipose cell receptor's sensitivity to glucose. As a result, glucose uptake is more efficient and plasma glucose lowered. In addition, it suppresses hepatic glucose production and hepatic glycogen output. A modest weight loss, usually 3–5 kilograms, is often seen during the first months with the use of metformin, as there is a reduction of glucose absorption from GI tract. There is little hypoglycemia risk with the use of metformin alone, though this may be noted when used with a sulfonylurea or insulin.

TABLE 10–1.
TREATMENT OPTIONS IN TYPE 2 DIABETES MELLITUS
For the obese, likely insulin-resistant person with type 2 diabetes mellitus
• First line products include metformin or thiazolidinediones (rosiglitazone, pioglitazone) • Consider using acarbose, miglitol
• Add a second insulin resistance-reducing agent if HbA1c not <7%
• Add sulfonylurea if HbA1c not <7%
• Discontinue sulfonylurea and start insulin with metformin or troglitazone if HbA1c not <7%
For the lean, insulin-deficient person with type 2 diabetes mellitus
• First line product include the sulfonylureas
• Add metformin or troglitazone if HbA1c not <7%
• Consider adding third oral agent if HbA1c not <7%
• Discontinue sulfonylurea and start insulin with metformin or troglitazone if HbA1c not <7%

Source: Fonseca, V. (1999). National Diabetes Education Initiative, available at www.ndei.org

The use of metformin can help improve lipid profile, decreasing LDL and triglycerides while increasing HDL. Metformin's major adverse effects are GI upset, avoidable by slowly increasing the dose. A rare but serious complication of metformin use is the development of lactic acidosis risk and is highest in those with complicating factors such as heart and liver disease, renal insufficiency, electrolyte imbalance as well as the use of radiographic imaging contrast dyes.

The thiazolidinediones (TZDs), a class of medications sharing the -glitazone suffix, are used in the treatment of diabetes mellitus. These products act by reducing insulin resistance and improving insulin sensitivity in muscle and adipose tissue. In addition, hepatic glucose output suppressed but somewhat less than with metformin use. Occasionally, modest weight loss and mild edema is reported with TZD use. There is little hypoglycemia risk when TZDs are used as monotherapy, but possible when coupled with sulfonylurea or insulin use. These products have a positive lipid effect, decreasing triglycerides by approximately 15% while increasing HDL by about 7% and decreasing LDL by about 10%. Periodic ALT monitoring is recommended in all patients on thiazolidinedione therapy; the medication should be discontinued if ALT reaches 3 times upper limit of normal.

Diabetes mellitus is the leading cause of chronic renal failure. After the diagnosis of diabetes mellitus is made, periodic screening of renal function should be done. Often the serum creatinine is used for this purpose. However, an increase in creatinine is not seen until at least 50% of the nephrons are not functioning. Thus elevated creatinine is a late rather than an early indicator of renal damage. A far more sensitive indicator of diabetic nephropathy is the presence of proteinuria, a harbinger for progressive renal failure. Urine protein consists of a number of forms, including the most abundant albumin as well as immunoglobulins, haptoglobin, and light chains. The standard dipstick test is sensitive to 100 to 150 mg/L of urine albumin, certainly an earlier marker of progressive renal failure than serum creatinine but still a later disease marker. However, the presence of a small amount of albumin (microalbumin or >20 mg/L albumin or >30 to 40 mg/day) is considered a predictor of glomerular dysfunction associated with diabetic nephropathy.

Microalbuminuria may precede development of diabetes mellitus by 10 years. With type 2 diabetes mellitus, the patient should be screened at onset of disease, with an annual recheck if normal. Correlation with creatinine collection of a first morning specimen is important because normal daily activity may cause a low level of protein spillage into the urine, creating a false-positive result. The diagnosis of microalbuminuria should be confirmed by obtaining at least two positives of three collections in a 3- to 6-month period. Intervention includes tightening of glycemic control, to HGBAIC <7% (see Table 10–2) controlling elevated BP (<130 mm Hg systolic and 85 mm Hg diastolic per the Joint National Committee on Prevention, Detection, Evaluation and Treatment of High Blood Pressure [JNC] 6 Guidelines), aggressive treatment of hyperlipidemia, and the addition of an agent to preserve renal function by reducing efferent arteriolar pressure (angiotensin-converting enzyme [ACE] inhibitor [drugs with the -pril suffix] angiotensin receptor blockers [drugs with the -sartan suffix], diltiazem, or verapamil).

The patient in Question 5 presents a situation in which a fair-skinned, overweight man who works outside and has significant hyperglycemia is in need of drug therapy. Because the sulfonylureas have photosensitizing

TABLE 10–2. RELATIONSHIP BETWEEN AVERAGE DAILY PLASMA GLUCOSE AND HgBAlc
For each 1% = add or subtract 30 mg/dL
4% = 60 mg/dL
5% = 90 mg/dL
6% = 120 mg/dL
7% = 150 mg/dL
8% = 180 mg/dL
9% = 210 mg/dL
10% = 240 mg/dL
11% = 300 mg/dL
13% = 330 mg/dL

potential, their use should be avoided in this situation. In addition, because of the sulfonylureas' action in enhancing insulin release, patients often note an increase in appetite and resulting weight gain after starting the medication. In contrast, metformin users often note a modest weight loss after initiating the use of this product. There is not a compelling reason to use insulin in this situation.

Discussion Sources

Hektor Dunphy, L. (1999). *Management Guidelines for Adult Nurse Practitioners*. Philadelphia: FA Davis. Pp. 415–422.
Price, M., Kent, D. Endocrine disorders: Diabetes mellitus. In Youngkin, E., Sawing, K., Kissinger, J., & Israel, D. (1999). *Pharmacotherapeutics; A Primary Care Clinical Guide*. Stamford, CT: Appleton & Lange. Pp. 709–729.

QUESTIONS

15. Risk factors for heat stroke include all of the following except:

    A. obesity

    B. use of beta adrenergic antagonists

    C. excessive activity

    D. use of a vasodilator

16. Possible adverse outcome from heat stroke includes:
    A. rhabdomyolysis
    B. anemia
    C. hypernatremia
    D. leukopenia

17. Laboratory findings in heat stroke may include:
    A. elevated creatine kinase
    B. anemia
    C. metabolic alkalosis
    D. hypokalemia

18. Intervention for patients with heat stroke includes:
    A. total body ice packing to ensure rapid cooling
    B. cautious fluid resuscitation because of pulmonary edema risk
    C. aggressive rehydration
    D. administration of potassium

ANSWERS

15. D
16. A
17. A
18. B

DISCUSSION

Heat stroke is a life-threatening emergency caused by a failure of the body's thermoregulatory system, usually in response to extreme environmental and personal factors. Risk factors for heat stroke include the use of medications that alter adrenergic activity and possibly decrease cardiac output (negative inotropes), such as tricyclic antidepressants (TCAs; triptyline drugs), beta adrenergic antagonists (beta blockers, drugs with the -ol suffix), and vasoconstrictors such as decongestants. The use of these products negates the body's normal attempts to decrease core temperature, such as increasing cardiac output and cutaneous vasodilatation.

Assessment of a patient with heat stroke includes a complete evaluation of electrolytes, hematologic parameters, and liver function. Creatine kinase (total CK) level is typically elevated, owing to this enzyme's being released by skeletal muscle injured by muscle cramping and convulsion. Because of the release of this intracellular electrolyte with tissue damage, hyperkalemia is common. Heat stroke can lead to a transient polycythemia caused by volume constriction, hyponatremia with Na^+ <120 mEq/L, and stress-induced leukocytosis.

Intervention for a patient with heat stroke includes controlled cooling by the use of tepid sprays and fanning or the application of cold packs to select areas such as the axillae, neck, and groin. Rapid cooling by ice packing is discouraged since it may stimulate cutaneous vasoconstriction inhibit heat loss. Fluid restriction should be aggressive but cautious because of the risk of pulmonary edema from reduced cardiac output.

Optimally, a patient with heat stroke should be admitted to the hospital for at least 24 hours after stabilization because of the risk of late complications that includes one of the most feared complications, rhabdomyolysis, a condition of rapid muscle tissue destruction.

As the muscle breaks down, large amounts of myoglobin and other cellular products are released into circulation to be excreted by the kidney. As a result, about 50% of patients with rhabdomyolysis develop acute renal failure. In heat stroke, the presence of myoglobinuria is an early indicator of rhabdomyolysis. Typically, the patient also has complaints of muscle pain and weakness. Treatment of rhabdomyolysis is largely supportive.

Discussion Sources

Hektor Dunphy, L. (1999). *Management Guidelines for Adult Nurse Practitioners*. Philadelphia: FA Davis. Pp. 422–427.
Hanson, P. (1998). Disturbances because of heat. In Rakel, R. *Conn's Current Therapy*. Philadelphia: WB Saunders. Pp. 166–1168.

QUESTIONS

19. A 62-year-old woman has hypertension, a 100-pack-year history of cigarette smoking, and intermittent claudication. Triglycerides = 320 mg/dL, HDL= 28 mg/dL, and LDL = 135 mg/dL. Which of the following represents the most appropriate pharmacologic intervention for this patient's lipid disorders?

    A. No further intervention is required.

    B. Probucol (Lorelco) should be prescribed.

    C. Cholestyramine (Questran) should be prescribed.

    D. Pravastatin (Pravachol) should be prescribed.

20. You examine a 46-year-old smoker with hypertension. His lipid profile is as follows: HDL = 48 mg/dL; LDL = 192 mg/dL; triglycerides = 110 mg/dL. He had been on a low-cholesterol diet for 6 months when this test was taken. Which of the following represents the best intervention for his lipid profile?

    A. No further intervention is required.
    B. Gemfibrozil (Lopid) should be prescribed.
    C. Atorvastatin (Lipitor) should be prescribed.
    D. Probucol (Lorelco) should be prescribed.

21. You examine a 64-year-old man who had a myocardial infarction (MI) 2 years ago. He has HBP and type 2 DM. His fasting lipid profile was obtained after following an appropriate diet for 8 months. Results are HDL = 38 mg/dL; LDL = 140 mg/dL; triglycerides = 180 mg/dL. Which of the following is the most appropriate advice?

    A. No further intervention is needed.
    B. His lipid profile should be repeated in 6 months.
    C. Lipid-lowering drug therapy should be initiated.
    D. Dietary therapy appears to be effective.

22. When providing care for a patient taking an HMG-CoA reductase inhibitor, periodic monitoring of which of the following is recommended?

    A. potassium
    B. aspartate aminotransferase (AST)
    C. CK
    D. blood urea nitrogen (BUN)

23. When prescribing gemfibrozil, the NP expects to see the following changes in lipid profile:

    A. decrease in LDL level
    B. increase in HDL level
    C. no effect on triglyceride level
    D. increase in very low density lipoprotein (VLDL) level

24. When prescribing niacin, the NP expects to see the following changes in lipid profile:

    A. decrease in LDL level
    B. increase in HDL level
    C. no effect on triglyceride level
    D. increase in VLDL level

25. In prescribing niacin therapy for a patient with hyperlipidemia, the NP considers that:

    A. post-dose flushing is often reported

    B. hepatic monitoring is not warranted

    C. low-dose therapy is usually effective

    D. drug-induced thrombocytopenia is a common problem

26. When prescribing estrogen replacement therapy for a post-menopausal woman, the NP expects to see the following changes in lipid profile:

    A. increase in LDL level

    B. increase in HDL level

    C. no effect on triglyceride level

    D. decrease in VLDL

ANSWERS

19. D
20. C
21. C
22. B
23. B
24. B
25. A
26. B

DISCUSSION

Treatment of hyperlipidemia is an important part of cardiovascular and cerebrovascular risk reduction. Dietary intervention is first line therapy; however most adults will achieve only a modest 5–10% reduction in LDL cholesterol with this as a single intervention. Further reduction may be seen if improved diet is coupled with exercise.

Pharmacologic intervention in hyperlipemia will likely be needed in patients with considerable cardiovascular and cerebrovascular risk, including patients with diabetes mellitus, hypertension and existing vascular disease. The choice of a lipid-lowering agent should be guided by the effect of the agent on the lipid profile, as well as the desired lipid levels (Table 10–3).

TABLE 10–3.
EFFECT OF MEDICATIONS ON LIPID LEVELS

Medication	Effect on Lipids	Cautions
Niacin (nicotinic acid)	>↑ HDL, ↓ LDL, ↓ triglycerides	Potentially hepatotoxic; monitor AST periodically Vasodilatation and flushing: Take 0.3 g ASA 1/2 hour before dose Potential increase in glucose: monitor periodically Hyperuricemia: Seen in ~ 1/5, may precipitate gout; Monitor uric acid periodically
Fibric acid derivatives (Gemfibrozil [Lopid])	↑ HDL, ↓ Triglycerides, sl ↓ LDL	Potentially hepatotoxic: Monitor AST periodically Myopathy risk when given concurrently with HMG-COA reductase inhibitors
Bile acid-binding resins (cholestyramine [Questran], colestipol, Colestid)	↓ LDL, sl ↑ triglycerides	Constipation common; may advise addition of psyllium May impair absorption of other medications if taken 1 h before or 2 h after medication Not suitable as single agent for many types of hyperlipidemia because of lack of positive effect on HDL, triglycerides
Probucol (Lorelco)	↓ sl LDL (modest)	Usually used as second- or third-line agent, antioxidant
Estrogen as part of hormone replacement therapy for postmenopausal women	↑ HDL, ↓ LDL, possible ↑ triglycerides	May increase thromboembolic rate About 50% of cardiovascular risk reduction attributable to positive lipid effect Use occasionally increases triglycerides in women with markedly elevated levels (> 400 mg/dL) Need to use conjugated equine estrogen (CEE, Premarin) equivalent = 0.625 mg to have cardioprotective effect

(continued)

TABLE 10–3. (continued)

Medication	Effect on Lipids	Cautions
HMG-COA reductase inhibitors (-statin medications, pravastatin [Pravachol], atorvastatin [Lipitor], others)	SI ↑ HDL, ↓ LDL, ↓ triglycerides (modest)	Most commonly used lipid-lowering drug Take at bedtime to enhance lipid-lowering effect Potentially hepatotoxic: Monitor AST periodically Drug interaction potential Myopathy on rare occasion with solo use; more common when statins used with cyclosporine, macrolides, danazol, niacin, others

Ms. Newton has a common lipid profile seen in the postmenopausal woman; low HDL with elevated triglycerides. Her LDL is elevated for a woman with vascular disease (intermittent claudication). Regardless of age, a patient such as Ms. Newton would benefit from pharmacologic intervention. The choice of the agent should be aimed at increasing HDL while lowering triglycerides and LDL. Niacin or an HMG-COA reductase inhibitor is appropriate. As an alternate, hormone replacement therapy (HRT) helps increase HDL and lower LDL. Mr. Carino has a history of myocardial infarction, therefore should have lipid lowering therapy initiated to reduce LDL< 100 mg/dl (Tables 10–4 and 10–5).

Discussion Sources

Hektor Dunphy, L. (1999). *Management Guidelines for Adult Nurse Practitioners.* Philadelphia: FA Davis. Pp. 427–430.

National Cholesterol Education Program Adult Treatment Panel II. (1993). Summary of the second expert panel on detection evaluation and treatment of high blood cholesterol in adults. *JAMA* 269. Pp. 3015–3036.

Sellers, J., Brubaker, M. (1999). Cardiovascular disorders. In Youngkin, E., Sawing, K., Kissinger, J. & Israel, D. (1999). *Pharmacotherapeutics; A Primary Care Clinical Guide.* Stamford, CT: Appleton & Lange. Pp. 309–367.

TABLE 10–4.
CHARACTERISTICS OF SECONDARY HYPERLIPIDEMIA

Cause	Lipid Abnormality
Inactivity	↓ HDL
Alcohol abuse	↑ Triglycerides, ↑ HDL, ↑ LDL
Diabetes mellitus	↑Triglycerides, ↓ HDL, ↑ TC
Hypothyroidism	↑ Triglycerides, ↑ TC
Higher-dose thiazide diuretics	↑ TC, ↑ LDL, ↑ triglycerides
High-dose beta blockers	↑ LDL, ↓ HDL
Chronic renal insufficiency	↑ TC, ↑ triglycerides

TABLE 10–5.
RISK CATEGORIES THAT MODIFY LDL-CHOLESTEROL GOALS

Risk Categories	LDL Goal
CHD and CHD risk equivalents	<100 mg/dl
Multiple (2+) risk factors	<130 mg/dl
Zero to one risk factor	<160 mg/dl

Reference: National Cholesterol Education Program AdultTreatment Panel III (ATP III) Guidelines. Available at www.nhlbi.nih.gov/ncep.

QUESTIONS

27. When counseling obese patients, the NP realizes that:

    A. A daily energy deficit of 500 to 1000 kcal/day leads to about a 1- to 2-lb weight loss per week.

    B. Each pound of body fat represents approximately 6000 stored calories.

    C. Exercise enhances insulin resistance.

    D. Thyroid dysfunction is found in the majority of cases.

28. Which of the following presents the most problematic pattern of obesity?

    A. female fat distribution pattern

    B. male with BMI < 28.5

    C. female with BMI 23 to 27

    D. male fat distribution pattern

ANSWERS

27. A

28. D

DISCUSSION

Patients with truncal distribution of excessive weight, often called male pattern or android obesity, carry a significant risk for increased rates of cardiovascular disease and diabetes mellitus in either gender as well as increased breast cancer risk in women. Obesity is defined as BMI of greater than 28.5 in men and greater than 27.5 in women. Although no specific endocrine disorder, including thyroid dysfunction, is usually found in obese individuals, the cause of obesity is likely a combination of environmental, genetic, and behavioral influences.

A pound of fat contains approximately 3500 stored calories. Thus, a deficit of 500 to 1000 calories per day will lead to a 1- to 2-lb weight loss per week. Exercise enhances insulin sensitivity.

Discussion Source

Hektor Dunphy, L. (1999). *Management Guidelines for Adult Nurse Practitioners*. Philadelphia: FA Davis. Pp. 430–433.

QUESTIONS

29. Risk factors for pancreatitis include all of the following except:

    A. hypothyroidism
    B. hyperlipidemia
    C. abdominal trauma
    D. thiazide diuretic use

30. A 28-year-old woman with a long-standing history of alcohol abuse presents with a 4-day history of a midabdominal ache that radiates through to the back, remains relatively constant, and includes nausea and three episodes of vomiting. She has tried taking antacids without relief. Abdomen, slightly hyperactive bowel sounds with upper abdominal tenderness without localization or rebound. Her skin is cool and moist with BP = 90/72; pulse 120; RR 24. The most likely diagnosis is:

    A. gastric ulcer
    B. pancreatitis
    C. acute alcohol poisoning
    D. viral hepatitis

31. Your next best action in caring for the patient in the previous question is to:

    A. Refer her to the hospital for admission.
    B. Attempt office hydration after administration of an analgesic agent.
    C. Initiate cimetidine and antacid regimen.
    D. Obtain serum electrolytes level.

32. Which of the following is true when evaluating a patient with acute pancreatitis?

    A. Elevated amylase level is a highly accurate marker for the condition.
    B. Abdominal ultrasound assists with the diagnosis.
    C. Measuring serum lipase level along with amylase level increases diagnostic specificity.
    D. Hypocalcemia is common.

33. Presentation of pancreatic cancer includes:

   A. jaundice
   B. polycythemia
   C. hematuria
   D. increased appetite

34. Which of the following is the most reliable test for the detection of pancreatic cancer?

   A. elevated alkaline phosphate level
   B. magnetic resonance imaging (MRI)
   C. abdominal ultrasound
   D. elevation of amylase level

ANSWERS

29. A
30. B
31. A
32. C
33. A
34. B

DISCUSSION

Pancreatitis, characterized by an acute or chronic inflammation of the organ, is a potentially life-threatening condition. The most potent risk factors are excessive alcohol use and gallstones. Less common risk factors are use of opioids, steroids, and thiazide diuretics; viral infections; and abdominal trauma. Hyperlipidemia, specifically with marked elevation of triglyceride level, is a risk factor for recurrent pancreatitis in the presence or absence of other influences.

In evaluating a patient with pancreatitis, serum amylase level is typically elevated. However, because elevated amylase level may be found in a number of other conditions, concurrently measuring serum lipase level increases diagnostic specificity. Abdominal ultrasound may assist in diagnosing contributing gallbladder disease; it does not typically help with diagnosing pancreatitis because of limited views of the organ.

Significant pain and volume constriction are common in patients with acute pancreatitis. Intervention includes parenteral hydration and analgesia as well as gut rest. Treatment of the underlying cause, such as gallbladder disease or hypertriglyceridemia, or discontinuation of the causative agent, such as alcohol, steroids, or thiazide diuretics, is also indicated (Table 10–6).

Pancreatic cancer most commonly presents with abdominal pain, weight loss, anorexia, nausea, and vomiting. In addition, jaundice is often present but usually without the localized right upper quadrant abdominal tenderness seen in hepatic and biliary disorders such as cholecystitis and acute hepatitis. Pancreatic cancer is an unfortunate condition with high mortality rates because presentation is usually with late disease and the spread of the cancer.

Magnetic resonance imaging is helpful in identifying pancreatic cancer. The usefulness of abdominal ultrasound is somewhat limited by the presence of intestinal gas. Alkaline phosphatase and amylase levels may be mildly elevated in patients with pancreatic cancer, but these elevations are not specific for this disease.

TABLE 10–6. CLASSIFICATION OF SERUM TRIGLYCERIDES
Normal <150 mg/dL
Borderline high 150–199 mg/dL
High 200–499 mg/dL
Very high ≥500 mg/dL

Reference: National Cholesterol Education Program Adult Treatment Panel III (ATPIII) Guidelines. Available at www.nhlbi.nih.gov/ncep.

Discussion Sources

Burch, J. (1998). Acute pancreatitis. In Rakel, R. *Conn's Current Therapy*. Philadelphia: WB Saunders. Pp. 506–510.

Hektor Dunphy, L. (1999). *Management Guidelines for Adult Nurse Practitioners*. Philadelphia: FA Davis. Pp. 436–437.

National Cholesterol Education Program Adult Treatment Panel II. (1993). Summary of the second expert panel on detection evaluation and treatment of high blood cholesterol in adults. *JAMA* 269. Pp. 3015–3036.

QUESTIONS

35. A 24-year-old woman presents with a new onset of nervousness, tremor, insomnia, and an involuntary 10-lb weight loss. Upon completing her history and physical examination, you suspect she has Graves' disease. Physical examination findings likely include a:

    A. diffusely enlarged thyroid gland
    B. single thyroid nodule
    C. firm, fixed thyroid lesion
    D. tender thyroid with pain radiating to the ears

36. Which of the following is a helpful treatment option for relief of tremor associated with hyperthyroidism?

    A. propanolol
    B. diazepam
    C. carbamazepine
    D. verapamil

37. Physical examination findings in patients with Graves' disease include:

    A. muscle tenderness
    B. coarse, dry skin
    C. eyelid retraction
    D. delayed relaxation phase of the patella reflex

38. Which is most likely found in Graves' disease?

    A. increased thyroid-stimulating hormone (TSH) level and free T_4
    B. decreased TSH level with elevated free T_4
    C. single "cold spot" on thyroid scan
    D. presence of a solid lesion on thyroid ultrasound

39. The mechanism of action of radioactive iodine in the treatment of Graves disease is to:

    A. destroy the overactive thyroid tissue
    B. reduce production of TSH
    C. alter the thyroid metabolic rate
    D. relieve distress caused by increased thyroid size

40. A 75-year-old woman who is feeling well has a 2.5-cm, relatively fixed painless mass on the right lobe of her thyroid. Ultrasound reveals a solid mass. The most likely diagnosis is:

    A. thyroid cancer
    B. Hashimoto's thyroiditis
    C. goiter
    D. thyroid cyst

41. As part of an evaluation of a 3-cm, round, mobile thyroid mass, you obtain a thyroid ultrasound revealing a fluid-filled structure. The most likely diagnosis is:

    A. adenoma
    B. thyroid cyst
    C. multinodular goiter
    D. vascular lesion

42. The most common cause of hypothyroidism is:

    A. primary pituitary failure
    B. thyroid neoplasia
    C. autoimmune thyroiditis
    D. radioactive iodine exposure

43. A 58-year-old woman presents with a 3-month history of progressive fatigue and memory problems. Her physical examination reveals delayed relaxation phase of the reflexes and coarse, dry skin. You consider a diagnosis of

    A. myxedema
    B. hypothyroidism
    C. organic depression
    D. multiple sclerosis

44. Pertaining to the use of thyroxine in the elderly, which of the following statements is true?

    A. The starting dose of thyroxine should be the anticipated therapeutic dose.
    B. The therapeutic dose of thyroxine needed by the elderly is approximately that needed by younger adults.
    C. Presentation of thyroxine excess in the elderly includes angina.
    D. TSH should be suppressed to nondetectable levels when seeking therapeutic effect.

45. Periodic monitoring for hypothyroidism is indicated in the presence of which of the following clinical conditions?

    A. digoxin use
    B. male gender
    C. Down syndrome
    D. alcoholism

46. Which of the following is consistent with subclinical hypothyroidism?

    A. low TSH level, elevated free T_4
    B. elevated total T_4 level with normal TSH level
    C. elevated TSH level with normal free T_4 level
    D. low total T_4 level with normal TSH level

ANSWERS

35. A
36. A
37. C
38. B
39. A
40. A
41. B
42. C
43. B
44. C
45. C
46. C

DISCUSSION

Thyroid hormone is essential to normal body function because it assists cells in energy-releasing activities. When assessing a patient with thyroid dysfunction, look for signs of excessive energy release in hyperthyroidism or decreased energy release in hypothyroidism. This may present in the history and physical examination (Table 10–7).

Although thyroid disease probably exists in less than 7% of the population, it is important to maintain a high index of suspicion in those at particular risk. Risk factors and associated conditions include:

- Down syndrome: Hypothyroidism
- The elderly: Hypothyroidism or hyperthyroidism with a high propensity for atypical presentation in either situation
- Use of certain medications causing an alteration in iodine metabolism (lithium, amiodarone): Hypothyroidism
- Female gender: Hyperthyroidism or hypothyroidism; as most is autoimmune in nature, thyroid dysfunction is more common in women than men, as are the majority of autoimmune diseases
- Postpartum: A transient hypothyroidism is common as is a transient thyroiditis

Because thyroid disease can produce low-level symptoms attributed to other conditions, especially stress, the issue of routine screening for thyroid disorders with determining TSH levels has been long debated. The Clinical Preventive Services Guidelines state that there is insufficient evidence to recommend for or against routine screening . However, a recent study (Danesse et al., 1996) developed a model of obtaining a sTSH level every 5 years for adults older than age 35 years. The authors state this is cost effective because it avoids complicated thyroid disorder sequelae such as lipid disorders, atrial fibrillation, and altered mental status that develop with untreated thyroid disease.

Subclinical hypothyroidism is diagnosed by the presence of an elevated sTSH level and a normal free T_4 level in the absence of symptoms. The estimated prevalence of this disorder is about 7% in women and 3% in men among community-dwelling individuals ages 60 to 89 years. There is a 5% likelihood of development of overt hypothyroidism per year if these findings are noted with the presence of antithyroid antibodies. If this is the case, intervention with levothyroxine is recommended, titrating the dose to reach a normal TSH level. If antithyroid antibody negative, repeat monitoring in 6 months is advisable. However, levothyroxine therapy should be initiated promptly if hypothyroid symptoms develop because then the situation is no longer considered subclinical (Table 10–8).

TABLE 10–7.
COMPARISON OF HYPERTHYROIDISM
WITH HYPOTHYROIDISM

	Hyperthyroidism	Hypothyroidism
Characteristics	Excessive energy release, rapid cell turnover	Reduced energy release, slow cell turnover
Causes	Graves disease, thyroiditis, metabolically active thyroid nodule	Postthyroiditis (> 90%), primary pituitary failure (rare)
Neurologic	Nervous, irritable, memory problems	Lethargy, disinterest, memory problems
Weight	Weight loss (usually modest, present in ~ 50%)	Weight gain (usually 5–10 lb)
Environmental response	Heat intolerance	Chills easily, cold intolerance
Skin	Smooth, silky skin	Coarse, dry skin
Hair	Fine hair with frequent loss	Thick, coarse hair with tendency to break
Nails	Thin nails that break with ease	Thick, dry nails
Gastrointestinal	Frequent, low-volume loose stools	Constipation
Menstrual	Amenorrhea or low-volume menstrual flow	Menorrhagia
Reflexes	Hyperreflexia with a characteristic "quick out-quick back" action	Hyporeflexia with a characteristic slow relaxation phase, the "hung-up" reflex
Muscle strength	Proximal muscle weakness	No change
Cardiac	Tachycardia	Bradycardia in severe cases

TABLE 10–8.
COMMON DIAGNOSTIC FINDINGS IN PATIENTS WITH THYROID DISEASE

Test	Significance of Findings	Comments
TSH (thyroid stimulating hormone, thyrotropin)	Increased in patients with hypothyroidism, decreased in patients with hyperthyroidism Sensitivity = 89–95% Specificity = 90–96%	In response to amounts of circulating thyroid hormone, the pituitary produces TSH Those taking a therapeutic levothyroxine dose should have a normal TSH level
Free T_4	Increased in patients with hyperthyroidism, decreased in patients with hypothyroidism	Unbound or metabolically active portion of thyroxine About 0.025% of all T_4; the remaining bound portion is metabolically inactive
Free thyroxine index (FTI)	$FTI = T_4 \times T_3 \ RU/100$	In ordinary circumstances, free T_4 preferred method of free thyroxine measure May be a more accurate measure for those with altered states of protein binding, such as oral contraceptive (OC) use, pregnancy, malnutrition
T_3	May be increased in patients with thyroidtoxicosis Rarely, T_3 thyroidtoxicosis can occur with normal T_4 measures	Under normal conditions, little produced directly by thyroid Most produced by peripheral deiodination of T_4 The most active thyroid hormone
Goiter	Thyroid enlargement	Etiology varies With tenderness, consider thyroiditis
Warm nodule	Metabolically functional lesion "Hot spot" at site lesion detectable on thyroid scan Distinct lesion palpable on examination	Usually benign

(continued)

TABLE 10–8. (continued)

Test	Significance of Findings	Comments
Cold nodule	Metabolically inactive lesion "Cold spot" detectable at site of lesion on thyroid scan Distinct lesion palpable on examination	High index of suspicion for malignancy, especially if fixed, nontender lesion
Fine-needle aspiration (FNA)	Preferred method of biopsy for thyroid nodules	Yields histologic diagnosis
Thyroid ultrasound	Detects cystic (fluid-filled) vs. solid (nodule, tumor) lesions	Thyroid cysts rarely malignant
Antithyroid antibodies	Elevated in thyroiditis Hashimoto's thyroiditis, an autoimmune disorder, most common type	Correlate with physical findings of swollen, possibly tender thyroid Initial symptoms of hyperthyroidism common; eventually hypothyroidism occurs
Radioactive iodine thyroid scan	The most metabolically active portion of the thyroid takes up the largest amounts of iodine, creating "hot" or "warm" spots Low uptake correlates with decreased metabolic activity	Increased radioactive iodine uptake in Graves disease, toxic nodular goiter, and early Hashimoto's thyroiditis Decreased radioactive iodine uptake in thyroid hormone use, thyroid damage Common finding in those with untreated hypothyroidism is finding of diffuse low radioactive iodine uptake

TABLE10–9.
TREATMENT OPTIONS FOR PATIENTS WITH
THYROID DISEASE

Treatment Option	Effect	Comments
Nonselective beta adrenergic blocker such as propanolol	Reduction of tachy-cardia, tremor, and > HBP commonly seen in hyperthyroidism	Use temporarily for symptom relief in early stages of antithyroid therapies
Methimazole (Tapazole), propyl-thiouracil (PTU)	Antithyroid medications that will help in management of hyperthyroidism	May be used before radioactive iodine therapy or as solo therapeutic agent ~ 50% recurrence of hyperthyroidism when medication withdrawn. Both have significant adverse reaction profiles
Radioactive iodine	Destroys overactive thyroid tissue. Used in treatment of hyperthyroidism	Posttreatment hypothyroidism common. Long-term study fails to demonstrate carcinogenesis or genetic mutations with its use
Levothyroxine	Thyroid replacement hormone	Easily converted to T_3 by body. Increased heart rate and inotrope in excessive amounts. Prescribing tips: Start the elderly on low dose because of angina risk (0.25–0.50 mg/d, increasing dose every 1–2 weeks to therapeutic level, likely 0.75–1.25 mg/d). Start younger adults on 0.50–0.75 mg daily increasing, dose every 1–3 weeks to therapeutic level. TSH should be normal when patient on appropriate levothyroxine dose. Excessive use of levothyroxine, demonstrated by suppressed TSH level, can lead to bone demineralization

Treatment options for patients with thyroid disease are aimed at relieving presenting symptoms as well as correcting the underlying thyroid problem. Examples of each are shown in Table 10–9.

Discussion Sources

Hektor Dunphy, L. (1999). *Management Guidelines for Adult Nurse Practitioners*. Philadelphia: FA Davis. Pp. 438–447.

Danesse, M., et al. (1996). Screening for mild thyroid failure at the periodic health exam: A decision and cost effectiveness analysis. *JAMA* 276: 285–292.

Report of the U.S. Preventive Services Task Force Guide to Clinical Preventive Services (2nd ed.) (1996) Baltimore: Williams and Wilkins.

11
CHAPTER

Hematologic and Immunologic Disorders

QUESTIONS

1. A 19-year-old man presents with sudden onset of edema of the lips and face as well as a sensation of "throat tightness and shortness of breath" after a bee sting. Physical examination reveals inspiratory and expiratory wheezing. Blood pressure (BP) = 78/44; heart rate (HR) = 102 bpm; RR = 24. The most likely diagnosis is:

   A. urticaria
   B. angioedema
   C. anaphylactic reaction
   D. reactive airway disease

2. Your priority in caring for the patient in Question 1 is to:

   A. administer a rapidly acting antihistamine
   B. assure airway patency
   C. initiate vasopressor therapy
   D. increase circulating volume

ANSWERS

1. C
2. B

DISCUSSION

Anaphylaxis is an acute, life-threatening systemic antibody-antigen reaction that is an example of a type I immune response or hypersensitivity reaction. This type of reaction occurs after a person had been exposed to an allergen and has developed antibodies. The resulting IgE antibodies occupy receptor sites on mast cells, causing a degradation of the mast cell and subsequent release of histamine, vasodilatation, mucous gland stimulation, and tissue swelling. Within the heading of type I hypersensitivity are two subgroups, atopy and anaphylaxis.

Atopy is a group of localized allergic reactions including allergic rhinitis and eczema. On the other hand, anaphylaxis typically causes a systemic IgE-mediated reaction in response to exposure to an allergen, often a drug such as penicillin, insect venom such as with a bee sting, or certain foods such as peanut allergy. Anaphylaxis is characterized by widespread vasodilatation, urticaria, angioedema, and bronchospasm, creating a life-threatening condition of airway obstruction coupled with circulatory collapse. First-line treatment includes avoiding or discontinuing the offending agent. Simultaneously, maintaining airway patency is the greatest priority. Maintaining adequate circulation is also critical. Angioedema and urticaria are subcutaneous anaphylactic reactions that are not life threatening unless tissue swelling impinges on the airway (see Table 3–5).

Discussion Source

Hektor Dunphy, L. (1999). *Management Guidelines for Adult Nurse Practitioners*. Philadelphia: FA Davis. Pp. 450–455.

QUESTIONS

3. The majority of the body's iron is obtained from:

   A. food sources
   B. recycled iron content from aged red blood cells (RBCs)
   C. endoplasmic reticulum production
   D. water supplies

4. Which of the following is most consistent with iron deficiency anemia?

   A. low mean corpuscular volume (MCV), normal mean corpuscular hemoglobin concentration (MCHC),
   B. low MCV, low MCHC
   C. low MCV, elevated MCHC
   D. normal MCV, normal MCHC

5. One of the earliest laboratory markers in iron deficiency anemia is a(n):

   A. increase in RBC distribution widths
   B. reduced hemoglobin level
   C. low mean corpuscular hemoglobin level
   D. increased platelet count

6. A 48-year-old woman developed an iron deficiency anemia after excessive perimenopausal bleeding, successfully treated by endometrial ablation. Her hematocrit level is 25%, and she is taking iron therapy. At 5 days into therapy, you expect to find a(n):

   A. correction of mean cell volume
   B. 10% increase in hematocrit level
   C. brisk reticulocytosis
   D. normal ferritin level

7. A healthy 34-year-old man asks if he should take an iron supplement. You respond:

   A. This is a prudent measure to assure health.
   B. Iron deficiency anemia is a common problem in men of his age.
   C. This may cause iatrogenic iron overload.
   D. Excess iron is easily excreted.

8. Which of the following is the best advice on taking ferrous sulfate?

   A. Take with other medications to enhance adherence.
   B. Take on a full stomach.
   C. Take on an empty stomach to enhance absorption.
   D. Do not take with vitamin C.

9. A 40-year-old woman with pyelonephritis on ciprofloxacin who is also being treated for iron deficiency anemia with ferrous sulfate asks about taking both medications. You advise that:

   A. She should take the medications with a large glass of water.
   B. An inactive drug compound may be formed if the two medications are taken together.
   C. She may take the medications together to enhance adherence to therapy.
   D. The ferrous sulfate may slow gastrointestinal (GI) motility and result in enhanced ciprofloxacin absorption

10. One month into therapy for pernicious anemia, you wish to check the efficacy of the intervention. The best laboratory test is:

    A. Schilling's test
    B. hematocrit
    C. reticulocyte count
    D. ferritin

11. A woman who is planning a pregnancy should increase her intake of which of the following to reduce the risk of neural tube defect?

    A. iron
    B. niacin
    C. folic acid
    D. vitamin C

12. Risk factors for folate deficiency anemia include:

    A. menorrhagia
    B. chronic ingestion of overcooked foods
    C. use of nonsteroidal anti-inflammatory drugs (NSAIDs)
    D. gastric atrophy

13. Folate deficiency anemia causes which of the following changes in the RBC indices?

    A. microcytic, normochromic
    B. normocytic, normochromic
    C. microcytic, hypochromic
    D. macrocytic, normochromic

14. Pernicious anemia is usually caused by:

    A. dietary deficiency of vitamin B_{12}
    B. lack of production of intrinsic factor by the gastric mucosa
    C. RBC enzyme deficiency
    D. a combination of micronutrient deficiencies caused by malabsorption

15. Pernicious anemia causes which of the following changes in the RBC indices?

    A. microcytic, normochromic
    B. normocytic, normochromic
    C. microcytic, hypochromic
    D. macrocytic, normochromic

16. Common physical examination findings in patients with pernicious anemia include:

    A. hypoactive bowel sounds
    B. stocking-glove neuropathy
    C. thin, spoon-shaped nails
    D. retinal hemorrhages

17. You examine a 47-year-old man with the following results on hemogram.

    - Hgb = 15 g
    - Hct = 45%
    - MCV = 108 fL

    The most likely diagnosis is:

    A. pernicious anemia
    B. alcohol abuse
    C. thalassemia
    D. Fanconi's disease

18. You examine a 22-year-old woman of Asian ancestry. She is without complaint. Hemogram results are as follows Hgb = 9.1 g (12 to 14 g); Hct = 28% (36–42%); RBC = 5 million (3.2 to 4.3 million); MCV = 68 fL (80 to 96 fL); red blood cell distribution width (RDW) = 13% (< 15%). The most likely diagnosis is:

    A. iron deficiency anemia
    B. Cooley's anemia
    C. alpha thalassemia minor
    D. hemoglobin Barts

19. A 68-year-old man is usually healthy but presents with new onset of "huffing and puffing" with exercise. Physical examination reveals conjunctiva pallor and a hemic murmur. Hgb = 7.6 g; MCV = 71 fL. The most likely problem is:

    A. poor nutrition
    B. occult blood loss
    C. malabsorption
    D. microcytosis

ANSWERS

3. B
4. B
5. A
6. C
7. C
8. C
9. B
10. B

11. C
12. B
13. D
14. B
15. D
16. B
17. B
18. C
19. B

DISCUSSION

Anemia is a decreased oxygen-carrying capability of the blood. It is not a disease but rather a symptom of an underlying process.

The clinical presentation of anemia is highly variable and compensation is common because most anemias are usually gradual in onset. In addition, the oxyhemoglobin-dissociation curve is moved to the right as the hemoglobin level decreases, with the oxygen molecule given up more freely by the RBC. As a result, symptoms of anemia seldom present unless the hemoglobin level decreases to below 10 g/dL.

The health history may reveal clues as to the cause of the anemia (i.e., excessive menstrual flow, acute blood loss). Patients may have complaints of deep, sighing respiration with activity, often associated with a sensation of rapid, forceful heart rate. This is likely a reflection of the decreased oxygen-carrying capability of the blood and a corresponding compensatory mechanism. Fatigue and headache may also present. In patients at risk of or who have coronary artery disease, angina may be reported.

The physical examination usually contributes little to the diagnosis of anemia unless anemia is severe. Pallor of the skin and mucous membranes is not a reliable indicator and is usually only seen when anemia is severe (hemoglobin <8 g/dL). In the elderly and in individuals with coronary artery disease, signs of congestive heart failure (i.e., distended neck veins, rales, tachycardia, right upper quadrant abdominal tenderness, hepatomegaly) may be seen in patients with severe anemia. An early systolic murmur may be heard because of the increase of blood flow over the heart valves. Neurologic findings such as paresthesia, stocking-glove neuropathy, and difficulty with balance, and, in extreme cases, confusion may be found in patients with vitamin B_{12} deficiency anemia.

When evaluating the hemograms of patients with anemia, the following questions should be answered in order to ascertain the origin of the anemia (Table 11–1):

TABLE 11-1.
DIFFERENTIAL DIAGNOSIS OF COMMON ANEMIA

- Hemoglobin comprises large portion of RBC and gives it color. Therefore, microcytic and hypochromic go together.
- RDW increase is an early marker of anemia because new, differently sized cells are formed.
- Anemia is the presentation of an underlying disease process that must be concurrently treated.

Type of Anemia	Risk Factors	Hemogram Results	Comments
Iron deficiency anemia	Increase iron needs during time of rapid growth • Pregnancy • Childhood, adolescence Blood loss • Excessive menstrual flow • Childbirth • GI bleeding Inadequate iron intake • Elderly • Vegans • Adolescents	Microcytic (MCV ↓ 80 fL) Hypochromic MCHC ↓ RDW ↑ 15% Ferritin ↓ TIBC ↑ Fe ↓	Iron therapy needed to correct anemia (1–3 months) and replenish stores (3+ months) Routine, unnecessary iron supplementation not recommended because of possible increased risk of iatrogenic iron overload and cardiovascular disease
Anemia of chronic disease	Chronic inflammation such as: • Rheumatoid arthritis • SLE Chronic infection such as: • HIV • Pressure ulcer	Normocytic (MCV 80–94 fL) Normochromic reticulocytes ↓ Fe ↓ TIBC ↓ Normal or ↑ ferritin	Hct usually greater than 25%; if less, consider additional cause for anemia such as occult blood loss or Fe, folate, or vitamin B_{12} deficiency

Vitamin B$_{12}$ deficiency	Decreased production of intrinsic factor (pernicious anemia, gastrectomy) • Dietary deficiency (rare)	Macrocytic (MCV ↑, usually marked at 110–140 fL) Normochromic (normal MCH) RDW ↑ RBC morphology • Anisocytosis • Poikilocytosis Leukopenia WBC morphology • Hypersegmented neutrophils Vitamin B$_{12}$ Positive Schilling test result	Anemia can be particularly severe with Hct as low as 10–15% because the disease is slow developing and compensation is common Oral irritation and icterus are common as are characteristic neurologic problems: peripheral neuropathy, difficulty with balance, memory changes; without treatment, neurologic changes may become permanent
Folate deficiency anemia	Inadequate dietary folic acid intake • Elderly • Alcoholics • Impoverished Decreased ability to absorb folic acid • Malabsorption syndromes such as sprue and celiac disease • Unusually high folic acid utilization • Pregnancy • Childhood growth spurts • Hemolytic anemia • Inflammation	Macrocytic (MCV ↑, usually not as dramatic as vitamin B$_{12}$ deficiency) Normochromic (normal MCH) RDW RBC morphology • Anisocytosis • Poikilocytosis Leukopenia WBC morphology • Hypersegmented neutrophils • RBC folate ↓ • Serum folate ↓	Folic acid is a water-soluble B complex vitamin found in abundance in peanuts, fruits, and vegetables Because it is heat labile, up to 90% of folic acid can be destroyed through excessive cooking or heating Those who eat little fresh food are at high risk

(continued)

TABLE 11–1. (continued)

Type of Anemia	Risk Factors	Hemogram Results	Comments
Aplastic anemia	Failure of bone marrow to produce stem cell (precursor to leukocytes, erythrocytes, platelets) • Drug induced • Idiopathic	Normocytic Normochromic Reticulocytopenia Thrombocytopenia Leukopenia (Pancytopenia)	Potentially life-threatening condition
Alpha thalassemia trait	Asian ancestry; occasionally seen in other ethnic groups	Microcytic Hypochromic Low Hct (24–33%), Hgb (8–11 g) with normal to high RBC Normal RDW Normal iron studies Normal hemoglobin electrophoresis	Diagnosis of exclusion; frequently confused with IDA Genetically based problem with hemoglobin synthesis so that many small pale cells are made No treatment needed
Beta thalassemia minor	Mediterranean or African ancestry; occasionally seen in other ethnic groups	Microcytic Hypochromic Low Hct (24–33%), Hgb (8–11 g) with normal to high RBC Normal RDW Normal iron studies Hgb A2↑ on hemoglobin electrophoresis	Frequently confused with IDA Genetically based problem with hemoglobin synthesis so that many small pale cells are made No treatment needed Differentiate from alpha thalassemia
G6PD deficiency	Mediterranean or African ancestry; occasionally seen in other ethnic groups	Normal markers in nonhemolytic state	Hemolysis with ingestion of certain oxidizing agents: fava beans, aspirin, sulfa drugs, nitrofurantoin, others

- *What is the cell size?* Is the RBC unusually small (microcytic or low MCV)? Because hemoglobin is a major contributor to cell size, microcytosis is usually seen in patients with anemia in whom hemoglobin synthesis is impaired, such as in those with iron deficiency anemia and the thalassemias. In addition, because hemoglobin gives RBCs their characteristic red color, small and pale go together. Thus, a microcytic cell can also be hypochromic (low MHC or mean hemoglobin concentration).
- *Is the RBC unusually large (macrocytic)?* Macrocytosis is most commonly caused by impaired RNA and DNA synthesis in young erythrocytes. Folic acid and vitamin B_{12} contribute significantly to this process. A lack of either or both of these micronutrients can cause a macrocytic anemia blood. Because hemoglobin synthesis is not the issue, macrocytic cells are usually of normal color (normochromic).
- *Is the RBC of normal size (normocytic)?* Generally in these anemias, there is no problem with RNA, DNA, or hemoglobin synthesis. Acute blood loss and anemia of chronic disease are examples of normocytic, normochromic anemia.
- *What is the RDW?* RDW is the degree of variation in RBC size. This may also be noted as anisocytosis on RBC morphology. RDW measurement is elevated when RBCs are of varying sizes, implying that cells were synthesized under varying conditions. For example, in an iron deficiency anemia, normal-sized cells produced before the iron depletion will continue to circulate until their 90- to 120-day lifespan ends. At the same time, the new, smaller, iron-deficient cells containing less hemoglobin are produced. Therefore, there will be wide variation in cell size and an increase in RDW. Because minor variation in cell size is normal, RDW is considered increased only when it is above 15%.
- *What is the hemoglobin content (color) of the cell?* The hemoglobin content of the cell is reflected in the MCHC mean (average) corpuscular hemoglobin concentration. It is reported as a percentage of the cell's volume. Because hemoglobin gives RBCs their characteristic red color, the suffix "-chromic" is used to describe the MCHC. Thus, when a cell has a normal MCHC, it is normal color, or normochromic. When there is an impairment of hemoglobin synthesis, such as in iron deficiency anemia or thalassemia, the cells are pale or hypochromic and the MCHC is low. RBCs are seldom hyperchromic or containing excessive amounts of hemoglobin.

Worldwide, iron deficiency is the most common reason for anemia. Because an estimated 8 years of poor iron intake is needed in adults before iron deficiency anemia occurs, diet is rarely its origin. Rather, chronic blood loss causing a wasting of the RBCs' recyclable iron is the most common cause. Occult GI blood loss, such as from an oozing gastritis or malignancy, is a common reason, as is excessive menstrual flow.

Men and postmenopausal women require 1 mg of iron each day. During reproductive years, women require 1.5 to 3 mg/day of iron, in part because of the monthly loss of RBCs with the menses. In all these circumstances, these iron requirements are achievable with a well-balanced diet. One ml of packed RBCs contains 1 mg iron, so even losses of 2 to 3 ml of blood through the GI tract can lead to iron deficiency.

The laboratory diagnosis of iron deficiency anemia is supported by the following findings.

- Early disease: Low to normal hemoglobin, and hematocrit, and total RBC count, normocytic, possible hypochromic, RDW > 15%
- Later disease: Microcytic, hypochromic anemia with low RBC count and elevated RDW > 15%
- Low serum Fe: Reflecting iron concentration in circulation; this level may be falsely elevated due to recent high iron intake
- Elevated total iron-binding capacity (TIBC): This is a measure of transferrin, a plasma protein that easily combines with iron; when more of transferrin is available for binding, the TIBC level increases, reflecting iron deficiency
- Iron saturation less than 15%: This is calculated by dividing the serum iron by the TIBC
- Low serum ferritin level: This is the body's major iron storage protein
- Absence of iron from bone marrow, if aspiration is done

In iron deficiency anemia, the order of the laboratory markers is as follows:

- Ferritin
- Marrow
- Serum iron
- RDW (increase)
- TIBC (increase)
- Hemoglobin
- Indices

Therefore, a decrease in hemoglobin or RBC indices is a late rather than an early marker of disease. Therapy for patients with iron deficiency anemia not only involves iron replacement but also treatment of the underlying cause.

Iron use without a distinct clinical indication is not recommended because this may lead to an iatrogenic iron overload. This includes the use of iron-fortified multiple vitamins. Iron overload has been hypothesized to be a cardiovascular risk factor. A lower rate of cardiovascular disease has been noted in frequent blood donors with relatively low levels of stored iron when compared with age controls. In addition, women's cardiovascular disease rates equal men's 5 to 10 years after menopause, a time when female and male ferritin levels are equal.

Reticulocytosis begins quickly after initiation of iron therapy, with the reticulocyte count peaking 7 to 10 days into therapy. Hemoglobin increases at a rate of 2 g/dL every 3 weeks in response to iron therapy and will likely take 2 months to correct. As a result, the following laboratory tests may be used to evaluate the resolution of iron deficiency anemia: reticulocytes at 1 to 2 weeks to ensure marrow response to iron therapy, hemoglobin at 6 weeks to 2 months to ensure anemia recovery, and ferritin at 2 months after measure of normal hemoglobin (or 4 months after initiation of iron therapy) to ensure documentation of replenished iron stores (Table 11–2).

Folic acid (pteroylglutamic acid) is a water-soluble B complex vitamin found in abundance in peanuts, fruits, and vegetables. Through a complex reaction, folic acid is reduced to folate. Folate donates one carbon unit to oxidation at various levels, reactions vital to proper DNA synthesis. During times of accelerated tissue growth and repair, such as in childhood, pregnancy, recovery from serious illness, and recovery from hemolytic anemia, folic acid requirements increase from the baseline of two- to fourfold. Folate deficiency causes a macrocytic, normochromic anemia.

The most common causes of folic acid deficiency anemia are inadequate dietary intake, seen in the elderly, alcoholic, and impoverished, and those with decreased ability to absorb folic acid, seen in those with malabsorption syndromes such as sprue and celiac disease. Folic acid deficiency can often be avoided with a healthy diet featuring folate-rich fruits and vegetables.

Folic acid transfers readily through the placenta to the fetus, with fetal levels usually higher than maternal levels; therefore, there is evidence that pregnancy is a maternal folate-depleting event. Repeated or multiple pregnancies, in particular, cause depletion of maternal folate stores. Folate deficiency during pregnancy can be largely avoided through the consistent use of prescriptive prenatal vitamins, each tablet usually containing 0.8 to 1.0 mg of folic acid. Over-the-counter prenatal vitamins contain significantly less of this micronutrient, usually about 0.4 mg per tablet. Supplementation should continue through lactation because approximately 0.5 mg/day of folic acid is transferred to breast milk. Accumula-

HEMATOLOGIC AND IMMUNOLOGIC DISORDERS

TABLE 11-2.
DRUG INTERACTIONS WITH IRON THERAPY

Drug	Effect	Comment
Al, Mg antacids	Decreased iron absorption	Calcium carbonate does not interact
Caffeine	Decreased iron absorption	Separate use by at least 2 hours
Fluoroquinolones (ciprofloxacin, norfloxacin, ofloxacin, lomefloxacin, gatifoxacin, moxifloxacin)	Decreased fluoroquinolone effect	Avoid concurrent use if possible
Levodopa	Decreased levodopa effect	May not be noted with carbidopa
Methyldopa (Aldomet)	Decreased antihypertensive effect	Monitor blood pressure
Tetracycline	Decreased tetracycline and iron effect	Do not use concurrently if possible Interaction not noted with doxycycline
Thyroid hormones	Decreased thyroxine effect	Take thyroid hormones at least 2 hours before or 4 hours after iron dose
Cimetidine	Decreased iron absorption	Avoid concurrent use; use an alternative H_2RA
Zinc	Decreased zinc absorption	Avoid concurrent use if possible

Reference: Rizack, M. (1996). *Handbook of Adverse Drug Interactions.* New Rochelle, NY: The Medical Letter. Pp. 215–216.

tion of the vitamin in human milk takes preference over maintaining maternal folate levels.

Maternal folic acid deficiency is a teratogenic state, particularly during neural tube formation. In order to reduce the rate of neural tube defects in their offspring, women planning a pregnancy should be advised take additional amount of folic acid, 0.4 mg/day for 3 months before conception. This recommendation should be extended to all women capable of conception. Over-the-counter multivitamin or diet supplementation with vitamin-fortified foods can easily supply the recommended folate dose. If a woman has a history of giving birth to a child with a neural tube defect, the folic acid dose should be increased to 4 mg/day 3 months before conception and continued at least through the first 12 weeks of pregnancy. If the pregnancy is unplanned or preconception counseling was not sought, initiating folic acid supplementation during the first 7 weeks of pregnancy appears to offer some neural tube protection. This can be supplied by a prescription prenatal vitamin supplement. However, if the pregnant woman cannot tolerate the prenatal vitamin supplement caused by nausea, a common condition, she will likely be able to take folic acid alone without difficulty.

Recommended doses for folic acid replacement in adults range from 0.5 mg/day to 1 mg/day to 5 mg/day, with the usual dose being 1 mg/day. The underlying cause of the folate deficiency must be also be treated.

Reticulocytosis occurs rapidly, with a peak at 7 to 10 days into folic acid therapy. The hematocrit level increases by 4–5% per week and generally returns to normal within 1 month. Leukopenia and thrombocytopenia resolve within 2 to 3 days of therapy. A repeat hemogram in 1 to 2 months assists in the monitoring of therapeutic effect. Resolution of the related signs and symptoms generally follows the time frame needed for the resolution of the anemia.

Vitamin B_{12}, a member of the cobalamin family, is found in abundance in foods of animal origin and is essential to the development of the RBC. When vitamin B_{12} is ingested orally, it binds with intrinsic factor, a glycoprotein produced by the gastric parietal cells and transported systematically. Within the portal blood flow, the vitamin is attached to transcobalamin II, a polypeptide synthesized in the liver and ileum. Intrinsic factor is not absorbed and the new compound is transported to the bone marrow and other sites, where it is available for use in RBC formation. Two additional glycoproteins, transcobalamin I and III, combine with B_{12} and are used in the formation of granulocytes. In synergy with folic acid, vitamin B_{12} plays a role essential to RBC DNA synthesis. When deficiencies of either of these micronutrients exist, DNA synthesis in the RBC is impaired, leading to the distinct changes in the RBC and bone marrow.

Vitamin B_{12} therapy should be initiated when the diagnosis is made. Usually there is a brisk hematologic response, and the anemia is resolved within 2 months. Reversal of neurologic abnormalities is generally slower, but improvement seen quickly.

Vitamin B_{12} is available generically and in oral and injectable form. The parenteral form is preferred because of its excellent absorption. In oral form, vitamin B_{12} is erratically absorbed in the distal portion of the small intestine, potentially leading to treatment failure. The usual initial B_{12} dose is 100 mcg/d intramuscularly for the first week, then weekly for the first month, and then monthly for the rest of the patient's life. Orally, a higher dose, 1000 mcg/d, is needed. When the cause of the macrocytic anemia has not yet been established, a prudent course of action is to initially give parenteral vitamin B_{12} while giving folic acid 1 to 2 mg/day. With this plan, no intervention time is lost. After the appropriate diagnosis is established, the correct vitamin supplement is continued (Table 11–3).

The hematologic response is generally rapid after therapy is begun. Reticulocytosis is brisk and peaks at 5 to 7 days. Hypokalemia, caused by serum-to-intracellular potassium shifts, is common if the anemia was particularly severe and is most likely seen with the peak of reticulocytosis. Full hematologic recovery usually takes about 2 months.

Reversal of the signs and symptoms of vitamin B_{12} deficiency are generally rapid. A sense of improved well-being is usually reported within

TABLE 11–3.
ORAL VITAMIN B_{12} DRUG INTERACTIONS

Drug	Effect
Aminoglycosides	With concomitant use, decreased vitamin B_{12} absorption
Colchicine	With concomitant use, decreased vitamin B_{12} absorption
Potassium supplements	With concomitant use, decreased vitamin B_{12} absorption
Ascorbic acid	May destroy vitamin B_{12} if taken within one hour

Reference: Rizack, M. (1996). *Handbook of Adverse Drug Interactions.* New Rochelle, NY: The Medical Letter. Pp. 94–96.

24 hours of the onset of treatment. Neurologic changes, if present for less than 6 months, reverse quickly. However, neurologic reversal is likely not possible if these changes have been present for a protracted period.

Discussion Sources

Fitzgerald, M. (1999). Hematologic disorders. In Youngkin, E., Savin, K., Kissinger, J., & Israel, D. *Pharmacotherapeutics: A Primary Care Clinical Guideline*. Stamford, CT: Appleton & Lange. Pp. 605–620.

Hektor Dunphy, L. (1999). *Management Guidelines for Adult Nurse Practitioners*. Philadelphia: FA Davis. Pp. 455–459.

QUESTIONS

20. You are examining a 21-year-old man with multiple risk factors for HIV infection. He asks you for an "AIDS test, but I do not want anyone to know I was tested." Which of the following represents your most appropriate response?

    A. Advise him to seek assistance at an anonymous test site.
    B. Obtain his test in your office in a confidential manner.
    C. Have him pay for the test in cash so his health insurance will not be billed.
    D. Counsel him about the high rate of false-positive test results and the possibility of misdiagnosis.

21. A 28-year-old man has recently been diagnosed as HIV positive. Before initiating antiretroviral therapy, his CD4 count was 545 cells uL. You realize that he is at increased risk for:

    A. cytomegalovirus retinitis
    B. *pneumocystis* pneumonia
    C. staphylococcal skin infections
    D. *Mycobacterium avium* complex

22. Which of the following places a woman at increased risk of contracting HIV infection from heterosexual vaginal intercourse?

    A. vaginal diaphragm use
    B. male partner using a latex condom
    C. being postmenopausal
    D. use of a spermicide

23. When a pregnant woman passes the HIV virus on to her unborn child, it is known as what kind of transmission?

    A. vertical
    B. chorionic
    C. placental
    D. horizontal

24. A 38-year-old woman has advanced HIV disease. She presents with a chief complaint of a painless rash over her trunk. Examination reveals umbilicated vesicular-form lesions scattered over her thorax. This is most consistent with:

    A. herpes zoster
    B. dermatitis herpetiformis
    C. molluscum contagiosum
    D. impetigo

25. Which of the following represents the NP's most appropriate response to this patient's statement? "I might as well just die now that I am HIV positive."

    A. "You sound frightened."
    B. "What makes you say that?"
    C. "I am concerned about your health and safety."
    D. "We need more tests before your prognosis can be known."

ANSWERS

20. A
21. C
22. C
23. A
24. C
25. C

DISCUSSION

Human immunodeficiency virus infection is a systemic disease that causes a wide clinical spectrum of diseases from asymptomatic state to fatal complications. Risk factors include close contact with blood and body fluids of a person with HIV. The risk of contracting HIV from a single contaminated hollow-bore needle stick is about 1 in 250, considerably less than that of contracting hepatitis B from the same needle. In addition, the unborn child can become infected by vertical transmission from the mother. This risk is considerably reduced by the use of antiretroviral therapy during pregnancy. Postmenopausal women are at particular risk for infection through horizontal transmission from heterosexual vaginal intercourse because of the thinning of the vaginal mucosa associated with a low estrogen state. Male and female condom use for insertive sexual practices is protective.

The presentation of HIV infection varies according to the point in the disease spectrum. Opportunistic infections are common. In addition, infections that can occur in an immunocompetent person, such as staphylococcal skin infections including impetigo and molluscum contagiosum, can also occur in immunocompromised patients. Impetigo often presents initially as a vesicular-form lesion that is mildly itchy followed by the formation of a honey-colored crust. Molluscum contagiosum usually presents as a painless vesicular-form lesion with an umbilicated center. However, the degree of severity is usually much worse for HIV-infected patients (Table 11–4).

TABLE 11–4.
RELATIONSHIP OF CD4 COUNTS TO OPPORTUNISTIC INFECTION*

Absolute CD4 Lymphocyte Count Cells uL	Associated Opportunistic Infection
> 350	Bacterial infections, tuberculosis, herpes simplex, herpes zoster, vaginal candidiasis, hairy leukoplakia, Kaposi's sarcoma
< 300	Pneumocystis pneumonia, toxoplasmosis, cryptococcosis, histoplasmosis, coccidioidomycosis, cryptosporidiosis
< 100	Disseminated MAC infection, CMV retinitis, CNS lymphoma

*A variety of opportunistic infections can occur at any point in the HIV infection continuum. This table gives general relationship for opportunistic infection and CD4 counts.

Unfortunately, prejudice against those who are infected with HIV exists. In addition, insurers and employers may make decisions based on a person's perceived HIV risk. To this end, an important part of primary care is counseling the patient about HIV testing. If testing is provided in a primary care office, held in a special manner during sampling and on the record, this usually qualifies as confidential testing. In this type of testing, the counselor or provider and the patient know one another's identity. The results are potentially traceable, helpful when the provider needs to find a patient who has not returned for results. However, insurers and others may be able to also trace the results, a potentially problematic situation. If testing is provided at an anonymous test site, the counselor does not know the patient's identity because a number or other designation is used. The result of this type of test is not traceable, thus protecting the patient's privacy. However, the drawback is that the patient cannot be identified. Therefore, if the patient does not return for results, no follow-up care is possible.

When counseling about HIV testing, inform patients that false-positive test results are rare and false-negative results are more common. This is caused by a "window period," the period from infection to development of antibodies. However, antibodies usually develop within 6 weeks of infection. Standard HIV testing includes an ELISA as a screening test. If the ELISA test result is positive, a confirming Western blot is obtained. A number of home testing options are also available.

A critically important part of care for patients infected with HIV is the ongoing support and counseling provided in the primary care relationship. As with other potentially life-threatening illnesses, patients display a range of emotions. However, NPs should maintain an objective stance and not attempt to assign feelings or badger the patient for additional information. Starting a counseling statement with "I" followed by a verb that conveys what you see or feel about a situation is very helpful when dealing with people in crisis. In the example given here, the patient states: "I might as well just die now that I am HIV positive." This may represent a suicidal statement. The NP must establish the safety, as well as health, status of this person.

Treatment of patients infected with HIV is a dynamic process with new therapies becoming available. As a result, it behooves NPs to be familiar with the latest therapies in order to afford the patient the best opportunity to achieve and maintain health.

Discussion Source

Hektor Dunphy, L. (1999). *Management Guidelines for Adult Nurse Practitioners.* Philadelphia: FA Davis. Pp. 462–468.

QUESTIONS

26. An 18-year-old woman has a chief complaint of a "sore throat and swollen glands" for the past 3 days. Her physical examination includes exudative pharyngitis, minimally tender anterior and posterior cervical lymphadenopathy, and maculopapular rash. Abdominal examination reveals right and left upper quadrant abdominal tenderness. Her most likely diagnosis is:

   A. group A beta hemolytic streptococcal pharyngitis
   B. infectious mononucleosis
   C. rubella
   D. scarlet fever

27. Which of the following is most likely to be found in the laboratory data in a person with infectious mononucleosis?

   A. neutrophilia
   B. lymphocytosis with atypical lymphocytes
   C. positive antinuclear antibody
   D. macrocytic anemia

28. You examine a 25-year-old man who has infectious mononucleosis with 4+ tonsillar hypertrophy, exudative pharyngitis, difficulty swallowing, and a patent airway. You prescribe the following:

   A. amoxicillin
   B. prednisone
   C. ibuprofen
   D. acyclovir

ANSWERS

26. B
27. B
28. B

DISCUSSION

Developing an accurate diagnosis of an acute febrile illness with associated rash and pharyngitis can be a daunting task. A few key points can help:

- Lymphadenopathy: Diffuse lymphadenopathy is most often seen in patients with diffuse infection, such as a systemic viral illness. When associated with a localized bacterial infection such as streptococcal pharyngitis, the affected lymph nodes are also localized (anterior cervical chain).
- Pharyngitis and associated symptoms: Systemic viral infection can cause pharyngitis but also involves other mucous membranes such as the conjunctiva and oral and respiratory mucosa. These signs and symptoms are usually absent from a more localized infection such as "strep throat."

Infectious mononucleosis is an acute systemic viral illness that frequently affects the liver and spleen; therefore, tenderness is usually found over these organs, and organomegaly is common. Treatment is usually supportive with recovery slow but complete. However, there is a potential for obstruction and respiratory distress when enlarged tonsils and lymphoid tissue impinge on the upper airway. Prednisone 40 to 60 mg/day for 3 days is the treatment of choice. Neither the use of antiviral agents such as acyclovir nor routine prescribing of corticosteroid agents is indicated in uncomplicated infectious mononucleosis. Diagnostic testing for patients with infectious mononucleosis usually includes obtaining a heterophil antibody test (Monospot). Characteristically, leukopenia with lymphocytosis is present. Darkly stained, usually large, atypical-appearing lymphocytes are seen. The presence of atypical lymphocytes is not unique to infectious mononucleosis and is commonly found in systemic viral infection (Table 11–5).

Discussion Source

Hektor Dunphy, L. (1999). *Management Guidelines for Adult Nurse Practitioners*. Philadelphia: FA Davis. Pp. 468–470.

QUESTIONS

29. A 29-year-old woman has a sudden onset of right-sided facial asymmetry. She is unable to tightly close her right eyelid or frown or smile on the affected side. Her examination is otherwise unremarkable. This represents paralysis of cranial nerve (CN):

    A. III
    B. IV
    C. VII
    D. VIII

TABLE 11–5.
DIFFERENTIAL DIAGNOSIS OF ACUTE RASH–PRODUCING ILLNESS ASSOCIATED WITH FEVER AND SORE THROAT

Clinical Condition with Causative Agent	Presentation	Comments
Infectious mononu-cleosis; agent: Epstein-Barr viruses (human herpesvirus 4)	Rash: Macropapular in ~ 20%, rare petechial rash Fever, "shaggy" purple-white exudative pharyngitis, malaise, marked diffuse lymph-adenopathy, hepatic and splenic tender-ness and occasional enlargement	Incubation period 20–50 days >90% of patients develop a rash if given amoxicillin or ampicillin during infec-tious mononucleosis Avoid contact sports for at least 1 month because of risk of splenic rupture
Acute HIV infection (human immuno-deficiency virus)	Macropapular rash Fever, mild pharyngitis, ulceration oral lesions, diarrhea, diffuse lymphadenopathy	Most likely to occur in re-sponse to infection with large viral load Consult with HIV specialist concerning initiation of antiretroviral therapies
Strep pyogenes (group A beta hemolytic strep-tococci) pharyn-gitis (scarlet fever)	Scarlatina-form, sand-paper-like rash occa-sionally present Severe sore throat usu-ally with exudate Fever; headache; tender, localized anterior cer-vical lymphadenopa-thy Occasional presenta-tion with mild sore throat and rash	When streptococcal pharyngitis presentation includes rash, usually called scarlet fever. Rash may peel during antibiotic therapy. Rate of long-term compli-cation or seriousness of illness same as when rash is absent Hoarseness, cough, nasal discharge rarely associ-ated with condition and suggest viral pharyngitis

(continued)

TABLE 11–5. (continued)

Clinical Condition with Causative Agent	Presentation	Comments
Rubella	Mild symptoms: fever, sore throat, malaise, nasal discharge Diffuse maculopapular rash lasting about 3 days Posterior cervical and postauricular lymphadenopathy 5–10 days before onset of rash Arthralgia in about 25% (most common in women)	Incubation period about 14–21 days with disease transmissble for ~ 1 week before onset of rash to ~ 2 weeks after rash appears Generally a mild self-limiting illness Greatest risk is effect of virus on the unborn child, especially with first trimester exposure (~ 80% rate congenital rubella syndrome) Prevent with immunization
Rubeola (measles)	Usually acute presentation with fever, nasal discharge, cough, generalized lymphadenopathy, conjunctivitis (copious clear discharge), photophobia, Koplik's spots (appear ~ 2 days before onset of rash as nearly pinpoint white lesions on mucous membranes, conjunctival folds) Pharyngitis is usually mild without exudate Macropapular rash onset 3–4 days after onset of symptoms, may coalesce to generalized erythema	Incubation period about 10–14 days with disease transmissible for ~ 1 week before onset of rash to ~ 2–3 weeks after rash appears CNS and respiratory tract complications common; prevent by immunization

Reference: Hektor Dunphy, L. (1999). *Management Guidelines for Adult Nurse Practitioners*. Philadelphia: FA Davis. Pp. 120–123.

30. From those listed below, which represents the most important diagnostic test for the patient in Question 29?

    A. complete blood count with white blood cell differential
    B. Lyme antibody titer
    C. computed tomography scan of the head with contrast enhancement
    D. serum protein electrophoresis

31. Which of the following symptoms does a person with stage 1 Lyme disease have?

    A. peripheral neuropathic symptoms
    B. high-grade atrioventricular heart block
    C. Bell's palsy
    D. single painless annular lesion

32. The preferred antibiotic for the treatment of adults with Lyme disease is a(n):

    A. tetracycline
    B. aminoglycoside
    C. cephalosporin
    D. penicillin

ANSWERS

29. C
30. B
31. D
32. A

DISCUSSION

Lyme disease is a multisystem infection caused by *Borrelia burgdorferi*, a tick-transmitted spirochete. Although original reports of this disease were clustered through select areas of the United States, primarily in the Northeast and Mid-Atlantic states, it has now been diagnosed in virtually every state. The origin of the disease's name comes from the town Old Lyme, Connecticut, where it was first diagnosed after a community epidemic of rash and arthritis. Lyme disease is the most common vector-borne disease in the United States.

Overdiagnosis of Lyme disease is a problem as is the issue of significant but understandable anxiety about any tick exposure. Infected ticks must feed on the human host for more than 24 hours in order to transmit the spirochete. In addition, not all ticks are infected, with rates varying from 15–65% in areas where Lyme disease is endemic.

Lyme disease is typically divided into three stages.

- Stage 1: A mild flulike illness typically with a single erythema migrans lesion. This is an annular skin lesion with a clearing center. The lesion is rarely pruritic or painful. These signs and symptoms can resolve without treatment.
- Stage 2: Typically months later, the classic rash may reappear with multiple lesions. Heart block, arthralgias and myalgia, and acute facial nerve paralysis (Bell's palsy) may also be present. Again, regression of symptoms can occur without treatment.
- Stage 3: Starting approximately 1 year after the initial infection, neuropsychiatric symptoms appear including memory problems, depression, and neuropathy.

Testing for Lyme disease can be problematic because of its relative lack of sensitivity. Careful correlation of patient history and physical examination along with laboratory diagnostics is critical to prevent both over- and underdiagnosing this condition.

The preferred antibiotic class for the treatment of uncomplicated Lyme disease is the tetracyclines. This group includes tetracycline as well as doxycycline. Be aware of the latest recommendation for dose as well as duration of treatment with these products.

Prevention of Lyme disease includes avoiding areas with known or potential tick infestation, wearing long-sleeved shirts and pants, and using insect repellents. Inspecting the skin and clothing for ticks is also helpful. A vaccine to prevent Lyme disease is available and should be offered to residents of areas where the disease is endemic as well as those who engage in activities that place them at increased risk for infection.

Discussion Source

Hektor Dunphy, L. (1999). *Management Guidelines for Adult Nurse Practitioners*. Philadelphia: FA Davis. Pp. 468–470.

QUESTIONS

33. Which of the following best describes the presentation of a person with rheumatoid arthritis?

    A. worst symptoms in weight-bearing joints later in the day
    B. symmetric early-morning stiffness
    C. sausage-shaped digits with associated skin lesions
    D. back pain with rest and anterior uveitis

34. Nonsteroidal anti-inflammatory drugs cause gastric injury primarily by:

    A. direct irritative effect
    B. slowing GI motility
    C. thinning of the protective mucosa
    D. enhancing prostaglandin synthesis

35. Of the following, who is at highest risk for NSAID-induced gastropathy?

    A. a 28-year-old man with an ankle sprain taking ibuprofen for the past week who drinks four to six beers every weekend
    B. a 40-year-old woman who smokes and takes about 6 doses of naproxen sodium per month to control dysmenorrhea
    C. a 43-year-old man with dilated cardiomyopathy who uses ketoprofen 1 to 2 times per week for low back pain
    D. a 72-year-old man who takes piroxicam (Feldene) daily for pain control of osteoarthritis

36. Which of the following is the preferred method of preventing NSAID-induced gastric ulcer?

    A. a high-dose histamine$_2$ receptor antagonist (H$_2$RA)
    B. timed antacid use
    C. sucralfate (Carafate)
    D. misoprostol (Cytotec)

37. Taking a high dose of aspirin or ibuprofen causes a(n):

    A. increase in drug's half-life
    B. enhanced renal excretion of the drug
    C. change in the drug's mechanism of action
    D. lowering of antiprostaglandin effect

38. Which of the following is most accurate concerning rheumatoid arthritis?

   A. Joint erosions may be evident on radiographs.
   B. Men are affected more frequently than women.
   C. Butterfly-shaped facial rash is common.
   D. Parvovirus B_{19} infection may contribute to its development.

39. Principles of treating patients with rheumatoid arthritis include:

   A. using a stepwise approach to care
   B. early use of disease antirheumatic modifying drugs (DMARD) to slow or stop joint damage
   C. pain relief as the chief therapeutic goal
   D. joint splinting is seldom advisable

40. Which of the following tests is most specific to the diagnosis of rheumatoid arthritis?

   A. elevated rheumatoid factor (RF)
   B. elevated erythrocyte sedimentation rate (ESR)
   C. depressed total white blood cell count
   D. elevated antinuclear antibody (ANA)

41. A 52-year-old woman has rheumatoid arthritis. She now presents with decreased tearing, "gritty"-feeling eyes and a dry mouth. You consider a diagnosis of:

   A. systemic lupus erythematosus (SLE)
   B. vasculitis
   C. Sjögren syndrome
   D. scleroderma

42. Cyclooxygenase 1 (COX-1) contributes to :

   A. inflammatory response
   B. pain transmission
   C. maintenance of gastric protective mucosal layer
   D. renal arteriole constriction

ANSWERS

33. B
34. C
35. D

36. D
37. A
38. A
39. B
40. A
41. C
42. C

DISCUSSION

Rheumatoid arthritis is a disease causing chronic systemic inflammation including the synovial membranes of multiple joints. As with most autoimmune diseases, rheumatoid arthritis is more common in women at a 3:1 ratio. Although new-onset rheumatoid arthritis can occur at any age, peak onset is from age 20 to 40 years. A family history of rheumatoid disease is often noted. Initial presentation may be with acute polyarticular inflammation. However, the slowly progressing picture of malaise, weight loss, and stiffness is more common. The stiffness is symmetric, typically worse upon arising, lasts about 1 hour, involves at least three joint groups, and can recur after a period of inactivity or exercise. The hands (sparing the distal interphalangeal joints), wrists, ankles, and toes are most often involved. Soft tissue swelling or fluid is also present, as are subcutaneous nodules. There are often periods of exacerbation and remission but little reduction in lifespan because of the disease.

Common diagnostic tests in rheumatoid arthritis include the ANA, ESR, RF, and radiographs. When interpreting results, bear in mind the following:

- Radiographs typically reveal joint erosion and loss of normal joint space.
- Erythrocyte sedimentation rate is a nonspecific test of inflammation. Generally, the higher the ESR, the greater the degree and intensity of the inflammatory process. Although frequently elevated in patients with rheumatoid arthritis, its presence is not diagnostic of the condition or other conditions. In addition, a single elevated ESR is seldom helpful; however, following trends during flare-up and regression of disease often aids in charting the therapeutic course and response.
- C-reactive protein (CRP) is also a nonspecific test of inflammation. It tends to increase more rapidly than ESR in patients with

rheumatoid arthritis but decreases an equivalent amount. Its usefulness and limitations are similar to those of ESR.

- Rheumatoid factor, an IgM antibody, is present in approximately 50–90% of patients with rheumatoid arthritis. The level of the titer may correspond to the severity of disease.
- Hemogram may reveal anemia of chronic disease.
- Antinuclear antibodies are antibodies against cellular nuclear components that act as antigens. ANA is occasionally present in healthy adults, but its presence is usually found in those with systemic rheumatic or collagen vascular disease. ANA testing is the most sensitive laboratory marker for SLE, detected in approximately 95% but only in 30–50% of those with rheumatoid arthritis. Patterns of immunofluorescence vary but have been given misplaced credence as to type of disease. Here are some examples of ANA patterns:

  - Homogeneous, diffuse or solid pattern to DNA: high titers strongly associated with SLE
  - Peripheral or rim pattern: associated with anti–double strained DNA and has a strong correlation with SLE
  - Nucleolar pattern: associated with anti-RNP and has a strong correlation with scleroderma
  - Speckled pattern: further antigen testing should be ordered with this result. This additional testing may be required in those with a variety of collagen-vascular or rheumatic diseases.

The program of treatment of patients with rheumatoid arthritis is to reduce inflammation and pain while preserving function and preventing deformity. Behavioral management is key because stress may precipitate a flare-up of rheumatoid arthritis. Allowing for proper rest periods is critical. Physical therapists can assist in the development of a reasonable activity plan. Maintenance of physical activity through appropriate exercise is of greatest importance. Water exercise in particular is helpful because it includes mild resistance as well as buoyancy. Splints may provide joint rest while maintaining function and preventing contracture.

Aspirin (ASA) and other NSAIDs have been the backbone of rheumatoid arthritis drug treatment for years. These medications are helpful in controlling inflammation and pain, both worthy therapeutic goals. Aspirin and ibuprofen are two of the more commonly used products. With many of the NSAIDs, the half-life of the drug is increased as the dose is raised.

A significant amount of peptic ulcer disease, in particular gastric ulcer and gastritis, is caused by NSAID use. NSAIDs inhibit synthesis of prostaglandins from arachidonic acid, yielding an anti-inflammatory effect. This is partly caused by the action of these products against cyclooxygenase. COX-1 is an enzyme found in gastric, small and large intestine mucosa, kidneys, platelets, and vascular epithelium. It contributes to the health of these organs through a number of mechanisms, including the maintenance of the protective gastric mucosal layer and proper perfusion of the kidneys. COX-2 is an enzyme that produces prostaglandins important to inflammatory cascade and pain transmission. The standard NSAIDs and steroids inhibit the synthesis of COX-1 and COX-2, thus controlling pain and inflammation but with gastric and renal complications. NSAIDs such as celecoxib (Celebrex) that spare COX-1 and are more COX-2-selective afford control of the potential for arthritis symptoms but have less risk of gastric and renal problems and minimal impact on platelet activity.

As helpful as NSAIDs are in symptom control, these products do not alter the underlying disease process, with joint destruction continuing despite excellent control of symptoms and reduction in swelling. Early use of DMARD can help slow or halt joint damage.

TREATMENT OF RHEUMATOID ARTHRITIS

Medication	Examples
Anti-inflammatory agents	NSAIDs, COX-2 inhibitors, corticosteroids
Analgesics	NSAIDs, COX-2 inhibitors, acetaminophen, opioids, topical agents
DMARDs (disease-modifying anti-rheumatic drugs)	Antimetabolites: Methotrexate, leflunomide, azathioprine Cytokine inhibitors: Cyclosporine, infliximab, etanercept FDA-approved miscellaneous DMARDs: Ridaura, injectable gold, hydroxychloroquine, penicillamine, sulfasalazine, minocycline, cyclophospamide

If a patient fails to achieve control of pain or symptoms with an adequate trial of DMARD and a NSAID, additional should be added. One option is intraarticular steroid injection. This can be quite helpful but should be limited to not more that two to three injections per joint per year to minimize risk of joint deterioration. Systemic corticosteroids can be most helpful in relieving inflammation, but use should not exceed 2 to 8 weeks because of their adverse reaction profile. Alternative, but more toxic, DMARDs include penicillamine and gold. Only those who have expertise with their use should prescribe them.

Sjögren syndrome is an autoimmune disease that usually occurs in conjunction with another chronic inflammatory condition such as rheumatoid arthritis or SLE. Complaints are usually related to problems related to decreased oral and ocular secretions. In addition, mouth ulcers and dental caries are common, and ESR is elevated in more than 90% of patients. A salivary biopsy for presence of mononuclear cells infiltration is useful. Intervention for those with Sjögren syndrome includes management of presenting symptoms with appropriate lubricants. Treating the underlying disease is critical.

Discussion Sources

Hektor Dunphy, L. (1999). *Management Guidelines for Adult Nurse Practitioners*. Philadelphia: FA Davis. Pp. 472–474, 476–478.

Hellman, D. Stone, J. (1999). Arthritis and musculoskeletal disorder. In Tierney, L., McPhee, S., & Papadakis, M. *Current Diagnosis and Treatment* (38th ed.). Stamford, CT: Appleton & Lange. Pp. 786–837.

12
CHAPTER

Psychosocial
Disorders

QUESTIONS

1. A 44-year-old man who admits to drinking a "few beers now and then" presents for examination After obtaining a health history and performing a physical examination, you suspect he is a heavy alcohol user. Your next best action is to:

   A. obtain liver enzymes
   B. administer the CAGE questionnaire
   C. confront the patient with your observations
   D. advise him about the hazards of excessive alcohol use

2. Which of the following blood alcohol level readings is most consistent with the diagnosis of alcohol abuse?

   A. 80 mg/100 mL obtained during a driving while intoxicated (DWI) arrest
   B. 200 mg/100 mL with clear intoxication
   C. 150 mg/100 mL without evidence of intoxication
   D. any level detected during a routine physical examination

3. Lorazepam is the preferred benzodiazepine for treating alcohol withdrawal symptoms when there is a concomitant history of:

   A. seizure disorder
   B. folate deficiency anemia
   C. multiple substance abuse
   D. hepatic disease

4. Which of the following is the most helpful approach in the care of a patient with alcoholism?

   A. Tell the patient to stop drinking.
   B. Counsel the patient that alcohol abuse is a treatable disease.
   C. Inform the patient of the long-term health consequences of alcohol abuse.
   D. Refer the patient to Alcoholics Anonymous.

5. A 42-year-old man who has a long-standing history of alcohol abuse presents for primary care. He admits to drinking 12 to 16 beers daily for 10 years. He states, "I really do not feel like the booze is a problem. I get to work every day." Your most appropriate response is:

   A. "Work is usually the last thing to go in alcohol abuse."
   B. "Your family has suffered by your drinking."
   C. "I am concerned about your health and safety."
   D. "Alcoholics Anonymous can help you."

6. Which of the following agents offers effective control of tremor and tachycardia associated with alcohol withdrawal?

   A. phenobarbital
   B. propanolol
   C. verapamil
   D. naltrexone

7. Which of the following is most likely to be noted in a 45-year-old woman with laboratory evidence of chronic excessive alcohol ingestion?

   A. alanine aminotransferase (ALT) = 202 U/L (0–31 U/L), MCV = 60 fL (80–96 fL)
   B. AST = 149 U/L (0–31 U/L), MCV = 81 fL (80–96 fL)
   C. ALT = 88 U/L (0–31 U/L), MCV = 140 fL (80–96 fL)
   D. AST = 80 U/L (0–31 U/L), MCV = 103 fL (80–96 fL)

ANSWERS

   1. B
   2. C
   3. D
   4. B
   5. C
   6. B
   7. D

DISCUSSION

Providing primary care for patients abusing alcohol presents a number of challenges because this is a complex disorder affecting family and social function and employment as well as health. Often patients minimize the effect of alcohol abuse, pointing out that employment has not been affected. In reality, alcoholism is a progressive disease that usually affects family and personal relationships first, then health and, much later, employment. The use of an effective screening tool for alcohol abuse such as the CAGE questionnaire (Box 12–1) is critical for disease detection. The National Institute on Alcohol Abuse and Alcoholism offers steps for alcohol screening and brief intervention (Fig. 12–1).

Counseling the patient and family about alcoholism as a lifelong but treatable disease is a helpful clinical approach. In addition, asking about current drinking habits and associated consequences to health with each visit is important. Consistently offering your assistance in accessing treatment conveys the seriousness of this life-threatening condition. As with other health problems with a behavioral component, using statements beginning with "I" is important—"I continue to be very concerned about your health and safety when I hear that you are drinking every day."

In providing primary care, the NP must maintain an attitude that, as with any substance abuse, the patient is capable of changing and achieving sobriety. Change occurs dynamically and often unpredictably. A commonly used change framework is based on the work of Prochaska, who notes five stages.

1. Pre-contemplation: The patient is not interested in change.
2. Contemplation: The patient is considering change and looking at its positive and negative aspects.

BOX 12–1
THE CAGE QUESTIONNAIRE*

Have you ever felt the need to **C**ut down on drinking?
Have you ever felt **A**nnoyed by criticism of drinking?
Have you ever had **G**uilty feelings about drinking?
Have you ever taken a morning **E**ye-opener?

---

*This questionnaire may be modified for use with other forms of substance abuse by substituting "N" (Normal) for "E" (Eye-opener). For example: Do you ever use heroin in order to keep from getting sick or withdrawing?

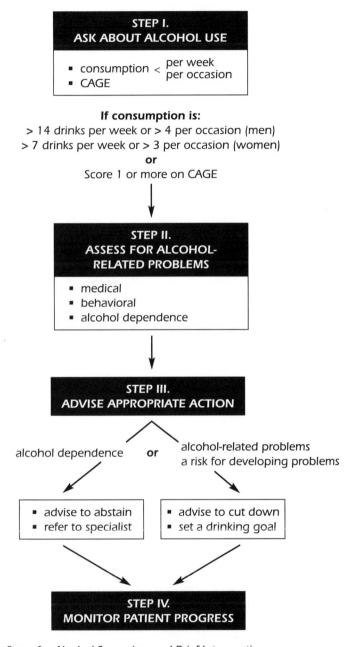

FIG. 12–1. Steps for Alcohol Screening and Brief Intervention
Source: The Physicians' Guide to Helping Patients with Alcohol Problems. National Institute on Alcohol Abuse and Alcoholism. NIH Publication No. 95–3769 National Institutes of Health, 1995.

3. Preparation: The patient exhibits some change behaviors or thoughts but may feel that he or she does not have the tools to proceed.
4. Action: The patient is ready to go forth with change.
5. Maintenance/relapse: The patient learns to continue the change and to deal with backsliding.

As counselor, the NP provides a valuable role in continually "tapping" the patient with a message of concern about health and safety, thus possibly moving the precontemplator to the contemplator stage. After the patient is at this stage, presenting treatment options and support for change is a critical part of an NP's role.

Benzodiazepines have long been used to treat alcohol withdrawal symptoms. Chlordiazepoxide (Librium) or diazepam (Valium), agents with a long half-life, are reasonable treatment options for a patient with adequate hepatic function, but lorazepam should be used in those with hepatic dysfunction. Alpha-adrenergic agonists (e.g., clonidine) or beta-adrenergic antagonists (e.g., propanolol, atenolol) are helpful in managing the distressing tachycardia and tremor associated with alcohol withdrawal (Box 12–2).

In a patient who drinks more than one half a bottle of hard liquor or six beers per day, alcohol withdrawal symptoms typically begin about 12 hours after the last drink. Peak symptoms are seen at 24 to 48 hours with

---

BOX 12–2
MEDICATION REGIMEN OPTIONS DURING OUTPATIENT ALCOHOL WITHDRAWAL

- Chlordiazepoxide (Librium) 50 mg every 6 hours for four doses, then 25 mg every 6 hours for eight doses
- Diazepam 10 mg (Valium) every 6 hours for four doses, then 5 mg every 6 hours for eight doses
- Lorazepam (Ativan) 2 mg every 6 hours for four doses, then 1 mg every 6 hours for eight doses
- NB: Chlordiazepoxide and diazepam have long half-life, but lorazepam (with a relatively short half-life) is the preferred agent in the elderly and those with hepatic insufficiency

---

Saitz, R., Valliant, G., Wolf, D. (1998, December 15). Recognizing and treating patients with drinking problems. *Patient Care*. Pp. 113–128. Available at www.patientcareonline.com

abatement over the next few days. Abrupt withdrawal of alcohol use in the addicted person can lead to potentially life-threatening problems with autonomic hyperactivity (i.e., agitation, hallucinations, disorientation) as well as seizures. Benzodiazepines are helpful in managing distressing symptoms as well as preventing seizures. Treatment of concurrent problems such as dehydration, malnutrition, and infection is also warranted. Inpatient detoxification is the safest treatment for high-risk individuals (Box 12–3).

A highly motivated patient with adequate support systems and a relatively low level of alcohol addiction may be a good candidate for outpatient detoxification. In this type of detoxification, the patient and support person contract with the health care provider about a safe plan of detoxification. This includes daily office visits or contact, ongoing involvement in Alcoholics Anonymous, and counseling services as well as use of a limited supply of medications for managing withdrawal symptoms.

Although it is tempting to rely on laboratory markers to make the diagnosis of alcoholism, few tests are helpful in reality. Tests of hepatic function are often ordered by providers who then have the dilemma of presenting the alcohol-abusing patient with a set of relatively normal test results. This may further reinforce the patient's denial or minimization of the effect excessive alcohol use has on health. All currently available hepatic testing indirectly measure liver function or capacity. The most commonly performed tests are hepatic enzymes, protein molecules acting as catalysts, and regulating metabolism within cells.

BOX 12–3
INPATIENT DETOXIFICATION CRITERIA

Inpatient detoxification is the safest treatment in individuals at high risk, including those who have the following:

- Other acute illness such as infection and cardiac disease
- Severe alcohol-related symptoms before detoxification
- Prior severe withdrawal characterized by delirium tremens or seizure
- Coexisting mental health problems such as depression

Saitz, R., Valliant, G., Wolf, D. (1998, December 15). Recognizing and treating patients with drinking problems. *Patient Care.* Pp. 113–128. Available at www.patientcareonline.com

Aspartate aminotransferase (AST formerly known as SGOT) is found in large quantities in hepatocytes. Small amounts are typically found in circulation for hepatic growth and repair. AST increases in response to hepatocyte injury, as may occur in alcohol abuse, the therapeutic use of HMG CoA reductase inhibitors (lipid-lowering drugs with -statin suffix such as lovastatin), and acetaminophen overdose. This enzyme is also found in skeletal muscle, myocardium, brain, and kidneys in smaller amounts, so damage to these areas may also cause an AST increase. AST has a circulatory half-life of approximately 12 to 24 hours, so levels increase in response to hepatic damage and clear quickly after damage ceases. AST elevation is generally found in only about 10% of problem drinkers. However, if AST is elevated with normal alanine aminotransferase (ALT) and mild macrocytosis (MCV > 100 fL, seen in about 30–60% of men who drink five or more drinks per day and in women at a threshold of three or more drinks per day), long-standing alcohol abuse is the likely cause.

Alanine aminotransferase (ALT formerly known as SGPT) is more specific to the liver, having limited concentration in other organs. This enzyme has a longer half-life than AST at 37 to 57 hours. Therefore, elevation persists longer after hepatic damage has ceased. The greatest elevation of this enzyme is likely seen in hepatitis caused by infection or inflammation. This enzyme is unlikely to increase in the presence of alcohol abuse.

When evaluating a patient with suspected substance abuse causing hepatic dysfunction, the NP must note both the degree of AST or ALT elevation as well as the AST-to-ALT ratio (Table 12–1; also see Table 6–6).

Discussion Sources

Hektor Dunphy, L. (1999). *Management Guidelines for Adult Nurse Practitioners*. Philadelphia: FA Davis. Pp. 481–484.

Landis, B.J., Bryant, S. (1999). Mental health disorders. In Youngkin, E., Sawin, K., Kissinger, J., & Israel, D., *Pharmacotherapeutics: A Primary Care Clinical Guide*. Stamford, CT: Appleton & Lange. Pp. 747–800.

National Institute on Alcohol and Alcoholism (1995). *The Physicians' Guide to Helping Patients with Alcohol Problems*. Rockville, MD: US Department of Health and Human Services. NIH Publication No. 95–3769.

Saitz, R., Valliant, G., Wolf, D. (1998, December 15). Recognizing and treating patients with drinking problems. *Patient Care*. Pp. 113–128. Available at www.patientcareonline.com

US Preventive Services Task Force. *1996 Guide to Clinical Preventive Services* (2nd ed). Baltimore: Williams and Wilkins.

TABLE 12–1.
HEPATIC ENZYMES ELEVATIONS AND THEIR SIGNIFICANCE

Enzyme Elevation	Associated Conditions	Comments
ALT increases to higher than AST	Hepatitis A, B, C, D, E, and so on Hepatitis associated with drugs or industrial chemicals	A memory jog for recalling reasons for increase is: "L" in "ALT" symbolizes *Liver* infection "T" symbolizes *troglitazone* (Rezulin) and other *therapeutic* agents
AST increases to higher than ALT	Alcohol-related hepatic injury (two times normal), HMG-CoA reductase inhibitor (-statin suffix) use, acetaminophen overdose	A memory jog for recalling reasons for increase is "AST" symbolizes *Alcohol, Statin, Tylenol*
AST/ALT elevation 1 to 5 times normal	Alcohol use Skeletal muscle injury secondary to seizure, protracted immobilization	Example: 38-year-old man with a 10-year history of increasingly heavy alcohol use AST = 83 U/L (0–31) ALT = 50 U/L (0–31)
AST/ALT elevation > 5 times normal	Infectious hepatitis	Example: 22-year-old woman who recently returned from a volunteer trip to a developing nation AST = 678 U/L (0–31 U/L) ALT = 828 U/L (0–31 U/L)

(continued)

TABLE 12–1. (continued)

Enzyme Elevation	Associated Conditions	Comments
Gamma glutamyl transferase (GGT)	Enzyme involved in the transfer of amino acids across cell membranes Found primarily in the liver and kidney In liver disease, usually parallels changes in alkaline phosphate Useful marker of hepatic disease in the following conditions, with marked elevation often noted in obstructive jaundice, hepatic metastasis, intrahepatic cholestasis In response to binge drinking, GGT leaks out of cells in greater amounts than other hepatic enzymes; GGT elevation is marked, sustained in high alcohol intake; will elevate modestly with lower consumption	Example: 40-year-old woman with cholecystitis AST = 25 U/L (0–31 U/L) ALT = 45 U/L (0–31 U/L) Alkaline phosphate = 155 U/L (0–125 U/L) GGT = 245 U/L (0–45 U/L) Example: 38-year-old man with a 10-year history heavy alcohol use with recent bingeing AST = 83 U/L (0–31 U/L) ALT = 50 U/L (0–31 U/L) GGT = 150 U/L (0–45 U/L)

Adapted from Nicoll, D., McPhee, S., Chou, T., Detmer, W. (1997). *Pocket Guide to Diagnostic Tests.* Stamford, CT: Appleton and Lange. Pp. 41, 54, 88, 330–331.

QUESTIONS

8. When providing primary care for a middle-aged woman with a history of prescription benzodiazepine abuse, you consider that:

   A. She is unlikely to have a problem with misuse of other drugs or alcohol.

   B. Rapid detoxification is the preferred method of treatment for this problem.

   C. There may be an underlying untreated psychiatric illness.

   D. She is at significant risk for drug-induced hepatitis.

9. Risk of benzodiazepine misuse can be minimized by use of:

   A. agents with a shorter half-life

   B. the drug as an "as-needed" rescue medication for acute anxiety

   C. more lipophilic products

   D. products with long duration of action

10. While counseling an adolescent about the risks of marijuana use, the NP considers that:

    A. Symptoms of physical and psychological dependency are rarely reported by regular users.

    B. Chronic obstructive airway disease is often associated with its regular use.

    C. Its use on a daily basis among teens is significantly less common than that of alcohol.

    D. Driving ability is minimally impaired with its use.

11. When assessing a person with acute opiate withdrawal, you expect to find:

    A. constipation

    B. hypertension

    C. hypothermia

    D. somnolence

12. When providing care for a middle-aged man with acute cocaine intoxication, you inquire about:

    A. feelings of anxiety

    B. poor sleeping patterns

    C. chest pain

    D. abdominal pain

13. Use of flunitrazepam (Rohypnol) has been associated with:

   A. agitation

   B. sexual assault

   C. increased appetite

   D. hallucination

ANSWERS

  8. C

  9. D

 10. B

 11. B

 12. C

 13. B

DISCUSSION

Substance abuse is a common problem, affecting 10–14% of primary care patients, with less than 10% being detected and appropriately treated. The *Diagnostic and Statistical Manual of Mental Disorders* (4th ed.) (DSM IV) describes substance abuse as a maladaptive pattern of use leading to clinically significant impairment or distress, manifested by one of more of the following, directly attributed to substance misuse, within a 12-month period:

- Failure to fulfill major obligations (person, professional, educational)
- Use during a time when physical harm may come to self or others
- Continued use despite persistent or recurrent problems caused or exacerbated by the effects of the substance

When rendering primary care, remember that substance abuse commonly means misuse of multiple agents, including alcohol, prescription drugs, and illegal agents. Many substance abusers have an underlying psychiatric problem such as a mood disorder. Substance abuse, including alcoholism, may be a method of self-treatment in patients with an undetected or untreated psychiatric illness.

Compared with men, women have higher rates of misuse of prescription medications, which is most likely caused by their more frequent use of the health care system. In addition, women are more likely to have disorders of mood, including anxiety and depression and, consequently, have potential drugs of abuse such as benzodiazepines prescribed by the primary care provider. However, benzodiazepine abuse is likely less common than perceived by prescribers who often fear that many patients receiving these anxiolytic agents will abuse or misuse the medications (Table 12–2). One issue that needs to be considered when prescribing benzodiazepines is the issue of their abuse and misuse. Indeed, prescribers often hesitate to use these highly effective agents because of fear of providing the patient with a potentially habituating drug with the possibility of needing increasing doses. In reality, psychological dependence does occur on occasion, but careful prescribing can help avoid this.

Psychological dependence on benzodiazepines is usually associated with a rapid-onset agent, one that possibly gives a sensation of intoxication. In addition, prescribing at dosing intervals beyond duration of action of the drug gives alternating periods of drug effect and withdrawal. The perception of difference is significant and possibly perceived as a buildup of unpleasant anxiety followed by a period of relief or rescue provided by the patient, with the cycle repeated with each drug dose. Interestingly, using a benzodiazepine as an "as-needed" product increases the likelihood of abuse because this heightens the patient's awareness of drug versus no-drug state. Psychological dependence on benzodiazepines can be avoided by using a slow-onset product with a long half-life, such as clonazepam. If using short-acting products, give adequate number of doses per day. If using on an as-needed basis, advise a maximum number of available or prescribed doses per week, such as 3 to 4 times per week rather than once or twice a day. This may help avoid benzodiazepine tolerance, a situation where the patient requires increasingly higher doses to reach therapeutic effect. Tolerance may lead to physical dependance.

Physical benzodiazepine dependence is a significant problem. When working with a patient to discontinue benzodiazepine use, consider reducing the dose by 25% per week. Rapid withdrawal can lead to tremors, hallucinations, seizures, and a delirium tremors-like state. The onset of withdrawal symptoms occurs a few days after the last dose in a benzodiazepine with a shorter half-life (e.g., lorazepam) and to up to 3 weeks in one with a longer half-life (e.g., clonazepam).

Benzodiazepines rarely cause hepatic or renal impairment. When taken alone in overdose, benzodiazepines have a rather favorable toxicity profile. However, sedation is enhanced when benzodiazepines are combined with alcohol and barbiturates, leading to a potentially life-threatening condition. Therefore, accidental and intentional fatalities often occur.

TABLE 12-2.
ANXIOLYTICS

Anxiolytic	Pharmacokinetics	Indications	Onset of Action	Comments
Buspirone (Buspar)	Slow onset of action (> 7 days), lipophilic, half-life of metabolite = 16 h	Generalized anxiety syndrome, social phobia May be used as adjunct in OCD, PTSD Less effective in panic disorder, acute anxiety Is not helpful in alcohol withdrawal	2–4 weeks for some relief of anxiety 4–5 weeks for full therapeutic effect	5-HT1A receptor site agonist, not a benzodiazepine Not effective as a PRN or sleep aid drug Nonsedating No tolerance, withdrawal syndrome No potentiation with alcohol Little abuse potential If anxiety is disabling, add short-term benzodiazepine while awaiting other agent's action
Lorazepam (Ativan)	Plasma peak in 1–6 h, about half as lipophilic as diazepam (Valium) No active metabolites Elimination half-life: 10–20 h	Generalized anxiety syndrome, social phobia, adjunct in OCD, PTSD, panic disorder Helpful in acute anxiety, alcohol withdrawal	Fairly slow onset of action, sustained effect	Benzodiazepine Abuse and habituation potential Upon discontinuation after long-term use, reduce dose by 25% per week to avoid withdrawal syndrome.

Oxazepam (Serax)	About half as lipophilic as diazepam, slower onset of action Plasma peak in 1–4 h No active metabolites Elimination half-life: 3–21 h	Generalized anxiety syndrome, social phobia, adjunct in OCD, PTSD, panic disorder Helpful in acute anxiety, alcohol withdrawal	Slow onset of action, relatively sustained effect	Benzodiazepine Abuse and habituation potential A good choice for anxious elderly patients because of short elimination half-life and lack of active metabolites
Alprazolam (Xanax)	Plasma peak in 1–2 h About half as lipophilic as diazepam Parent compound half-life: 12–15 h Active metabolite half as active as parent compound	Generalized anxiety syndrome, social phobia, adjunct in OCD, PTSD, panic disorder Helpful in acute anxiety, alcohol withdrawal	Slow onset of action, relatively sustained effect	Benzodiazepine Abuse and habituation potential Upon discontinuation after long term use, reduce dose by 25% per week to avoid withdrawal syndrome.

(continued)

TABLE 12-2. (continued)

Anxiolytic	Pharmacokinetics	Indications	Onset of Action	Comments
Clonazepam (Klonopin)	Plasma peak in 1–2 h About one-quarter as lipophilic as diazepam No active metabolites Elimination half-life: 18–50 h	Generalized anxiety syndrome, social phobia, adjunct in OCD, PTSD, panic disorder Helpful in acute anxiety, alcohol withdrawal Absence and petit mal seizures Anxiety and panic	Slow onset of action, highly sustained effect	Benzodiazepine Abuse and habituation potential Protracted half-life may pose a problem when used in the elderly Upon discontinuation after long term use, reduce dose by 25% per week to avoid withdrawal syndrome
Diazepam (Valium)	Plasma peak in 0.5–2.0 h Highly lipophilic Three active metabolites with various half-life Desmethyldiazepam: 30–200 h Oxazepam (Serax): 3–21 h 3-Hydroxydiazepam: 5–20 h	Generalized anxiety syndrome, social phobia, adjunct in OCD, PTSD, panic disorder Helpful in acute anxiety, alcohol withdrawal Anxiety Seizures Musculoskeletal pain	Rapid onset of action, relatively sustained effect	Benzodiazepine Abuse and habituation potential Protracted half-life may pose a problem when used in the elderly Upon discontinuation after long term use, reduce dose by 25% per week to avoid withdrawal syndrome

Maxmen, J., Ward, N. (1995). *Psychotropic Drugs Fast* (2nd edition). W. W. Norton and Company. New York. Pp. 255–312.

Opioid withdrawal shares many common characteristics with alcohol withdrawal. Hypertension, tachycardia, diarrhea, nausea, hyperthermia, restlessness, myalgia, lacrimation, and rhinorrhea are often reported. Although most distressing, the condition is not life-threatening and usually resolves within a few days. Clonidine, an alpha$_2$-adrenergic antagonist, helps minimize opioid withdrawal symptoms. As with any chemical dependence, long-term rehabilitation therapy is usually needed, necessitating a high level of patient desire for sobriety. The use of methadone, a long-acting opioid, may help curb the use of illegal drugs.

Marijuana has historically been considered a drug that has potential for psychological dependence but with little potential for physical addiction. For teens in many communities, its daily use is more common than that of alcohol. However, the marijuana currently used is potent because of its high tetrahydrocannabinol (THC) content. After a period of abstinence, physical withdrawal symptoms are often reported among daily marijuana users. Chronic marijuana use can lead to airway obstruction such as that found in heavy tobacco users. Driving and activities requiring concentration or physical skills show significant impairment during marijuana intoxication.

Cocaine is a potent sympathomimetic. With its use, the user has an increase in heart rate and myocardial contractility as well as generalized vasoconstriction, causing an increase in blood pressure. In addition, cocaine preferentially constricts the coronary and cerebral vessels, creating significant risk for cerebral ischemia and stroke as well as myocardial ischemia and infarction. Inquiring about chest pain is prudent in caring for a patient with cocaine abuse.

Flunitrazepam (Rohypnol) is a benzodiazepine, also know as Ruffies or the date rape drug. Particularly potent with a rapid onset of action, this product is not available for prescription use in North America. However, it is available and commonly used as a sleep aid in other countries. It had been misused, particularly on college campuses, as a drug given to reduce sexual inhibition, usually given without the knowledge of the recipient. Flunitrazepam's use is often associated with amnesia. Thus, sexual assault can take place, possibly without the victim's recalling the event.

Discussion Sources

Hektor Dunphy, L. (1999). *Management Guidelines for Adult Nurse Practitioners*. Philadelphia: FA Davis. Pp. 484–488.

Gold, M. (1998). Drug abuse. In *Conn's Current Therapy* (50th ed.). Philadelphia: WB Saunders. Pp. 1123–1132.

QUESTIONS

14. Which of the following is true concerning anorexia nervosa?

    A. It affects men and women equally.
    B. Onset is usually in the mid-twenties for both men and women.
    C. Depression is often found concomitantly.
    D. Individuals with anorexia nervosa are aware of the extreme thinness associated with the disease.

15. Treatment for anorexia nervosa often includes:

    A. referral for parenteral nutrition evaluation
    B. antidepressant therapy
    C. use of psychostimulants
    D. psychoanalysis

16. Physical examination findings in patients with bulimia nervosa typically include

    A. obesity
    B. dental surface erosion
    C. tachycardia
    D. easily pluckable hair

17. Which of the following is most consistent with the diagnosis of bulimia nervosa?

    A. Patients with bulimia nervosa usually present asking for treatment.
    B. Periods of anorexia may occur.
    C. Hyperkalemia often results from laxative abuse.
    D. Most patients with bulimia nervosa are significantly obese.

18. All of the following pharmacologic interventions are used in the treatment of patients with bulimia nervosa except:

    A. fluoxetine (Prozac)
    B. desipramine (Norpramin)
    C. bupropion (Wellbutrin)
    D. paxil (Paroxetine)

ANSWERS

14. C
15. B
16. B
17. B
18. C

DISCUSSION

Aorexia nervosa is a potentially life-threatening disease. DSM IV criteria for anorexia nervosa includes

- An inability or refusal to maintain body weight
- 85% of normal weight for age and height
- Intense fear of gaining weight and becoming fat despite low body weight
- A disturbance in perception of body weight and shape.

A denial of seriousness of the low body weight is often found in patients with anorexia nervosa. Often despite extreme thinness, a patient with anorexia nervosa will look in the mirror and comment on the need to lose "just a few more pounds." Amenorrhea common in patients with anorexia nervosa contributes to establishing the diagnosis. The usual onset of anorexia nervosa in women is during the teens to early twenties, with ages 14 and 18 years being the most common; men present a few years later. This is an overwhelmingly female disease (90%), with either gender often involved in an activity that has an emphasis on weight and shape. These include wrestling, modeling, dancing, gymnastics, and swimming.

Those with anorexia nervosa usually demonstrate one of two types of behavior. With the restricting type, a patient with anorexia nervosa severely limits food intake but does not use binge eating or purging. In the binge-purging type, a patient with anorexia nervosa has cycles of these behaviors.

Unlike bulimia nervosa, which is a secretive disease with relatively few findings, anorexia nervosa is usually easy to identify clinically. Besides the marked reduction in weight, muscle wasting; abdominal distention with hepatomegaly; cheilosis; oral and gum disease; coarse, dry skin; and hypotension with bradycardia and hypothermia are common.

Treating anorexia nervosa usually includes cognitive-behavioral as well as pharmacologic therapy. In cognitive-behavioral therapy, the focus is the disturbed eating and the patterns of thinking that help perpetuated the binge-purge cycle. To be effective, a clinician who is expert in eating disorders should provide this form of treatment.

Pharmacologic therapy usually involves the use of antidepressants, which may have an effect because of the high rate of comorbid depression. All antidepressants can be used. The choice of a specific agent should be guided by the principles used in choosing therapy in the treatment of depression. Benzodiazepines are also sometimes used to reduce anxiety associated with eating. Cyproheptadine (Periactin) may be used before meals to enhance appetite and reduce anxiety.

Bulimia nervosa is more common in women and typically is present for many years before the patient presents for treatment or before the disorder is noted by a health care provider. Because this tends to be a secretive disease, few with bulimia nervosa present directly requesting intervention.

According to DSM IV criteria, a patient with bulimia nervosa has episodes of binge eating characterized by eating excessive quantities of food in a discrete period, such as 2 hours. During this period, the patient feels a lack of control over the eating for both the amount and type of food ingested. In addition, there is a recurrent compensatory behavior used to prevent excessive weight gain from a binge, such as self-induced vomiting, excessive exercise, laxative or diuretic abuse, or fasting. Body weight and shape excessively influence self-worth.

Bulimia nervosa may be identified in the clinical setting by problems with erosion of the lingual surface of the upper teeth because of excessive exposure to gastric contents during induced vomiting, hypokalemia caused by laxative and diuretic use, and ipecac-induced cardiomyopathy. Body weight provides few clues because a patient is typically of average to slightly above average weight.

Treatment of a patient with bulimia nervosa usually includes cognitive-behavioral as well as pharmacologic therapy. In cognitive-behavioral therapy, the focus is the disturbed eating and the thinking patterns that help perpetuate the binge-purge cycle. To be effective, a clinician who is expert in eating disorders should provide this form of treatment.

Pharmacologic therapy usually involves the use of antidepressants. This is usually highly successful in reducing both the frequency and amount of binges, in part because of their activity at the 5-HT1A-receptor site. All antidepressants can be used except for bupropion (Wellbutrin), which may induce further bingeing or seizures in patients with bulimia nervosa. The choice of a specific agent should be guided by the principles used in choosing depression therapy. Fluoxetine has been extensively studied and used in treating patients with bulimia nervosa.

Discussion Sources

Hektor Dunphy, L. (1999). *Management Guidelines for Adult Nurse Practitioners*. Philadelphia: FA Davis. Pp. 488–493.
Walsh, B.T. (1998). Bulimia nervosa. In *Conn's Current Therapy* (50th ed.). Philadelphia: WB Saunders. Pp. 1135–1137.

QUESTIONS

19. Which patient presentation is most consistent with the diagnosis of depression?

    A. recurrent diarrhea and cramping
    B. difficulty initiating sleep
    C. diminished cognitive ability
    D. consistent early morning wakening

20. Of the following in need of antidepressant, who is the best candidate for fluoxetine (Prozac) therapy?

    A. an 80-year-old woman with depressed mood 1 year after the death of her husband
    B. a 45-year-old man with mild hepatic dysfunction
    C. a 28-year-old woman who occasionally "skips a dose" of her pre- scribed medication
    D. a 44-year-old woman with decreased appetite

21. In caring for the elderly, an NP considers that all of the following is true except:

    A. Many older patients with dementia have a component of depres- sion.
    B. Dementia signs and symptoms usually evolve over months, but depression has a more rapid onset.
    C. With dementia, a patient is aware of difficulties with cognitive ability.
    D. Treating concurrent depression may help improve symptoms of dementia.

22. Which of the following is most consistent with the diagnosis of dysthymia?

    A. a 23-year-old man with a 2-month episode of depressed mood after a job loss
    B. a 45-year-old woman with "jitteriness" and difficulty initiating sleep for the past 6 months
    C. a 38-year-old woman with fatigue and anhedonia for the past 2 years
    D. a 15-year-old boy with a school adjustment problem and weekend marijuana use for the past year

23. Drug treatment options for a patient with bipolar disorder typically include all of the following except:

    A. fluoxetine (Prozac)
    B. lithium
    C. carbamazepine (Tegretol)
    D. valproic acid (Depakote)

24. Which of the following drugs is likely to be the most dangerous when taken in overdose?

    A. a 4-week supply of fluoxetine
    B. a 2-week supply of nortriptyline
    C. a 3-week supply of nefazodone
    D. a 3-day supply of diazepam

25. One week into sertraline (Zoloft) therapy, a patient complains of a recurrent dull frontal headache that is relieved with acetaminophen. Which of the following is true in this situation?

    A. This is a common, transient side effect of selective serotonin reuptake inhibitor (SSRI) therapy.
    B. She should discontinue the medication.
    C. Fluoxetine should be substituted.
    D. Desipramine should be added.

26. A patient has been taking fluoxetine for 1 week and complains of mild nausea and diarrhea. You advise that:

    A. This is a common, long-lasting side effect of SSRI therapy.
    B. He should discontinue the medication.
    C. Luvox should be substituted.
    D. He should be taking the medication with food.

27. Which of the following medications is most likely to cause sexual dysfunction?

    A. nefazadone (Serzone)

    B. fluoxetine (Prozac)

    C. nortriptyline

    D. bupropion (Wellbutrin)

28. SSRI withdrawal syndrome is best characterized as:

    A. bothersome but not life threatening

    B. potentially life threatening

    C. most often seen with agents that have a long half-life

    D. associated with seizure risk

29. Which of the following is most consistent with the presentation of a patient with bipolar I disorder?

    A. increased need for sleep

    B. impulsive behavior

    C. fatigue

    D. anhedonia

30. According to the Agency for Health Care Policy and Research (AHCPR) treatment guidelines, pharmacologic intervention for patients with depression should:

    A. generally be given for about 4 to 6 months

    B. continue for at least 6 months after remission is achieved

    C. be continued indefinitely with a first episode of depression

    D. be titrated to a lower dose after symptom relief is achieved

ANSWERS

19. D
20. C
21. C
22. C
23. A
24. B
25. A
26. D

27. B
28. A
29. B
30. B

DISCUSSION

Depression is a common health problem with a minimum of 15% lifetime occurrence rate. DMS IV criteria for depression includes the presence of the particular symptoms and findings for more than 2 weeks. There must be a disorder in mood, usually with diurnal variation, with morning being the worst with a lack of interest present. Five or more of the following symptoms must be present:

- Problems with sleep: Initiating sleep usually is not a problem; rather, early morning wakening is the issue
- Change in appetite: Decreased appetite with loss of food enjoyment common
- Low energy: Fatigue is nearly universal
- Loss of interest in life and in usually enjoyable activities and events (anhedonia)
- A change in cognition
- Lack of motivation

Depression is sometimes mistaken for new-onset dementia. However, a patient with dementia typically has cognitive changes that are slowly progressive over months to years. The cognitive changes reported by patients with depression have usually evolved over a much shorter period.

Other symptoms of depression are often reported. Hypochondria is found in about 30% of patients; such patients are unable to process objective information that he or she has no health problems. Suicidal thoughts are often present, most often passive ideas without a plan. The patient often agrees with the statement "If I could just die in my sleep, it would be all right." As with anyone with suicidal ideation, a thorough safety evaluation should be completed.

Anxiety is often reported by the depressed person and is an important differential diagnosis. However, in depression patients, mood disturbance occurs first, followed in a number of weeks by the addition of anxiety-related symptoms. Consider depression as the diagnosis rather than anxiety if the patient reports feeling worse while taking benzodiazepines.

Psychomotor agitation with fidgeting and irritability is often found in patients with depression, especially in children and adolescents. In these age groups, this presentation is more likely than psychomotor retardation. This type of increased activity is also found in type A adults with depression.

Intervention for patients with depression includes a combination of support, counseling, and antidepressants. Interpersonal therapy, including counseling and support, alone has a 40–60% efficacy with high relapse. As a single therapeutic modality, this is most effective for those with reactive depression. Combined therapy of pharmacologic intervention along with interpersonal therapy allows the patient to have effective therapy for what is now recognized as a biochemical disorder while acquiring the cognitive skills that are helpful in dealing with what is often a chronic, relapsing condition.

Dysthymia is found in approximately 3% of the general population and is characterized by low-level daily depression with at least of two of the previously identified depressive symptoms for at least 2 years in adults and 1 year in children. As with those who are depressed, patients with dysthymia respond well to a combination of interpersonal and pharmacologic intervention. In fact, a patient who reports a life-changing feeling with antidepressant use, often described as, "feeling good to be alive for the first time," is likely dysthymic. The person's underlying personality emerges after being suppressed or altered by the debilitating effects of the low-level depression that characterizes dysthymia.

Depressed mood may follow a significant life stressor such as death of a loved one or loss of a job. If criteria for depression last longer than 3 months after the precipitating event, the diagnosis of major depression should be considered. Treatment for adjustment disorder with depressed mood lasting beyond 3 months is the same as that for major depression, recognizing that interpersonal therapy can be highly effective in assisting patients in dealing with loss.

Eighty percent of all antidepressant prescriptions are written by primary care providers, making the acquisition of skill in prescribing these helpful medications crucial to practice. All prescription antidepressants are about equally effective if taken in therapeutic doses for sufficient lengths of time. However, primary care providers tend to underdose antidepressants and prescribe the product for an insufficient length of therapy. The AHCPR offers guidelines for length of therapy (Box 12–4). Long-term antidepressant therapy should be considered when there is a high risk of depression relapse (Box 12–5).

When prescribing an antidepressant, encourage psychotherapy to work on skills building needed to help manage this usually long-term

---

BOX 12-4
LENGTH OF PHARMACOLOGIC INTERVENTION FOR PATIENTS WITH DEPRESSION PER AHCPR GUIDELINES

A minimum of 6 to 9 months therapy total

- Acute phase treatment to bring symptoms under control and into remission; lasts up to 3 months
- Continue medication for a minimum of 6 months after depression remission achieved
- Relapse highest in first 2 months after discontinuation of therapy
- With more than two episodes, 80% relapse in 1 year without treatment
- Consider maintenance therapy as with any chronic illness

Adapted from Health Care Policy and Research (1993) Depression in Primary Care. Vol. 2. Available at http://text.nlm.nih.gov/ftrs/gateway

---

BOX 12-5
RISKS IN DEPRESSION RELAPSE

- Dysthymia preceding episode
- Poor recovery between episodes
- Current episode > 2 years
- Onset depression < age 20 years, > 50 years
- Family history of depression
- Severe symptoms such as suicide and psychosis

---

health problem. In particular, convey the message to the patient that the use of antidepressants can help facilitate therapy.

When choosing an antidepressant, the prescriber should ask the following questions:

- What has worked in the past? Unless now contraindicated, this is should be the agent of choice.
- What has worked for relatives? Besides having heard positive comments about the medication from family members, certain medications appear to have greater activity at given serotonin receptor sites. Relatives often have similar serotonin receptor site activity.

- What are the most bothersome signs and symptoms of the depression? Choose an antidepressant with activity against these, or at minimum, one that will not make these worse. For example, if insomnia and anxiety bother a depressed person, using a highly energizing SSRI is a poor choice (Table 12–3).

When choosing an antidepressant, the side effect profile is critical. Often a given agent has a desirable side effect, such as sedation in a patient having difficulty with sleep or anxiety (Table 12–4). In addition, the drug's half-life influences the therapeutic choice, with shorter half-life products being desirable in the elderly and in the presence of hepatic disease.

Another consideration in choosing an antidepressant is its toxicity when taken in overdose. The suicidal patient clearly needs hospitalization to ensure safety and appropriate treatment. However, as with many disease states, depression is a disease with episodes of improvement and deterioration. Therefore, the prescriber should consider the risk of an intentional overdose.

A 2-week supply of a tricyclic antidepressant (TCA) in full therapeutic dose will likely be lethal, with significantly smaller amounts capable of causing seizures and dysrhythmias. In comparison, the SSRIs and atypical antidepressants have a significantly better safety profile when taken in overdose: usually more than a 2-month supply of a full therapeutic dose is needed to cause life-threatening effects (see Table 12–3).

When antidepressants are taken by a patient who is depressed and undergoing an ongoing significant life stressor, such as family or marital discord or abuse, depressive symptoms usually subside as the medication takes effect. However, if the stressor continues, the antidepressant may appear to lose its initial effectiveness. Ongoing interpersonal therapy can be highly effective in augmenting pharmacologic treatment in such situations.

Antidepressants generally work by causing an increase in availability of select neurotransmitters, such as serotonin, norepinephrine, and dopamine. This allows for greater activity at the neurotransmitter's respective receptor sites. Interestingly, there is evidence that interpersonal therapy also increases serotonin availability.

The SSRIs are a heterogenous group of drugs with a common mechanism of action, blocking reuptake of serotonin in the central nervous system and increasing amounts of serotonin available to postsynaptic neuron. The end effect is that more serotonin is available for action at select receptors. Serotonin is active at a number of receptor sites (Table 12–5).

With all antidepressants, receptor site–induced effect is immediate when therapy is initiated. However, the length of onset of therapeutic action is usually a number of weeks. This length of onset is likely associated

TABLE 12–3.
THE SELECTIVE SEROTONIN REUPTAKE INHIBITORS (SSRIS)

SSRI	Half-life	Labeled Indications	Adverse Reaction Profile	Comments
Paxil (Paroxetine)	26 h No active metabolites	Panic disorder, depression, OCD	Rather sedating (HS dosing likely best) Some anticholinergic effect More constipation (13%) than diarrhea (11%) Antihistamine-like activity may increase appetite	Helpful in anxious depression Elimination via renal and hepatic routes Less problem with limited renal or hepatic function Low mania induction in bipolar With relatively short half-life and lack of active metabolites, helpful in treating depression in the elderly
Fluvoxamine (Luvox)	16 h No active metabolites	Depression, panic disorder, OCD	High rate of nausea (40%) and insomnia (21%)	Commonly used in treating OCD
Sertraline (Zoloft)	25–65 h Metabolite half-life = 52–102 h	Depression panic disorder, OCD	Equal numbers find it sedating and energizing Low rate of nervousness, anorexia	Take with food to enhance absorption

Citalopram (Celexa)	Parent compound half-life = 24–48 h Metabolite half-life = 2 days for one, 4 days for another	Depression	Equal numbers report somnolence and insomnia (18%) 21% nausea rate Low rates of agitation and anorexia	Used outside the United States for many years
Prozac (Fluoxetine)	24–72 h Metabolite half-life $t_{1/2} = 4\text{–}16$ days	Depression, OCD, bulimia nervosa	Energizing Anorexia common	AM dosing recommended Protracted half-life may present problem in elderly Missed doses less of problem because of protracted half-life ~3–5-lb weight loss common in first months of use

Maxmen, J., Ward, N. (1995). *Psychotropic Drugs Fast* (2nd edition). W. W. Norton and Company. New York. Pp. 77–143.

TABLE 12–4.
THE ATYPICAL TRICYCLICS AND TETRACYCLIC ANTIDEPRESSANTS

Agent	Half-life	Adverse Reactions	Comments
Nefazadone (Serzone)	4 h	Low anxiety, insomnia rate Excellent GI side effect profile Low rate of nausea, diarrhea Problems with somnolence, dry mouth, dizziness Take with food for slower absorption and less drowsiness Excellent sexual function profile	Inhibits neuron reuptake of serotonin and norepinephrine 5-HT2 antagonist Antidepressant and anxiolytic agent Alternative for SSRI nonresponder or when SSRI sexual dysfunction an issue
Venlafaxine (Effexor)	5 h (4–24 h)	Stimulating in higher doses. May need trazodone or other agent to help with sleep Significant nausea with rapid onset of high dose Dose-dependent increases in DBP: Average response of 5mmHg	Serotonin, Norepinephrine and Dopamine effect, especially at higher doses Withdrawal syndrome similar to that of SSRIs

| Bupropion (Wellbutrin) | 9.8 h (3.9–24 h) | Few anticholinergic effects
Energizing
Possible increased libido, agitation (25%)
Avoid with significant manifestation of anxiety, agitation, insomnia | Possibly blocks reuptake of dopamine at the presynaptic neuron, especially in high doses, some increase in norepinephrine transmission
Dopamine receptor sites are likely stimulated in substance abuse, making bupropion a helpful antidepressant for patients with a history of substance abuse
Nonaddicting and nonintoxicating
Avoid use in presence of eating disorder or if anorexia is a major component of the depression
Weight loss often seen (28% > 5 lb) after initiation of therapy
Do not give if history of or risk for seizure, closed-head injury history, history of quiescent epilepsy
Seizure risk worsens if dose increased rapidly |
| Mirtazapine (Remeron) | | Potent H$_1$ inhibitors
Weight gain common
Major side effect is sedation that is worse in lower doses
Little sexual dysfunction or GI side effect | A designer antidepressant
Effect likely caused by increase in central noradrenergic and serotonergic activity
Selectively stimulates 5-HT1A while blocking 5-HT2 and 5-HT3
Higher doses more receptor site selective and associated with fewer side effects |

(continued)

TABLE 12–4. (continued)

Agent	Half-life	Adverse Reactions	Comments
TCAs (-ine suffix; Includes nortriptyline [Pamelor, active precursor of amitriptyline], desipramine [Norpramin, active metabolic of imipramine])	24–32 h	Weight gain Anticholinergic activity (blurred vision, dry mouth, memory loss, sweating, anxiety, postural hypotension, dizziness, and tachycardia) Constipation is a problem but infrequent Nausea Little sexual dysfunction	Inexpensive More effective than SSRIs in more severe depression, likely because of its norepinephrine as well as serotonin activity More bothersome side-effect profile leads to high dropout rate Primary care providers seldom prescribe sufficient doses to relieve depression Wean off over 2–4 weeks to avoid TCA withdrawal symptoms: sleep disturbance, nightmares, GI upset, malaise, irritability
Trazodone	5h (3–9 h)	Highly sedating, dizziness, favorable GI side-effect profile Priapism risk found in 1 in 6000 males using drug Patient should be informed to go to ED promptly for painful erection > 30 minutes Frequent issue in litigation	Anxiolytic and antidepressant activity 5-HT2 antagonist Clinical use limited by marked sedation Effective hypnotic with little AM drowsiness at 25–100 mg at HS May use in low, frequent doses as benzodiazepine alternative for generalized anxiety

Adapted from Maxmen, J., Ward, N. (1995). *Psychotropic Drugs Fast* (2nd Edition). W. W. Norton and Company. New York. Pp. 77–143.

TABLE 12–5.
SEROTONIN ACTIVITY

Serotonin Receptor Sites	Activity When Stimulated	Comments
5-HT1A	Antidepressant, anti-OCD behavior, antipanic, antisocial phobia action, antibulimia effect	Action at this site is the basis of most antidepressant, antipanic therapy Reason that shyness often lifts with SSRI use
5-HT1C, 5-HT 2C	Influence cerebrospinal fluid production, cerebral circulation Regulation of sleep Perception of pain Cardiovascular function	Reason tachycardia, dizziness, alteration of sleep patterns and change in pain perception occurs with SSRI use
5-HT1D	Antimigraine activity	Triptan preparation such as Sumatriptan (Imitrex) work by stimulating this receptor site TCAs also agonize this site and are therefore helpful in preventing migraine headache
5-HT2	Agitation, akathisia, anxiety, panic, insomnia, sexual dysfunction Excessively unregulated in those with depression	Receptor site highly stimulated in activating SSRIs such as fluoxetine Activity at this receptor site causes sexual dysfunction associated with SSRI use Nefazodone (Serzone) and trazodone (Desyrel) antagonize action at this site and are helpful in treating anxious depression
5-HT3	When stimulated, nausea, GI distress, diarrhea, headache	Particularly stimulated with antidepressants with poor GI side-effect profile Products such as Zofran (a 5-HT3 antagonist) block activity at this site

with time needed for change in receptor site activity. A withdrawal syndrome may be seen with SSRI use longer than 5 weeks when the product is rapidly discontinued. In SSRI withdrawal syndrome, there is a sudden change in the amount of serotonin available and an alteration in receptor site action. Its onset is related to the half-life of the drug, with 5 to 7 half-lives before the drug clears fully. Therefore, symptoms occur more rapidly after SSRI discontinuation with a drug with a short half-life and may not occur at all in one with a protracted half-life (e.g., fluoxetine).

Symptoms of SSRI withdrawal syndrome include dizziness, paresthesia, anxiety, nausea, sleep disturbance, and insomnia. Although disturbing and uncomfortable, this syndrome, unlike benzodiazepine withdrawal, is not dangerous or life threatening, generally resolving within days to a few weeks.

In early SSRI therapy, the patient often complains of drug-related side effects; these resolve within 2 to 6 weeks and include headache, nausea, and diarrhea. Advising the patient that these are easily treatable and expected, yet transient, problems helps avoid the problem of self-discontinuation of this important therapeutic agent. The headache is usually frontal in location and resolves with acetaminophen. Using a nonsteroidal anti-inflammatory drug (NSAID) may contribute further to the gastrointestinal upset often found in the first weeks of SSRI use. Taking the medication with food can minimize nausea and diarrhea. Taking any medication with an antacid may limit its effectiveness.

Use of SSRIs is often associated with sexual function problems. Decreased libido, anorgasmy, and erectile dysfunction are often reported. If this is a problem, switching the patient to an atypical antidepressant or TCA may be indicated because the use of these products is much less often associated with sexual dysfunction.

The TCAs are a group of helpful but often misunderstood and underused medications. The TCAs have a more problematic side effect profile compared with the SSRIs. In addition, they require considerable prescriber skill and patient cooperation. These medications are likely superior to the SSRIs when depression is moderate to severe and characterized by emotional withdrawal, guilt, anorexia, and middle to late insomnia. In addition, they are effective in depressed patients who also have chronic pain, fibromyalgia, migraine, or the need for sedative or hypnotic agents. Choosing a TCA (e.g., nortriptyline [Pamelor] or desipramine [Norpramin]) with less anticholinergic effect and slowly increasing the dose helps enhance patient adherence.

If a patient with depression also has episodes of mania, bipolar I disorder is present. Bipolar disorders occur in approximately 1% of the general population. In bipolar I disorder, the patient usually presents with cycles of elevated or irritated mood lasting longer than 1 week. As part of this, reports of marked diminished sleep need ("2 to 3 hours, and I am just fine") are the norm. When such patients are interviewed, grandiosity, flight of ideas, pressured speech, and distractibility are evident. Bipolar I disorder is most common in women, with an onset around puberty.

If a patient with depression has episodes of mania lasting less than 4 days with little social incapacitation, the diagnosis of bipolar II disorder is made. In patients with bipolar II disorder, the episodes of mania are relatively mild (hypomania) and may be rather productive in contrast to the low point of depression.

Further descriptors of bipolar disease include rapid cycling and cyclothymic disorder. In rapid-cycle bipolar disorder, there are four or more hypomanic manic, mixed, or major depressive episodes in a 1-year period. In cyclothymic disorder, the mood disorder has been present for at least 2 years with episodes of mania lasting less than 4 days, too brief to fit standard criteria of mania or hypomania. If a TCA is given to a person with bipolar disorder, approximately 15% will develop mania. This may also happen when an energizing SSRI such as fluoxetine is given.

Discussion Sources

Dunner, D. (1998). Mood disorders. In *Conn's Current Therapy* (50th ed.). Philadelphia: WB Saunders. Pp. 1141–1148.

Hektor Dunphy, L. (1999). *Management Guidelines for Adult Nurse Practitioners.* Philadelphia: FA Davis. Pp. 494–496.

Landis, B. J., Bryant, S. (1999). Mental health disorders. In Youngkin, E., Sawin, K., Kissinger, J., & Israel, D., *Pharmacotherapeutics: A Primary Care Clinical Guide.* Stamford, CT: Appleton & Lange. Pp. 747–800.

QUESTIONS

31. Which of the following is most consistent with the diagnosis of anxiety?

    A. nausea

    B. difficulty initiating sleep

    C. diminished cognitive ability

    D. consistent early morning wakening

32. When prescribing a benzodiazepine, the NP considers that:

    A. The drugs are virtually interchangeable, with similar durations of action and therapeutic effect.

    B. The onset of therapeutic effect is usually rapid.

    C. These drugs have a low abuse potential in substance abusers.

    D. The elderly may use doses similar to those needed by younger adults.

33. Buspirone (Buspar) has:

    A. low abuse potential
    B. significant antidepressant action
    C. a withdrawal syndrome when discontinued, similar to the benzo-
       diazepines
    D. rapid onset of action

34. A 24-year-old woman has a new onset of panic disorder. As part
    of her clinical presentation, you expect to find all of following, *except*:

    A. peak symptoms at 10 minutes into the panic attack
    B. history of agoraphobia
    C. report of chest pain during panic attack
    D. history of thought disorder

35. As you develop the treatment plan for the patient in Question 34, you
    consider prescribing:

    A. carbemazipine (Tegretol)
    B. risperidone (Risperdal)
    C. paroxetine (Paxil)
    D. bupropion (Wellbutrin)

36. Diagnostic criteria for generalized anxiety disorder includes all of the
    following except:

    A. difficulty concentrating
    B. consistent early morning wakening
    C. apprehension
    D. irritability

37. Which of the following is often reported by anxious patients?

    A. constipation
    B. muscle tension
    C. hive-form rash
    D. somnolence

38. According to the AHCPR treatment guidelines, pharmacologic inter-
    vention in anxiety should be:

    A. generally given for about 4 to 6 months
    B. continued for at least 6 months after remission is achieved
    C. continued indefinitely with a first episode of anxiety
    D. titrate to a lower dose after symptom relief is achieved

39. The use of which of the following drugs often mimics generalized anxiety disorder?

    A. sympathomimetics
    B. benzodiazepines
    C. anticholinergics
    D. alpha beta antagonists

40. When prescribing a benzodiazepine, an NP should consider that:

    A. The ingestion of as little as 3 to 4 day's therapeutic dose can be life threatening.
    B. The medication must be taken at the same hour every day.
    C. Concomitant use of alcohol should be avoided.
    D. Onset of therapeutic effect takes a number of days.

41. A middle-aged woman who has taken therapeutic dose of lorazepam for the past 6 years wishes to stop taking the medication. You advise her that:

    A. She may discontinue the drug immediately if she thinks it no longer helps with her symptoms.
    B. Rapid withdrawal in this situation can lead to tremors and hallucinations.
    C. She should taper down the dose of the medication over the next week.
    D. Gastrointestinal upset is typically reported during the first week of benzodiazepine withdrawal.

42. Risk of benzodiazepine misuse is minimized by use of:

    A. agents with a shorter half-life
    B. the drug as an as-needed rescue medication for acute anxiety
    C. more lipophilic products
    D. products with long durations of action

43. Concomitant health problems found in a patient with panic disorder often include:

    A. irritable bowel syndrome
    B. thought disorders
    C. hypothyroidism
    D. *Helicobacter pylori* colonization

44. In providing primary care for a patient with posttraumatic stress disorder (PTSD), you consider that all of the following will likely be reported except:

A. agoraphobia
B. feeling of detachment
C. hyperarousal
D. poor recall of the precipitating event

45. Preferred pharmacologic treatment options for patients with PTSD include:

A. methylphenidate (Ritalin)
B. oxazepam (Serax)
C. lithium carbonate
D. buspirone (Buspar)

46. Which of the following medications is used to assist in treating irritability and impulsivity often found in patients with PTSD?

A. carbamezepine
B. trazodone
C. kava kava
D. diazepam

47. Which of the following is an over-the-counter herbal preparation used to relieve symptoms of depression?

A. valerian root
B. melatonin
C. kava kava
D. St. John's wort

48. Patients with treatment-resistant panic disorder may respond to the use of:

A. imipramine
B. bupropion
C. clonidine
D. a monoamine oxidase inhibitor (MAOI)

49. In treating a person with panic disorder using a SSRI, an NP should consider that there is:

A. considerable abuse potential with the medications
B. no significant therapeutic advantage over the TCAs
C. a reduction in number and severity of panic attacks
D. significant toxicity in overdose

ANSWERS

31. B
32. B
33. A
34. D
35. C
36. B
37. B
38. B
39. A
40. C
41. B
42. D
43. A
44. D
45. D
46. A
47. D
48. D
49. C

DISCUSSION

Anxiety is a normal human emotion that is an important part of fear response. It helps a patient focus on the issue at hand, such as anxiety associated with taking an important examination or making a presentation. Anxiety can also be protective, heightening senses when an individual encounters a dangerous situation. It should be a rational, expected emotion when present for appropriate reason and should dissipate with the cessation of the stressor. However, anxiety becomes problematic when it is exaggerated, prolonged, or interferes with daily function.

Generalized anxiety disorder (GAD) is present in approximately 2–4% of the population. The typical age of onset is usually in the teen to young adult years; 15% have a first-degree relative with GAD. DMS IV criteria for GAD include the following:

- Excessive anxiety or worry, despite information to the contrary. This must be present on most days for at least 6 months.

- A report of difficulty controlling worry, with physical or mental distress causing impairment in social or occupational function.
- These problems cannot be attributed to use of medications or alcohol, disease, or other conditions.
- The above-mentioned criteria are associated with three or more of the following: muscle tension, restlessness, fatigue, difficulty concentrating, irritability, difficulty initiating sleep.

Anxiety often occurs in patients with depression, making the differentiation between these two common disorders problematic. However, a patient with depression that has an anxious component usually reports nervous feelings after the onset of depressed mood. Also in depression, the patient has feelings of worthlessness and the feeling that situations are hopeless; patients with anxiety often report feeling "worried sick" and helpless.

The cardinal presenting signs of anxiety disorder are related to the hypersympathetic state. Physical manifestations include tachycardia, hyperventilation, palpitations, tremors, and sweating. Therefore, when establishing the diagnosis of GAD, it is important to rule out a number of clinical conditions that can mimic the disorder, including thyroid toxicosis, alcohol withdrawal, or abuse of sympathomimetic drugs such as caffeine, amphetamines, and cocaine.

Treatment recommendations for pharmacologic intervention in anxiety disorders are similar to the AHCPR guidelines for depression. You should begin with a 3-month trial period of working with the patient to find the correct medication and dose that help abate symptoms. Encourage psychotherapy to work on skills building needed to help manage a long-term health problem. In particular, convey the message to the patient that the use of anxiolytic agents can help facilitate therapy. This acute care phase should be followed with a 6- to 12-month maintenance period, although longer-term therapy should be considered, especially if symptoms recur.

Choice of a therapeutic agent is guided by a number of factors, including asking about what has worked in the past and what has worked in the treatment of relatives with similar conditions.

Neurotransmitters implicated in anxiety include GABA, the brain's major inhibitory chemical, and serotonin (5-HT). Norepinephrine, dopamine, and epinephrine likely play a role as well. Drug therapy for patients with anxiety disorders includes agents that enhance GABA function, such as the benzodiazepines, and products that enhance the availability of serotonin, such as the SSRIs.

The benzodiazepines' mechanism of action is as a mediator of GABA, enhancing its activity. Benzodiazepines are highly effective in the treatment of anxiety disorders. Given that a number of benzodiazepines are available, choosing the appropriate agent may appear to be a daunting task. However, critical differences can be found in these agents. Some agents, such as diazepam (Valium), are more lipophilic, entering the brain more rapidly and igniting an effect promptly. Although this may appear to be a desired therapeutic effect for severely anxious patients, this rapid ignition can also be rather intoxicating. More-hydrophilic benzodiazepines such as lorazepam give reasonable therapeutic effect while having a slower onset of action and tend to be less intoxicating. In addition, with a highly lipophilic agent, excess is stored in body fat; this leaves a large repository for the drug and gives a longer half-life.

As with any drug, the half-life should be considered. Products such as diazepam and clonazepam with a long half-life give sustained effect without periods of withdrawal. With a shorter half-life, such as with oxazepam (Serax), therapeutic gaps can occur. However, the use of drugs with a shorter half-life without active metabolites should be considered when treating the elderly.

One issue that needs to be considered when prescribing benzodiazepines is their abuse and misuse. Indeed, prescribers often hesitate to use these highly effective agents because of fear of providing the patient with a potentially habituating drug with the possibility of needing increasing doses. In reality, psychological dependence does occur on occasion, but careful prescribing can help avoid this.

Psychological benzodiazepine dependence is usually associated with a rapid-onset agent, possibly giving a sensation of intoxication. In addition, prescribing at dosing intervals beyond the duration of action of the drug gives alternating periods of drug effect and withdrawal. The perception of difference is significant and possibly perceived as a buildup of unpleasant anxiety followed by a period of relief or rescue provided by the patient, with the cycle repeated with each drug dose. Interestingly, using a benzodiazepine as an as-needed product increases the likelihood of abuse because this heightens the patient's awareness of drug versus no-drug state. Psychological benzodiazepine dependency can be avoided by using a slow-onset product such as clonazepam that has a long half-life. If using short-acting products, give adequate number of doses per day. If using on an as-needed basis, advise a maximum number of available or prescribed doses per week such as 3 to 4 times per week rather than once or twice a day. Increasing tolerance to high therapeutic dose, usually at a level 2 to 4 times the prescribed level, creates physical dependence on benzodiazepines.

When taken alone in overdose, benzodiazepines have a rather favorable toxicity profile. However, sedation is enhanced when benzodiazepines are combined with alcohol and barbiturates, leading to a potentially life-threatening condition. As a result, accidental and intentional fatalities often occur.

Physical benzodiazepine dependence is a significant problem. When working with the patient to discontinue benzodiazepine use, consider reducing the dose by 25% per week. Rapid withdrawal can lead to tremors, hallucinations, seizures, and a delirium tremors-like state. Onset occurs a few days after the last dose in a benzodiazepine with a shorter half-life (e.g., lorazepam) to up to 3 weeks in one with a longer half-life (e.g., clonazepam).

Panic disorder affects 2–4% of the general population. Average age of onset is age 27 years; new onset is rare after age 45 years. There is a strong comorbidity with depression. The female-to-male ratio for panic disorder is approximately 1:1 if seen without agoraphobia. However, panic disorder with agoraphobia is decidedly more common in women, outnumbering men two to one. A strong family history of agoraphobia is often also reported.

DSM IV criteria for panic disorder includes a history of at least one attack followed by at least 1 month of worry about an additional attack, pondering implications of attacks or significant change of behavior related to attack.

The panic attack is central to panic disorder. This is a period of intense fear or discomfort developing abruptly and peaking within 10 minutes with at least four characteristic symptoms present. Panic attack symptoms include palpitations, tachycardia, sweating, trembling, shortness of breath, choking, chest pain, chills, nausea, dizziness, and a sensation of de-realization and depersonalization. Additional symptoms include fear of losing control or dying, paresthesia, and hot flashes. In addition to the characteristics mentioned, many individuals with panic disorder have problems with alcohol abuse, depression, dizziness, and chronic fatigue. Irritable bowel syndrome is often found in patients with panic disorder.

Because of the low abuse potential and favorable side effect profile, SSRIs have become the treatment of choice for those with panic disorder. Their use helps decrease the number and severity of panic attacks and, to a lesser degree, phobia and anxiety related to the attacks. They are significantly more effective against panic disorders than TCAs.

When using an SSRI for treating a patient with panic disorder, keep in mind that "start low, go slow" should guide therapy. Those with panic disorder usually do not tolerate a rapid induction or change in any therapy because of their heightened sympathetic state. Pick an agent with an early side-effect profile that the patient is likely to tolerate, such as a product that is less rather than more energizing with a lower rate of insomnia, nervousness, and akathisia, such as paroxetine (Paxil). Also realize that SSRI use may precipitate panic attacks with early use but prevent them after the full therapeutic effect is realized.

Tricyclic antidepressants may also be used in treating patients with panic disorder. Because patients with panic disorder are sensitive to the sensation of tachycardia, choose a product with serotonergic rather than norepinephrine activity, such as clomipramine (Anafranil) or nortriptyline (Pamelor). As with SSRIs, start with a low dose and increase it slowly.

Monoamine oxidase inhibitors are the most potent drugs available for treating patients with panic disorder. Because of side effects and the need for dietary restriction while patients take the medications, their use is generally limited to those with treatment-resistant panic disorder.

Posttraumatic stress disorder is an anxiety disorder that occurs after a significant single event such as a natural disaster or being the victim of a crime. It may also be precipitated by recurrent trauma such as serving in combat, living in a war-torn area, or domestic abuse. Horror and helplessness are expected emotions in response to a traumatic life event for at least 1 month afterward. However, these emotions last significantly longer in patients with PTSD and are coupled with intrusive recall of the event, numbing of emotions, detachment, hyperarousal, and impaired social and occupational function.

Treatment of patients with PTSD requires an interdisciplinary approach of expert providers. Pharmacologic intervention often includes the use of an SSRI or a TCA. Benzodiazepines should be used with caution because substance abuse is a common co-condition in patients with PTSD. Buspirone (Buspar), with its anxiolytic action and low abuse potential, provides a reasonable therapeutic option for the anxiety usually associated with this condition. Carbamazepine (Tegretol) and valproic acid (Depakote) have been used with some success in treating irritability, aggression, and impulsiveness. Clonidine and propanolol may be helpful in minimizing hyperarousal. Trazodone offers a nonaddicting option to enhance sleep.

Patients often choose to treat anxiety and depression with herbal products, which are available over the counter in unlimited supply. Although encouraging and facilitating patient self-care is an important part of the role of NPs, the use of herbal products should be approached with some caution. Herbal medications are considered nutritional supplements and are therefore not subject to the regulatory process common to prescription and over-the-counter medication. As a result, quality control in their production may be lacking, leading to inconsistent amounts of herbs per dose. In addition, when a patient takes an herb to treat symptoms of anxiety and depression, he or she is self-medicating a potentially life-threatening disease. Using herbs with prescription medications may lead to problems with drug interactions or additive effects, such as when St. John's wort is used concurrently with an SSRI. The NP and patient both need to be aware of the effects, efficacy, and side-effect profiles of these products (Table 12–6).

Discussion Sources

Hektor Dunphy, L. (1999). *Management Guidelines for Adult Nurse Practitioners*. Philadelphia: FA Davis. Pp. 499–506.

Landis, B. J., Bryant, S. (1999). Mental health disorders. In Youngkin, E., Sawin, K., Kissinger, J., & Israel, D., *Pharmacotherapeutics: A Primary Care Clinical Guide*. Stamford, CT: Appleton & Lange. Pp. 747–800.

Maxmen, J., Ward, N. (1995). *Psychotropic Drugs Fast* (2nd ed.). New York, NY: WW Norton and Company.

QUESTIONS

50. You note that a 25-year-old woman has bruises on her right shoulder. She states: "I fell up against the wall." The bruises appear finger-shaped. She denies that another person injured her. What is your best choice of statement in response to this?

    A. "Your bruises really look as if they were caused by someone grabbing you."
    B. "Was this really an accident?"
    C. "I notice the bruises are in the shape of a hand."
    D. "How did you fall?"

51. The patient in Question 50 is in the office for a visit with you and brings her partner. He watches her hang up her coat and says, "Are you stupid? Can't you tell it's going to fall off that hanger?" Your best response is to say:

    A. "I will put the coat on the chair."
    B. "I am offended by your speaking like that."
    C. "The clinic has a policy about using insulting language."
    D. "You seem angry. Would you like to talk about it?"

52. Which of the following is true concerning domestic violence?

    A. It is found largely among those of lower socioeconomic status.
    B. The person in an abusive relationship usually seeks help.
    C. Routine screening is indicated during pregnancy.
    D. A predictable cycle of violent activity followed by a period of calm is the norm.

TABLE 12–6.
OVER-THE-COUNTER HERBAL PRODUCTS FOR ANXIETY AND DEPRESSION

Agent	Mechanism of Action	Comments
St. John's wort	? Similar to MAOIs, SSRIs, TCAs Likely > 10 active compounds	When compared with TCAs: Less anticholinergic effect, weight gain, less efficacy in more severe depression When compared with SSRIs: Similar potential for energizing such as fluoxetine, similar efficacy in mild to moderate depression with limited study TID-QID dosing needed; 6–8 weeks before clinical effect is seen; little information on drug interactions; likely prudent to avoid concurrent use of SSRIs, TCAs, MAOIs Potentially photosensitizing, peripheral neuropathy in high doses
Kava kava	Action at GABA receptors similar to benzodiazepines	Satisfactory response when compared with placebo, low-dose oxazepam (Serax) Sedating, can potentiate effects of alcohol Cross-allergenic with pepper Potentially hepatotoxic
Valerian root	Action similar to benzodiazepines	5–10% with paradoxical stimulating effect Available in a rather aromatic tea, but weaker, shorter duration of action Less drug hangover than with benzodiazepines

ANSWERS

50. A
51. B
52. C

DISCUSSION

Interpersonal violence among family members (i.e., domestic violence) is found in all socioeconomic and ethnic groups. However, because providers working with lower income and select ethnic groups usually are more vigilant about domestic violence, there is often an appearance that the abuse is more a problem in certain groups.

Abuse can take a number of forms: psychological, financial, emotional, and physical. Acts of violence are typically thought to be against the victim but may include destruction of property, intimidation, and threats. A cycle of tension building including criticism, yelling, and threats followed by violence and then a quieter period of apologies and promises to change is often seen. However, this cycle usually accelerates over time, with the violence being less predictable. Love for the perpetrator, hope that things will change, and fear of the consequences of leaving the relationship help to keep the victim in the relationship. These items also usually prevent victims from coming forth and asking for help.

As with counseling and screening for other health problems, using objective statements beginning with "I" is helpful. When a patient denies that finger-shaped bruises are caused by intentional injury by another person, an NP can simply state what is seen. This reinforces the assessment of abuse and allows the patient to offer more information. In a situation in which a patient is verbally abused in your present, reinforce your role as patient advocate by stating that the behavior is unacceptable in your presence. Some may fear that this can possibly precipitate another episode of abuse. However, this is unlikely.

Discussion Sources

Hektor Dunphy, L. (1999). *Management Guidelines for Adult Nurse Practitioners*. Philadelphia: FA Davis. Pp. 496–500.
Peace at Home, Inc. (1995). *Domestic Violence: The Facts*. Boston: Harvard Community Health Plan Foundation.

13
CHAPTER

Female Reproductive and Genitourinary Systems

QUESTIONS

1. Which of the following is a contraindication to combined oral contraception (COC) use?

   A. mother with a history of breast cancer
   B. personal history of hepatitis A at age 10 years
   C. currently casted healing femur fracture
   D. cigarette smoking

2. A 22-year-old woman taking COC calls after forgetting to take her pills for 3 consecutive days. She is 2 weeks into the pack. You advise her to:

   A. Take two pills today and two pills tomorrow.
   B. Discard two pills and take two pills today.
   C. Discard the rest of the pack and start a new pack with the first day of her next menses.
   D. Continue taking the pills for the rest of the cycle but expect some breakthrough bleeding (BTB).

3. When counseling a woman about COC use, you advise that:

   A. Long-term use is discouraged because the body needs a "rest" from birth control pills from time to time.
   B. Fertility is often delayed for a number of months after their discontinuation.
   C. There is an increase in the rate of breast cancer after protracted use.
   D. Premenstrual syndrome symptoms are often improved.

4. Noncontraceptive benefits of oral contraceptives include a decrease in all of the following except:

   A. iron deficiency anemia
   B. pelvic inflammatory disease (PID)
   C. cervicitis
   D. ovarian cancer

5. Which of the following women is the best candidate for progestin-only pill (POP) use?

   A. an 18-year-old woman who frequently forgets to take prescribed medications
   B. a 28-year-old woman with multiple sexual partners
   C. a 32-year-old woman who is breast feeding a 3-week-old infant
   D. a 26-year-old woman who wants to use the pill to help regulate her menstrual cycle

6. A 38-year-old nulliparous woman who smokes two packs a day is in an on-and-off relationship. The woman presents seeking contraception. Which of the following represents the most appropriate method?

   A. intrauterine device (IUD)
   B. oral contraceptives
   C. tubal ligation
   D. cervical cap

7. Which of the following statements is true concerning vaginal diaphragm use?

   A. When in place, the woman is aware that the diaphragm fits snugly against the vaginal walls.
   B. It is a suitable form of contraception for women with recurrent cystitis.
   C. After insertion, the cervix should be smoothly covered.
   D. The device should be removed within 2 hours of coitus to minimize the risk of infection.

8. All of the following are relative contraindications to the use of an IUD except:

   A. valvular heart disease
   B. multiple sexual partners
   C. hypertension
   D. lack of availability for follow-up care

9. Which of the following is the most appropriate response to a 27-year-old woman who is taking phenytoin (Dilantin) for the treatment of a seizure disorder and is requesting hormonal contraception?

   A. It is preferable for you to use a barrier method.
   B. COC use is acceptable.
   C. Depo-Provera will not interact with your seizure medication.
   D. IUD use is contraindicated.

10. Which of the following is commonly found after 1 year of using Depo-Provera (medroxyprogesterone acetate in a depot injection [DMPA])?

    A. weight gain
    B. hypermenorrhea
    C. acne
    D. rapid return of fertility when discontinued

ANSWERS

1. C
2. C
3. D
4. C
5. C
6. D
7. C
8. C
9. C
10. A

DISCUSSION

Despite the availability of numerous methods of highly reliable contraception, nearly one half of all pregnancies are unplanned. Rates of continued contraception use vary greatly according to the method (Table 13–1). Helping a woman choose an effective and acceptable form of family planning is an important part of providing health care.

Available for more than three decades, COC has been used by millions of women. This highly reliable form of contraception usually results in 1

TABLE 13–1. RATE OF SATISFACTION AFTER 1 YEAR OF USE OF VARIOUS CONTRACEPTIVE METHODS	
Type of Contraception	Satisfaction, %
COC	71
DMPA injection (Depo-Provera)	70
IUD	80
Norplant	88
Male condom	61
Female condom	56
Cap/diaphragm	60

pregnancy in 1000 women with perfect use and 50 in 1000 with typical use.

Contraceptive effect is achieved through the action of the COC's progesterone and estrogen components. Progestational effects help to inhibit ovulation by suppressing luteinizing hormone (LH), thickening endocervical mucus, and hampering implantation by endometrial atrophy. Through its estrogenic effects, ovulation is inhibited by suppression of follicle-stimulating hormone (FSH) and LH and through altering endometrial cellular structure.

When COC is discontinued, fertility usually returns promptly. Contrary to common belief, there is no need to delay conception after discontinuing COCs; prolonged COC use is not associated with future infertility or other health problems.

Noncontraceptive COC benefits include a lower rate of benign breast tumors and dysmenorrhea. Menstrual volume is reduced by about 60%, resulting in decreased rates of iron deficiency anemia. Decreased rates of endometrial, ovarian, and breast cancer are particularly noted among long-term users (> 5 years). Although not protective against sexually transmitted diseases (STDs), COC users have decreased frequency of PID, which results from thickened endocervical mucus; this results in lower rate of future ectopic pregnancy. Decreased rates of acne, hirsutism, and ovarian cyst; reduction in premenstrual syndrome; and improvement in rheumatoid arthritis symptoms are also noted among COC users.

The highest dropout rates with COC and progestin-only pill (POP) use is in the first 3 months of use. The most frequently mentioned reasons are (breakthrough bleeding BTB) and inconvenience of use. Although BTB is bothersome, it is not harmful and does not indicate lower contraceptive benefit. BTB can be minimized by taking the COC or POP within the same 4-hour period every day. Cigarette smoking, a relative contraindication to COC use, increases the likelihood of BTB and should therefore be discouraged (Box 13–1).

Nausea with COC and hormone replacement therapy (HRT) is often reported. This is usually a transient problem noted in the first months of

---

BOX 13–1
ABSOLUTE AND RELATIVE CONTRAINDICATIONS TO THE USE OF COMBINED ORAL CONTRACEPTION (COC)

Absolute contraindications to COC use (refrain from prescribing COCs to women with the following conditions):

- Pregnancy
- Current or past history cerebrovascular or cardiovascular disease
- Known or suspected breast cancer
- Unexplained or undiagnosed vaginal bleeding
- Estrogen-dependent cancer
- Prolonged immobilization or surgery to the leg
- Age >35 yrs when a cigarette smoker (especially in those who smoke more than 20 cigarettes per day)
- Current or past history of benign or malignant liver tumor

Relative contraindications to COC use (exercise caution with the use of COCs in women with the following conditions):

- Migraine headache or recurrent tension-type headache
- Hypertension
- Renal disease
- Diabetes mellitus
- Gallbladder disease
- Active hepatitis
- Acute mononucleosis
- Sickle cell disease
- Depression
- Lactation
- Recent surgery, fracture, or severe injury without prolonged immobilization

---

Reference: Hatcher, R., Guillebaud, J. (1998). The pill: Combined oral contraceptives. In Hatcher, R., Trussell, J., Stewart, F., et al. *Contraceptive Technology* (17th ed.). New York: Ardent Media. Pp. 420–423.

use and can be minimized by taking the medication with food or at bedtime. If vomiting occurs within 2 hours of taking COC, the dose should be repeated.

Combined oral contraception can interact with a limited number of drugs. However, interaction is noted with a number of antiepileptic drugs (AEDs), including phenytoin, carbamazepine, phenobarbital, and primidone, potentially causing a reduction in therapeutic levels of these important medications. In addition, seizure threshold can be altered with COC use. A woman with a seizure disorder who wishes to use hormonal contraception will likely have a reduction in frequency and severity of seizures while using Depo-Provera. In addition, Depo-Provera does not interact with AED. Norplant (levonorgestrel implants) may have the same effect. Barrier methods or IUD use does not interfere with AED and has no effect on seizure threshold.

Although not consistently suppressing ovulation, POP likely provides contraception through thickening of endocervical mucus as well as through the alteration of the endometrium. POP use offers certain advantages and disadvantages compared with COC. With failure rates of 1–4%, POP is a less effective contraceptive than COC. The nausea rate with its use is significantly lower than with COC use owing to the lack of estrogen. POPs are taken daily, a schedule many women find more convenient than the typically 3-weeks-on, 1-week-off schedule with COCs. However, POP must be used daily for maximum efficacy. For lactating women who wish to use an oral hormonal contraceptive, POP use is highly effective and does not alter the quality or quantity of breast milk. One significant disadvantage with POP use is bleeding irregularity, ranging from prolonged flow to amenorrhea.

Medroxyprogesterone acetate in a depot injection (Depo-Provera) given every 90 days is a highly reliable form of contraception (99.7% efficacy). DMPA injection is best suited for women who do not wish a pregnancy for at least 18 months because resumption of fertility is frequently delayed by 6 to 12 months. When the injection is given within first few days of menses, the contraceptive effect is immediate. When started at 5 days after the onset of menses, it is prudent to use a backup method for 1 week. Depo-Provera may be started immediately postpartum if the woman is not breast feeding and initiated at 3 to 6 weeks postpartum if she is breast feeding. Earlier use may diminish quantity but not quality of breast milk.

Irregular bleeding, a common problem during the first few months of DMPA injection use, can be minimized by the use of a prostaglandin inhibitor such as ibuprofen 400 mg TID or naproxen sodium 375 to 500 mg BID for 3 to 5 days. Estrogen supplements may also be helpful such using a 0.1-mg estrogen patch for 7 to 10 days. After 1 year of use, 30–50% of women have amenorrhea.

TABLE 13–2.
ABSOLUTE AND RELATIVE CONTRAINDICATIONS TO USE
OF INTRAUTERINE DEVICES

Absolute contraindications to IUD use	Pelvic infection
	Pregnancy
	Undiagnosed vaginal bleeding
	Distorted uterine cavity (leiomyomata, bicornuate uterus, others)
	Malignant disease of the cervix or uterus
Relative contraindications to IUD use	History of PID
	History of ectopic pregnancy
	Recent abnormal Pap test results
	Valvular heart disease
	Endometriosis
	Dysmenorrhea or hypermenorrhea
	Impaired coagulation or immune response

Reference: Brown, K. (2000). *Management Guidelines for Women's Health Nurse Practitioners.* Philadelphia: FA Davis. Pp. 108–110.

Based on observation from limited study, bone density may be reduced in women using DMPA. However, this is unlikely to be a long-term problem. Calcium supplementation should be recommended at 1000 to 1500 mg/day.

Intrauterine devices are an effective form of contraception and have a failure rate of 0.5–2.9%. Their mechanism of activity is not entirely understood, but it is unlikely that they are abortifacients. Because there may be an increase in menstrual bleeding and upper reproductive tract infection with their use and because there are a number of absolute and relative contraindications (Table 13–2), IUDs are not widely used.

The diaphragm, a barrier method of contraception, is placed in the vagina before intercourse. This device, which has an effectiveness rate of 80–95%; it should be used in conjunction with a spermicide and removed no sooner than 6 hours after coitus. When properly fitted and in the appropriate position, the woman and partner should be unaware of the diaphragm's presence. If either partner can feel the diaphragm, it is either the wrong size or not properly inserted.

Discussion Sources

Brown, K. (2000). *Management Guidelines for Women's Health Nurse Practitioners.* Philadelphia: FA Davis. Pp. 111–119.
McKay, H. (1999). Gynecology. In Tierny, L., McPhee, S., & Papadakis, M. *Current Medical Diagnosis and Treatment* (38th ed.). Stamford, CT: Appleton & Lange. Pp. 703–736.

QUESTIONS

11. An 18-year-old woman presents requesting emergency contraception after having unprotected intercourse approximately 18 hours ago. Today is day 12 of her normally 27- to 29-day menstrual cycle. You advise her:

    A. Emergency contraception use reduces the risk of pregnancy by approximately 33%.
    B. All forms of emergency contraceptive must be used within 12 hours after intercourse.
    C. The likelihood of conception is minimal.
    D. Taking COCs in multiple doses offers an effective emergency contraceptive option.

12. Which of the following is likely not among the proposed mechanisms of action of COC when used for emergency contraception?

    A. inhibits ovulation
    B. is an abortifacient
    C. slows sperm transport
    D. slows ovum transport

13. A 24-year-old woman who requests emergency contraception with COC wants to know its effects if pregnancy does occur. You respond that there may be an increase in the likelihood of:

    A. spontaneous abortion
    B. ectopic pregnancy
    C. birth defects
    D. placental insufficiency

ANSWERS

11. **D**
12. **B**
13. **B**

DISCUSSION

More than 3 million unintended pregnancies occur annually. Emergency contraception (EC) is used after coitus to minimize the risk of unintended pregnancy when a contraceptive method fails or is not used (Box 13–2). An estimated 800,000 annual pregnancy terminations could be avoided if knowledge of and access to emergency contraception were widely available.

A number of methods are available, including the use of COCs, POPs, and IUDs (Table 13–3).

Emergency contraception using oral hormonal agents is highly effective, reducing the risk of pregnancy by 75% based on the following model: If 100 fertile women have unprotected heterosexual intercourse in the second to third weeks of their cycles, eight typically become pregnant. Only two typically become pregnant when using emergency contraception. Its mechanism of action is not clearly established but may help reduce pregnancy risk by multiple methods, including inhibiting or delaying ovulation or impairing ova or sperm transport. Emergency contraception is unlikely to prevent pregnancy by preventing implantation of a fertilized ovum because the resulting minor endometrial changes would likely not be sufficient to prevent implantation. Oral hormonal emergency contraception use will not interrupt an established pregnancy nor increase risk of early pregnancy loss. If pregnancy does occur, use of emergency contraception does not appear to be teratogenic but is associated with an increased risk of ectopic pregnancy.

A copper-containing IUD such as the Paragard T can be inserted within 5 to 7 days after intercourse as a form of emergency contraception. Because of the risk of upper reproductive tract infections, its use is

---

BOX 13–2
INDICATIONS FOR EMERGENCY CONTRACEPTIVE USE

No use of contraception
Barrier contraception problem such as condom tear or slippage or
    inappropriate diaphragm placement
Sexual assault
Two or more oral contraceptive pills (COC or POP) missed
Two or more days late starting oral contraceptive pills
Late for Depo-Provera injection

Reference: Oral contraceptives used for emergency contraception in the United States. Available at http//opr.princeton.edu/ec/dose.html

TABLE 13–3.
EXAMPLES OF EMERGENCY CONTRACEPTION OPTIONS

Drug	Dosage	Instructions
Plan B (levonorgestrel 0.75 mg)	One pill q 12 h x 2 doses	Start within 72 hours after inter-course
Oval (50 μg estra-diol with 0.25 mg levonorgestrel)	Two pills q 12 h x 2 doses	Start within 72 hours after inter-course
LoOvral/Nordette/ Levelen (30 μg es-tradiol with 0.15 mg levonorgestrel)	Four pills q 12h x 2 doses	Start within 72 hours after inter-course
Ovrette (POP for total 0.75 mg levonorgestrel)	Twenty pills q 12 h x 2 doses	Start within 72 hours after inter-course
Preven (50 μg estra-diol with 0.25-mg levonorgestrel)	Two pills taken q 12 h x 2 doses	Start within 72 hours after inter-course
Paragard T (copper containing)		Start within 5 to 7 days after in-tercourse

Reference: Oral contraceptives used for emergency contraception in the United States. Available at http//opr.princeton.edu/ec/dose.html

contraindicated in the presence of a STD. IUD insertion also provides a hormone-free emergency contraception option as well as ongoing contraception.

Menstrual bleeding should be expected within 3 to 4 weeks of using emergency contraception. If none occurs, a pregnancy test should be done.

Discussion Sources

McKay, H. (1999). Gynecology. In Tierny, L., McPhee, S., & Papadakis, M. *Current Medical Diagnosis and Treatment* (38th ed.). Stamford, CT: Appleton & Lange. Pp. 703–736.
Oral contraceptives used for emergency contraception in the United States. Available at http//opr.princeton.edu/ec/dose.html
Van Look, P., Stewart, F. (1998). Emergency contraception. In Hatcher, R., Trussell, J., Stewart, F., et al. *Contraceptive Technology* (17th ed.). New York: Ardent Media. Pp. 277–296.

QUESTIONS

14. In advising a woman about menopause, you offer the following information.

   A. The average age at menopause is 47 to 48 years.
   B. Hot flashes and night sweats occur in about 80% of women.
   C. Women with surgical menopause usually have milder symptoms.
   D. FSH and LH levels are suppressed.

15. Findings in estrogen deficiency (atrophic) vaginitis include:

   A. malodorous vaginal discharge
   B. increased number of lactobacilli
   C. reduced number of white blood cells
   D. pH > 5

16. A 53-year-old woman who is taking HRT with conjugated equine estrogen (CEE) 0.625 mg/day with progesterone has bothersome atrophic vaginitis symptoms. You advise that:

   A. Her oral estrogen dose should be increased.
   B. Topical estrogen may be helpful.
   C. Progesterone should be discontinued.
   D. Baking soda douche should be used.

17. Relative contraindications to postmenopausal estrogen therapy include all of the following except:

   A. unexplained vaginal bleeding
   B. seizure disorder
   C. dyslipidemia
   D. migraine headache

18. Absolute contraindications to postmenopausal estrogen therapy include:

   A. endometrial cancer
   B. seizure disorder
   C. dyslipidemia
   D. migraine headache

19. In advising a perimenopausal woman about HRT, you consider that it may:

    A. increase serum high-density lipoprotein (HDL) level and lower low-density lipoprotein (LDL) level
    B. significantly lower serum triglyceride levels
    C. worsen hypertension in most women
    D. increase bone density

20. Postmenopausal HRT may cause:

    A. a reduction in the rate of thromboembolic disease
    B. an increase in the rate of Alzheimer's disease
    C. a reduction in the frequency of spinal and hip fracture
    D. a disturbance in sleep patterns

21. The progesterone component of HRT is given to:

    A. counteract the negative lipid effects of estrogen
    B. minimize endometrial hyperplasia
    C. help with vaginal atrophy symptoms
    D. prolong ovarian activity

22. Concerning raloxifene (Evista) therapy, which of the following is correct?

    A. Concurrent progestin opposition is needed.
    B. Hot flashes are reduced in frequency and severity.
    C. Its use is contraindicated when a woman has a history of breast cancer.
    D. Osteoporosis risk is reduced with its use.

ANSWERS

14. B
15. D
16. B
17. A
18. A
19. A
20. C
21. B
22. D

DISCUSSION

Menopause marks a transition in a woman's reproductive life and the cessation of the menses. Perimenopause is the time surrounding menopause; its onset is marked by the beginning symptoms of menopause and ends with the cessation of menses. The average age at menopause is 50 to 51 years, with a woman living up to one third of her life after this time.

With menopause, LH and FSH levels increase dramatically. Hot flashes occur in about 80%, from mildly bothersome to debilitating. When compared with naturally occurring menopause, women with surgical menopause usually have more severe symptoms because hormonal shifts are more rapid and dramatic.

The use of postmenopausal HRT can significantly reduce a woman's risk of developing osteoporosis and Alzheimer's disease and other forms of dementia.

Estrogen deficiency is a potent risk factor in the development of osteoporosis, which is most common in postmenopausal woman. By age 80, the average woman has lost greater than 30% of her premenopausal bone density. When taken with calcium supplements, postmenopausal HRT can help reduce the risk of postmenopausal fracture by as much as 50% by minimizing further bone loss. HRT use can help improve verbal memory and cognitive function as well as have a positive effect on mood. In addition, skin thinning is reduced by approximately 50%. Because the vaginal introitus remains colonized with protective flora when HRT is used, there are lower rates of urogenital atrophy and UTIs. However, some women using HRT may continue to need topical estrogen in the form of a vaginal cream or estrogen-impregnated ring (Estring) to help minimize urogenital atrophy symptoms.

Endometrial cancer risk with unopposed estrogen use is considerable, with the rate of 4 to 5 per 1000 users per year, with a year 5 risk of 2% and year 10 risk of 4%. There has been an observed increase risk of breast cancer with HRT use. HRT use in women with a history of breast cancer has been considered contraindicated; recent studies may contradict this (Table 13–4).

Estrogen typically acts at target-particular sites found in the breast, brain, reproductive tract, and cardiovascular system. As a result, postmenopausal estrogen use acts on body systems where its effects are positive, such as enhanced endothelial function and reduced risk of certain types of dementia. In addition, it acts in areas where its effects are not desirable, such as by increasing breast and endometrial cancer with unopposed estrogen use.

TABLE 13–4. CONTRAINDICATIONS TO POSTMENOPAUSAL ESTROGEN THERAPY	
Contraindication	**Disease State**
Absolute contraindications	Unexplained vaginal bleeding
	Acute liver disease
	Chronic impaired liver function
	Thrombotic disease
	Endometrial cancer
	Neuro-ophthalmologic vascular disease
	Breast cancer (controversial)
Relative contraindications	Seizure disorder
	Dyslipidemia
	Migraine headache
	Thrombophlebitis
	Gallbladder disease

Estrogen-deficiency or atrophic vaginitis is a noninfectious disease that affects postmenopausal women. During the process, there is a rise in vaginal pH (> 5), thinning of vaginal tissue, and loss of vaginal lubrication. Urinary frequency and burning without UTI is often reported. On physical examination, the vaginal tissue appears fragile. and vaginal rugae are lost.

Intervention for atrophic vaginitis includes using lubricants during sexual activity to minimize tissue trauma. Avoiding tight-fitting clothing and wearing cotton underwear can be helpful. Topical estrogen in the form of a cream or through the use of an estrogen-impregnated ring can also be used and are highly effective. However, many women who use oral HRT continue to have symptoms of atrophic vaginitis; the addition of topical estrogen can be helpful. Increasing the dose of oral estrogen is seldom helpful and likely increases HRT adverse effects.

Tamoxifen is a selective estrogen receptor modulator (SERM) that locks out estrogen's effects on the breasts. It is useful as both primary prevention of breast cancer in high-risk women as well as a means to lower breast cancer recurrence. Because endometrial sites are not antagonized, there is a small increase in endometrial cancer rate when tamoxifen is used. Evaluation of unexplained vaginal bleeding is critical during tamoxifen use.

Raloxifene (Evista) is a SERM with activity in the cardiovascular system and the bone but little to no activity in breast, uterine, or brain tissue.

Raloxifene's cardioprotective benefits occur in part because of a change in vessel response as well as its ability to lower total cholesterol and fibrinogen levels. In addition, it is helpful in preventing osteoporosis because of its ability to preserve bone density. Because it lacks breast tissue effect, raloxifene may be a reasonable treatment option for cardiovascular and bone protection in postmenopausal women with a history of or at high risk for breast cancer. Hot flashes are among the most commonly reported side effect with raloxifene use, with little report of breast tenderness and bloating often noted with estrogen therapy.

Discussion Sources

Brown, K. (2000). *Management Guidelines for Women's Health Nurse Practitioners*. Philadelphia: FA Davis. Pp. 78–80.
Kennedy-Malone, L., Fletcher, K., Plank, L. (2000). *Management Guidelines for Gerontological Nurse Practitioners*. Philadelphia: FA Davis. Pp. 292–295.
McKay, H. (1999). Gynecology. In Tierny, L., McPhee, S., & Papadakis, M. *Current Medical Diagnosis and Treatment* (38th ed.). Stamford, CT: Appleton & Lange. Pp. 703–736.

QUESTIONS

23. Patients with urge incontinence often report urine loss:

    A. with exercise

    B. at night

    C. associated with a strong sensation of needing to void

    D. as dribbling after voiding

24. Patients with urethral stricture often report urine loss:

    A. with exercise

    B. during the day

    C. associated with urgency

    D. as dribbling after voiding

25. Patients with stress incontinence often report urine loss:

    A. with lifting

    B. at night

    C. associated with a strong sensation of needing to void

    D. as dribbling after voiding

26. Factors that contribute to stress incontinence include:

   A. detrusor overactivity
   B. pelvic floor weakness
   C. urethral stricture
   D. UTI

27. Factors that contribute to urge incontinence include:

   A. detrusor overactivity
   B. pelvic floor weakness
   C. urethral stricture
   D. UTI

28. Pharmacologic intervention for patients with urge incontinence includes:

   A. doxazosin (Cardura)
   B. terodiline (Detrol)
   C. finasteride (Proscar)
   D. pseudoephedrine (Dexatrim)

29. Pharmacologic intervention for patients with stress incontinence includes:

   A. doxazosin (Cardura)
   B. terodiline (Detrol)
   C. finasteride (Proscar)
   D. phenylpropanolamine (Dexatrim)

30. Behavioral intervention for patients with stress incontinence includes:

   A. establishing a voiding schedule
   B. gentle bladder-stretching exercises
   C. Kegel exercises
   D. restricting fluid intake

31. Which form of urinary incontinence is most common in the elderly?

   A. stress
   B. urge
   C. iatrogenic
   D. overflow

ANSWERS

23. C
24. D
25. A
26. B
27. A
28. B
29. D
30. C
31. B

DISCUSSION

Urinary incontinence (UI) is the involuntary loss of urine sufficient to be a problem. This condition is often thought by many women to be a normal part of aging. In reality, numerous treatment options are available after the cause of UI is established (Table 13–5). In all cases, urinalysis and urine culture and sensitivity should be obtained. If UTI is present, treatment with antibiotics is indicated.

Urge incontinence is the most common form of UI in the elderly. Behavioral therapy, including a voiding schedule and gentle bladder stretching, is helpful. Pharmacologic intervention is indicated in conjunction with behavioral therapy (Table 13–6). Terodiline is a selective muscarinic receptor antagonist that blocks bladder receptors and limits bladder contraction. Helpful in the treatment of urge incontinence, its use is associated with a decrease in the number of micturations as well as incontinent episodes along with an increase in voiding volume. Oxybutynin is a nonselective muscarinic receptor antagonist that blocks both receptors in the bladder and oral cavity, with activity similar to terodiline; its use is somewhat limited because of the side effects of dry mouth and constipation.

Discussion Sources

Brown, K. (2000). *Management Guidelines for Women's Health Nurse Practitioners.* Philadelphia: FA Davis. Pp. 147–150.

Kennedy-Malone, L., Fletcher, K., Plank, L. (2000). *Management Guidelines for Gerontological Nurse Practitioners.* Philadelphia: FA Davis. Pp. 525–529.

Presti, J., Stoller, M., Carrol, P. (1999). Urology. In Tierny, L., McPhee, S., & Papadakis, M. *Current Medical Diagnosis and Treatment* (38th ed.). Stamford, CT: Appleton & Lange. Pp. 894–931.

QUESTIONS

32. Which of the following is not a normal finding in a woman during the reproductive years?

    A. vaginal pH of 4.5 or less
    B. lactobacillus as the predominant vaginal organism
    C. thick, white vaginal secretions during the luteal phase
    D. vaginal epithelial cells with adherent bacteria

33. Which of the following findings is most consistent with vaginal discharge during ovulation?

    A. dry and sticky
    B. milky and mucoid
    C. stringy and clear
    D. tenacious and odorless

34. Physical examination on a 19-year-old woman with a 3-day history of vaginal itch reveals moderate perineal excoriation; vaginal erythema; and a white, clumping discharge. Expected microscopic examination findings include:

    A. pH > 6.0
    B. increased number of lactobacilli
    C. hyphae
    D. abundance of white blood cells

35. Women with bacterial vaginosis typically present with:

    A. vulvitis
    B. pruritus
    C. dysuria
    D. malodorous discharge

36. Treatment of vulvovaginitis caused by *Candida albicans* includes:

    A. metronidazole gel
    B. clotrimazole cream
    C. hydrocortisone ointment
    D. clindamycin cream

TABLE 13–5.
CLINICAL ISSUES IN URINARY INCONTINENCE

Type of Urinary Incontinence	Cause and Population Most Often Affected	Clinical Presentation	Treatment Options
Urge incontinence	Detrusor overactivity causing uninhibited bladder contractions Most common form of incontinence in the elderly	Strong sensation of needing to empty the bladder that cannot be suppressed, often coupled with involuntary loss of urine	Avoiding stimulants, gentle bladder stretching by increasing voiding interval by 15 to 30 minutes after establishing a 1- to 2-hour voiding schedules Add agent to reduce bladder contraction: tolterodine (Detrol) or oxybutynin (Ditropan)
Stress incontinence	Weakness of pelvic floor and urethral muscles Most common form of incontinence in women; rare in men	Loss of urine with activity (e.g., coughing, sneezing, exercise) that causes increase in intraabdominal pressure	Kegel exercises Support to the area through the use of a vaginal tampon, urethral stents, injections, and pessary use Topical and systemic estrogen if associated with postmenopausal urogenital atropic changes Phenylpropanolamine (alpha adrenergic agonist) Surgical intervention can be helpful in 75–85%

Urethral obstruction	Obstruction of bladder outflow through urethral obstruction (prostatic, stricture, tumor) resulting in urinary retention with overflow and detrusor instability Most commonly found in older men	Dribbling after voiding coupled with urge incontinence presentation	Treatment of urethral obstruction
Transient incontinence	Associated with acute event such as delirium, UTI, medication use, restricted activity	Presentation consistent with underlying process	Treatment of underlying process, discontinuation of offending medication

References: Kennedy-Malone, L., Fletcher, K., Plank, L. (2000). *Management Guidelines for Gerontological Nurse Practitioners.* Philadelphia: FA Davis. Pp. 525–529.

Presti, J., Stoller, M., Carrol, P. (1999). Urology. In Tierny, L., McPhee, S., & Papadakis, M. *Current Medical Diagnosis and Treatment* (38th ed.). Stamford, CT: Appleton & Lange. Pp. 894–931.

TABLE 13–6.
SELECT MEDICATIONS AND THEIR EFFECTS
ON URINARY CONTINENCE

Type of Medication	Effect on Urinary Continence
Diuretics	Increase in volume and frequency of voiding
Drugs with anticholinergic activity, such as first-generation antihistamines, tricyclic antidepressants, antipsychotics	Urinary retention, overflow incontinence, alteration in sensorium, fecal impaction
Opioids	Urinary retention, overflow, alteration in sensorium, fecal impaction
Alcohol	Increase in volume, frequency, and urgency of voiding; alteration in sensorium
Sedatives, hypnotics, benzodiazepines	Alteration in sensorium, reduced mobility
Alpha adrenergic antagonists (prazosin, doxazosin, terazosin)	Relaxing internal urethral sphincter; this may be a desired effect in men with BPH

References: Kennedy-Malone, L., Fletcher, K., Plank, L. (2000). *Management Guidelines for Gerontological Nurse Practitioners.* Philadelphia: FA Davis. Pp. 525–529.

Presti, J., Stoller, M., Carrol, P. (1999). Urology. In Tierny, L., McPhee, S., & Papadakis, M. *Current Medical Diagnosis and Treatment* (38th ed.). Stamford, CT: Appleton & Lange. Pp. 894–931.

37. A 24-year-old woman presents with a 1-week history of thin, green-yellow vaginal discharge with perivaginal irritation. Physical examination findings include vaginal erythema with petechial hemorrhages on the cervix, numerous white blood cells, and motile organisms on microscopic examination. These findings most likely represent:

   A. motile sperm with irritative vaginitis

   B. trichomoniasis

   C. bacterial vaginosis

   D. condylomata acuminata

38. The preferred treatment option for trichomoniasis is:

    A. oral metronidazole
    B. clindamycin cream
    C. acyclovir
    D. azithromycin

39. Treatment options for bacterial vaginosis include all of the following except:

    A. oral metronidazole
    B. clindamycin cream
    C. oral clindamycin
    D. azithromycin

40. A 30-year-old woman presents without symptoms but states that her male partner has dysuria without penile discharge. Examination reveals a friable cervix covered with thick yellow discharge. This description is most consistent with an infection caused by:

    A. *Chlamydia trachomatis*
    B. *Neisseria gonorrhea*
    C. human papilloma virus (HPV)
    D. *Trichomonas vaginalis*

41. Which of the following is an effective, single-dose treatment for uncomplicated gonorrheal infection?

    A. cefixime 400 mg
    B. metronidazole 2 g
    C. azithromycin 1 g
    D. amoxicillin 2 g with probenecid

42. Which of the following is an effective, single-dose treatment for uncomplicated chlamydial infection?

    A. ciprofloxacin 500 mg
    B. metronidazole 2 g
    C. azithromycin 1 g
    D. ceftriaxone 125 mg

43. Gram stain of the vaginal discharge in a 27-year-old woman with purulent vaginal discharge reveals gram-negative cocci. This most likely represents:

    A. *C. trachomatis*
    B. *Ureaplasma* spp.
    C. *N. gonorrhoeae*
    D. *Escherichia coli*

44. Treatment options for a patient with uncomplicated gonococcal proctitis include:

    A. ceftriaxone 125 mg IM as a single dose
    B. erythromycin 500 mg BID for 7 days
    C. norfloxacin 400 mg BID for 3 days
    D. azithromycin 1 g as a single dose

45. Which of the following is true of gonococcal infection?

    A. The risk of transmission from an infected woman to male sexual partner is about 80%.
    B. Most men have symptomatic infection.
    C. The incubation period is about 2 to 3 weeks.
    D. The organism rarely produces beta-lactamase.

46. Complications of gonococcal and chlamydial genitourinary infection in women include all of the following except:

    A. PID
    B. tubal scarring
    C. pyelonephritis
    D. peritonitis

ANSWERS

32. **D**
33. **C**
34. **C**
35. **D**
36. **B**

37. B
38. A
39. D
40. A
41. A
42. C
43. C
44. A
45. B
46. C

DISCUSSION

Vulvovaginitis is one of the most common gynecologic problems. Treatment is guided by presentation and causative organism (Table 13–7). Chlamydial infection is one of the most common STDs, primarily affecting adolescents and adults younger than age 25 years. The causative organism, *C. trachomatis* immunotype D-K, is an obligate intracellular parasite closely related to gram-negative bacteria. This infection causes cervicitis in the majority of infected women. About one half have urethral infection, and one third have endometrial involvement. Despite this, many women are asymptomatic, but mucopurulent vaginal discharge, dysuria, dyspareunia and postcoital bleeding may be reported (Table 13–8).

Clinical presentation of *C. trachomatis* genitourinary infection in women typically includes the presence of mucopurulent discharge, often adherent to a friable cervix. Cervical motion and adnexal tenderness may be present when there is endometrial involvement. Diagnostic testing includes DNA probe endocervical testing or urinalysis for ligase chain reaction.

Treatment options in *C. trachomatis* infection include antibiotics that act against intracellular organisms. This includes doxycyline, erythromycin, and azithromycin. Azithromycin is given in a highly efficacious, well-tolerated, single-dose oral therapy.

Gonorrhea, caused by the gram-negative diplococci *N. gonorrheae*, is one of the most common STDs. It has a short incubation period of 1 to 5 days and is likely to cause infection in approximately 20% of men who have sexual contact with an infected woman and approximately 80% of women who have sexual contact with an infected man.

TABLE 13–7.
DIFFERENTIAL DIAGNOSIS OF INFECTIVE VULVOVAGINITIS

Condition and Causative Organism	Clinical Presentation	Microscopic Examination Findings	Treatment Options
Bacterial vaginosis caused by overgrowth of anaerobes, including *Gardnerella* species and *Mycoplasma hominis*	Increased volume of vaginal secretions, thin, gray, homogeneous discharge, burning, pruritus	Vaginal pH > 4.5, clue calls, positive whiff test	• Metronidazole gel (MetroGel) 0.75% vaginally QD or BID for 5 days • Metronidazole 500 mg BID for 7 days • Metronidazole 2 g as a one time dose (85% efficacy) • Clindamycin 300 mg BID for 7 days • Clindamycin cream vaginally at hs x 7 days
Nongonococcal cervicitis caused by *C. trachomatis*	Cervicitis, irritative voiding symptoms, occasional mucopurulent discharge	Numerous white blood cells	In uncomplicated infection • Azithromycin 1 g PO as a single dose • Doxycycline 100 mg po BID x 7 days • Erythromycin 500 mg PO QID x 7 days • Ofloxacin 300 mg BID x 7 days
Gonoccocal vaginitis caused by *N. gonorrhoeae*	Irritative voiding symptoms, occasional purulent discharge	Numerous white blood cells	In uncomplicated infection • Cefixime 400 mg • Ceftriaxone 125 mg IM • Ciprofloxacin 500 mg • Ofloxacin 400 mg • Concurrently treat with azithromycin 1 g as a single dose or Doxycyline 100 mg BID x 7 days due to risk of con current gonococcal urethritis

TABLE 13–7.
DIFFERENTIAL DIAGNOSIS OF
INFECTIOUS VULVOVAGINITIS

Condition and Causative Organism	Clinical Presentation	Microscopic Examination Findings	Treatment Options
Trichomoniasis caused by *T. vaginalis*	Dysuria, itching, vulvovaginal irritation, dyspareunia, yellow-green vaginal discharge, cervical petechial hemorrhages ("strawberry spots")	Large motile organisms, numerous white blood cells	Metronidazole 2 g as a one time dose or 500 mg PO BID x 7 days
Candidiasis caused by Candida albicans, Candida glabrata, Candida tropicalis	Itching, burning, thick white to yellow adherent, curd-like discharge, vulvovaginal excoriation, erythema, excoriation	Ph ≤ 4.5, hyphae and spores	Miconazole Butoconazole Terconazole Tioconazole

References: Brown, K. (2000). *Management Guidelines for Women's Health Nurse Practitioners.* Philadelphia: FA Davis. Pp. 75–77.

Chambers, H. (1999). Infectious disease: Bacterial and chlamydia. In Tierny, L., McPhee, S., & Papadakis, M. *Current Medical Diagnosis and Treatment* (38th ed.) Stamford, CT: Appleton & Lange. Pp. 1291–1331.

Whereas the majority of women are asymptomatic, men are typically symptomatic. In women, presentation typically includes dysuria with a milky to purulent, occasionally blood-tinged, vaginal discharge. With anal-insertive sex, rectal infection leading to proctitis is often seen. Because the organism frequently produces beta-lactamase, the choice of a therapeutic agent should include agents with beta-lactamase stability and include select fluoroquinolones, ceftriaxone, and cefixime (see Table 13–8).

TABLE 13–8.
GUIDELINES FOR ASSESSING AND TREATING PATIENTS WITH GENITOURINARY INFECTIONS

Condition	Causative Organism	Clinical Presentation	Treatment Options
Chancroid	*Haemophilus ducreyi*	Painless genital ulcer	Azithromycin 1 g PO OR ceftriaxone 250 mg IM or ciprofloxacin 500 mg PO BID x 3 days OR erythromycin 500 mg PO QID x 7 days
Herpes simplex	Herpes simplex virus 1 or 2	Painful ulcerated lesions, lymphadenopathy	For initial infection: Acyclovir 400 mg PO TID x 7 to 10 days OR acyclovir 200 mg five times per day x 7 to 10 days OR famciclovir 250 mg PO TID x 7 to 10 days OR valacyclovir 1 g PO BID x 7 to 10 days For episodic recurrent infection: Acyclovir 400 mg PO TID x 5 days OR famciclovir 250 mg PO BID x 5 days OR valacyclovir 1 g PO QD x 5 days OR valacyclovir 500 mg PO BID x 5 days For suppression of recurrent infection: Acyclovir 400 mg PO BID OR famciclovir 250 mg PO BID OR valacyclovir 1 g PO QD OR valacyclovir 500 mg PO for extended period of time

Lymphogranuloma venereum	Invasive serovar L1, L2, L3 of *C. trachomatis*	Vesicular or ulcerative lesion on the external genitalia with inguinal lymphadenitis or buboes	Doxycyline 100 mg PO BID x 21 days OR erythromycin 500 mg QID x 21 days
Nongonococcal urethritis and cervicitis	*C. trachomatis*	Cervicitis, irritative voiding symptoms, occasional mucopurulent discharge	Azithromycin 1 g PO as a single dose OR doxycycline 100 mg PO BID x 7 days OR erythromycin 500 mg PO QID x 7 days OR ofloxacin 300 mg BID x 7 days
Gonococcal urethritis and vaginitis	*N. gonorrhoeae*	Irritative voiding symptoms, occasional purulent discharge	Single-dose therapy for uncomplicated infection: Cefixime 400 mg Ceftriaxone 125 mg IM OR ciprofloxacin 500 mg OR ofloxacin 400 mg Concurrently treat with azithromycin 1 g as a single dose OR doxycyline 100 mg BID x 7 days because of the risk of concurrent nongonococcal urethritis
PID	*N. gonorrheae, C. trachomatis, E. coli, Mycoplasma* spp. and *Ureaplasma* spp., others	Irritative voiding symptoms; fever; and abdominal pain and cervical motion tenderness	Ceftriaxone 250 mg IM as a single dose plus doxycyline 100 mg BID x 14 days With penicillin or cephalosporin allergy or when oral regimen desired: Ofloxacin 400 mg with metronidazole 500 mg PO BID x 14 days

(continued)

TABLE 13–8. (continued)

Condition	Causative Organism	Clinical Presentation	Treatment Options
Trichomoniasis	*Trichomonas vaginalis*	Dysuria, itching, vulvo-vaginal irritation, dyspareunia, yellow-green vaginal discharge, cervical petechial hemorrhages ("strawberry spots"), motile organisms and white blood cells on microscopic examination	Metronidazole 2 g as a one-time dose OR 500 mg PO BID x 7 days
Genital warts (condyloma acuminata)	HPV	Verruca-form lesions or may be subclinical or unrecognized	For treatment of visible lesions: Podofilox OR imiquimod OR trichloroacetic acid OR cryotherapy OR interferon or surgery

Reference: Centers for Disease Control and Prevention (1998). 1998 Guidelines for Treatment of Sexually Transmitted Disease. Available at http://www.cdc.gov.epo/mmwr/preview/mmwrhtml/00050909.htm

Discussion Sources

Brown, K. (2000). *Management Guidelines for Women's Health Nurse Practitioners*. Philadelphia: FA Davis. Pp. 75–77.

Chambers, H. (1999). Infectious disease: Bacterial and chlamydia. In Tierny, L., McPhee, S., & Papadakis, M. *Current Medical Diagnosis and Treatment* (38th ed.). Stamford, CT: Appleton & Lange. Pp. 1291–1331.

Presti, J., Stoller, M., Carrol, P. (1999). Urology. In Tierny, L., McPhee, S., & Papadakis, M. *Current Medical Diagnosis and Treatment* (38th ed.). Stamford, CT: Appleton & Lange. Pp. 894–931.

QUESTIONS

47. Women with PID typically present with all of the following except:

   A. dysuria

   B. low back pain

   C. cervical motion tenderness

   D. diffuse abdomen pain

48. The most likely causative pathogen in a 26-year-old woman with PID is:

   A. *E. coli*

   B. *Enterobacteriaceae* spp.

   C. *C. trachomatis*

   D. *Pseudomonas* spp.

49. Which of the following is a treatment option for a 30-year-old woman with PID and severe penicillin allergy?

   A. ofloxacin with metronidazole

   B. amoxicillin with gentamicin

   C. cefixime with vancomycin

   D. clindamycin with azithromycin

ANSWERS

47. B

48. C

49. A

DISCUSSION

Pelvic inflammatory disease is an infectious disease consisting of endometritis, salpingitis, and oophoritis. It is caused by a variety of pathogens, including C. trachomatis, N. gonorrhea, Hemophilus influenzae, Streptococcus spp., select anaerobes, Mycoplasma spp., and Ureaplasma spp., with approximately 60% acquired through sexual transmission. Clinical presentation includes lower abdominal pain, abnormal vaginal discharge, dyspareunia, fever, gastrointestinal upset, and abnormal vaginal bleeding. An adnexal mass may be palpable when tubo-ovarian abscess is present. Supporting laboratory tests may include elevated sedimentation rate or C-reactive protein, as well as leukocytosis with neutrophilia. Although diagnosis can usually be made by clinical findings, transvaginal ultrasound may demonstrate tubal thickening with or without free pelvic fluid or tubo-ovarian abscess.

Treatment options differ according to patient presentation. When a woman with PID is severely ill, pregnant, or has tubo-ovarian abscess, hospitalization for hydration and parenteral antibiotic therapy is indicated. In most situations, outpatient therapy with oral or parenteral antibiotics is sufficient. Ceftriaxone 250 mg IM as a one-time dose followed by doxycycline 100 mg BID for 2 weeks is likely the most commonly used treatment regimen and is highly effective. Ofloxacin 400 mg BID with metronidazole 500 mg BID for 2 weeks offers an effective oral treatment option that is a reasonable alternative in the face of severe penicillin allergy.

As with all STDs, a critical part of care is the discussion of preventive strategies, including condom use and limiting the number of sexual partners. NPs should offer and encourage testing for other STDs, including HIV.

Discussion Sources

Brown, K. (2000). *Management Guidelines for Women's Health Nurse Practitioners*. Philadelphia: FA Davis. Pp. 78–80.

McKay, H. (1999). Gynecology. In Tierny, L., McPhee, S., & Papadakis, M. *Current Medical Diagnosis and Treatment* (38th ed.). Stamford, CT: Appleton & Lange. Pp. 703–736.

Center for Disease Control and Prevention (1998). 1998 Guidelines for Treatment of Sexually Transmitted Disease. Available at http://www.cdc.gov.epo/mmwr/preview/mmwrhtml/00050909.htm

QUESTIONS

50. Sequelae of genital condyloma acuminata may include:

A. cervical carcinoma
B. PID
C. vaginal fistula
D. Reiter syndrome

51. Which of the following best describes the lesions associated with condyloma acuminata?

A. verruca form
B. plaquelike
C. vesicular form
D. bullous

52. Treatment options for patients with condyloma acuminata include:

A. imiquimod (Aldara)
B. azithromycin
C. acyclovir
D. metronidazole

ANSWERS

50. A
51. A
52. A

DISCUSSION

Condyloma acuminata, verruca-form lesions seen in genital warts, is an STD. The causative agent is HPV, with infection with multiple virus types usually seen with genital infection. Anal, penile, and cervical carcinoma can be consequences of HPV infection. However, not all HPV types are correlated with malignancy.

About 50% will have a spontaneous regression of warts without intervention. Treatment options include podofilox, imiquimod, trichloroacetic acid, or cryotherapy; the patient, saving the cost and inconvenience of office visits, may administer podofilox and imiquimod cream. Interferon therapy or surgery is typically reserved for complicated, recalcitrant lesions (see Table 13–8).

As with all STDs, a critical part of care is the discussion of preventive strategies, including condom use and limiting the number of sexual partners. NPs should offer and encourage testing for other STDs, including HIV.

Discussion Source

Brown, K. (2000). *Management Guidelines for Women's Health Nurse Practitioners.* Philadelphia: FA Davis. Pp. 81–82.

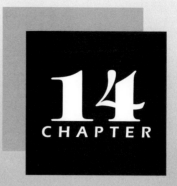

14
CHAPTER

Pediatrics

QUESTIONS

1. Which of the following is appropriate advice to give to a mother who is breastfeeding her 10-day-old infant?

   A. Your milk will come in today.
   B. To minimize breast tenderness, the baby should not be kept on each breast for more than 5 to 10 minutes.
   C. A pacifier should be offered between feedings.
   D. The baby's urine should be light or colorless.

2. Which of the following is appropriate advice to give to a mother who is breastfeeding her 12-hour-old infant?

   A. You will likely have enough milk to feed the baby within a few hours of birth.
   B. The baby may need to be awakened to be fed.
   C. Supplemental feeding is needed unless the baby has at least 4 wet diapers in the first day of life.
   D. A seedy yellow stool is anticipated.

3. When compared with the use of infant formula, advantages of breast-feeding include all of the following except:

   A. lower incidence of diarrheal illness
   B. greater weight gain in the first few weeks of life
   C. reduced risk of allergic disorders
   D. lower occurrence of constipation

4. At 3 weeks of age, the average weight formula-fed infant should be expected to take:

   A. 2 to 3 oz every 2 to 3 hours
   B. 2 to 3 oz every 3 to 4 hours
   C. 3 to 4 oz every 2 to 3 hours
   D. 3 to 4 oz every 3 to 4 hours

5. Solid foods are best introduced no earlier than:

   A. 1 to 3 months
   B. 3 to 5 months
   C. 4 to 6 months
   D. 6 to 8 months

6. Nursing infants generally receive about which percentage of the maternal dose of a drug?

   A. 1
   B. 3
   C. 5
   D. 10

7. Most drugs pass into breast milk through:

   A. active transport
   B. facilitated transfer
   C. simple diffusion
   D. creation of a pH gradient

8. In order to remove a drug from breast milk through "pump and dump," the process must be continued for:

   A. two infant feeding cycles
   B. approximately 8 hours
   C. 3 to 5 half-lives of drugs
   D. a period of time that is highly unpredictable

9. When counseling a breastfeeding woman about alcohol use during lactation, you describe the following:

   A. It enhances the let-down reflex.
   B. Because of its high molecular weight, relatively little alcohol is passed into breast milk.
   C. Maternal alcohol use causes a reduction in the amount of milk ingested by the infant.
   D. Infant intoxication may be seen with as little as 1 to 2 maternal drinks.

10. A 23-year-old woman is breastfeeding her newborn. She wishes to use hormonal contraception. Which of the following represents the best regimen?

   A. combined oral contraception initiated at 2 weeks
   B. progesterone-only oral contraception initiated at 3 weeks
   C. Depo-Provera given day 1 postpartum
   D. all forms are contraindicated during lactation

11. The anticipated average daily weight gain during the first 3 months of life is approximately:

   A. 15 g
   B. 20 g
   C. 25 g
   D. 30 g

12. The average required caloric intake in an infant from age 0 to 3 months is usually:

   A. 40 to 60 kcal/kg/d
   B. 60 to 80 kcal/kg/d
   C. 80 to 100 kcal/kg/d
   D. 100 to 120 kcal/kg/d

ANSWERS

1. D
2. B
3. B
4. A
5. C
6. A
7. C
8. C
9. C
10. B
11. D
12. D

DISCUSSION

Breastfeeding provides the ideal form of nutrition during infancy. In the United States, nearly 60 percent of all infants are breast-fed at birth, with only about 25 percent continuing by 6 months. NPs can help influence successful breastfeeding.

The content of commercially prepared formula available in the developed world continues to be improved to be closer in composition to breast milk. However, infant formula continues to lack critically important components. Breast milk contains immunoactive factors that help protect infants against infectious disease and may reduce the frequency of allergic disorders. Nutritionally, formula lacks a number of micronutrients found in breast milk. If a baby is formula-fed, the parents and caregivers should be encouraged to hold the child during feeding in order to have the interaction inherent in breastfeeding.

Frequency, amount, and type of feedings are a frequent question asked during well-child visits. Counseling should be offered to help ensure optimal nutrition (Box 14–1 and Table 14–1).

If a nursing mother becomes ill or has a chronic health problem, she is often erroneously encouraged to discontinue breastfeeding based on the

---

BOX 14–1
GUIDELINES FOR NUTRITION IN
THE FIRST MONTHS OF LIFE

- Frequency of feeding during months 1 and 2
  - Breast-fed infants: A minimum of 10 minutes at each breast every 1½ to 3 hours
  - Formula-fed infants: 2–3 oz every 2 to 3 hours
- Fluoride supplementation is advisable for the breast-fed infant and if formula is not mixed with fluoridated water
- Solid foods are best introduced at age 4 to 6 months
- Signs that a baby is ready for solid food
  - Doubled birth weight
  - More than 32 oz formula per day
  - More than 8 to 10 feedings per day

Reference: Hill, N., & Sullivan, L. (1999). *Management Guidelines for Pediatric Nurse Practitioners*. Philadelphia: FA Davis. Pp. 32–33.

TABLE 14-1.
ANTICIPATED WEIGHT GAIN AND CALORIC
REQUIREMENTS IN THE FIRST THREE YEARS OF LIFE

Age	Anticipated Average Weight Gain per Day (in grams)	Required Kilocalorie per Kilogram per Day
0–3 months	26–31	100–120 kcal
3–6 months	17–18	105–115 kcal
6–9 months	12–13	100–105 kcal
9–12 months	9	100–105 kcal
1–3 years	7–9	100 kcal

incorrect assumption by the health care provider that most medications are not safe to use. In fact, most medications can be used during lactation, but the benefit of improved maternal health should be balanced against the risk of exposing an infant to medication.

Postpartum contraception is usually an important concern of new mothers. Some women may opt not to breastfeed, fearing an inability to access reliable hormonal contraception while lactating. In fact, a number of options are available, including the use of progestin-only pill (POP) and Depo-Provera. For lactating women who wish to use an oral hormonal contraceptive, POP is highly effective and does not alter the quality or quantity of breast milk. One significant disadvantage of POP use is bleeding irregularity, ranging from prolonged flow to amenorrhea. Medroxyprogesterone acetate (DMPA) in a depot injection (Depo-Provera) given every 90 days is a highly reliable form of contraception at 99.7 percent efficacy. Depo-Provera use may be started immediately postpartum if the woman is not breastfeeding and started at 3 to 6 weeks postpartum if she is breastfeeding. Earlier use may diminish the quantity but not quality of breast milk.

Nearly all breastfeeding mothers use some type of medications (most often analgesic agents such as nonsteroidal anti-inflammatory drugs [NSAIDs], acetaminophen, opioids, and antibiotics) in the first 2 weeks after giving birth. About 25 percent need to use medication intermittently to manage episodic disease. These medications usually include analgesics, antihistamines, decongestants, and antibiotics.

About 5 percent of breastfeeding women have a chronic health problem necessitating daily use of a medication; the most common chronically used are for treating asthma, mental health problems, seizure disorder, and hypertension. Nursing infants usually get about 1 percent, often less, of the maternal dose, and only a small number of drugs are contraindicated (Box 14–2).

The "pump and dump" procedure is a less-than-helpful way to reduce drug levels in mother's milk because this creates an area of lower drug concentration in the empty breast. This encourages the drug to diffuse from the area of high concentration (maternal serum) to the area of low concentration (breast milk). If the mother takes a medication that may be problematic for the nursing infant, pumping while discarding the milk needs to continue for 3 to 5 half-lives of the medication.

Alcohol has a low molecular weight and is highly lipid-soluble; both of these characteristics allow it to have easy passage into breast milk. Even in small amounts, alcohol ingestion by a nursing mother can cause a smaller amount of milk produced and reduction in let-down reflex as well as less rhythmic and frequent sucking by the infant. This results in a smaller volume of milk ingested. Cigarette smoking is similarly problematic. Nicotine, a highly lipid-soluble substance with a low molecular weight, passes easily into breast milk. Maternal cigarette smoking may reduce milk supply as well as expose an infant to passive smoke. Infant crankiness, diarrhea, tachycardia, and vomiting have been reported with high maternal nicotine dose.

Discussion Source

Hill, N., & Sullivan, L. (1999). *Management Guidelines for Pediatric Nurse Practitioners.* Philadelphia: FA Davis, Pp. 1–31

BOX 14–2
MEDICATIONS CONTRAINDICATED IN BREASTFEEDING MOTHERS

- Cocaine
- Ergotamine
- Lithium
- Phencyclidine (PCP)
- Select antineoplastic and immunosuppressive agents (including cyclosporine, doxorubicin, cyclophosphamide, and methotrexate)

QUESTIONS

13. Which of the following is most consistent with a normal developmental examination for a 3-month-old full-term infant?

    A. sits briefly with support
    B. experiments with sound
    C. rolls over
    D. has a social smile

14. Which of the following is most consistent with a normal developmental examination for a thriving 5-month-old infant born at 32 weeks' gestation?

    A. sits briefly with support
    B. experiments with sound
    C. rolls over
    D. performs hand-to-hand transfers

15. A healthy baby between the age of 3 to 5 months should be able to:

    A. recognize parents
    B. bring hands together
    C. reach with one hand
    D. feed self biscuit

16. A healthy baby between the ages of 9 to 11 months is expected to:

    A. roll back to stomach
    B. imitate "bye-bye"
    C. imitate peek-a-boo
    D. hand toy on request

17. The typical 2-year-old child is able to:

    A. speak in phrases of two or more words
    B. throw a ball
    C. scribble spontaneously
    D. ride a tricycle

18. At which age will a child likely start to imitate housework?

    A. 15 months
    B. 18 months
    C. 24 months
    D. 30 months

19. A healthy 3-year-old child is expected to:

    A. give his or her first and last name
    B. use pronouns
    C. kick a ball
    D. name a best friend

20. A healthy 6-month-old infant is able to:

    A. pull to sit without head lag
    B. feed self cracker
    C. reach for object
    D. crawl on abdomen

21. You examine a healthy 9-month-old infant from a term pregnancy and expect to find that he or she:

    A. sits without support
    B. cruises
    C. has the ability to recognize his or her own name
    D. imitates a razzing noise

22. A healthy 3-year-old child is in your office for well-childcare. You expect this child to be able to:

    A. name three colors
    B. alternate feet when climbing stairs
    C. speak in two-word phrases
    D. tie shoelaces

23. Which of the following would not be found in newborns?

    A. best vision at a range of 8 to 12 inches
    B. presence of red reflex
    C. light-sensitive eyes
    D. lack of defensive blink

24. Which of the following do you expect to find in an examination of a 2-week-old infant?

    A. a visual preference for the human face
    B. a preference for low-pitched voices
    C. indifference to the cry of other neonates
    D. poorly developed sense of smell

25. Which of the following is the most appropriate response in the developmental examination of the average 5-year-old child?

   A. has the ability to name a best friend
   B. gives gender appropriately
   C. names an intended career
   D. hops on one foot

ANSWERS

13. **B**
14. **B**
15. **B**
16. **C**
17. **A**
18. **A**
19. **A**
20. **A**
21. **C**
22. **B**
23. **D**
24. **A**
25. **A**

DISCUSSION

Performing a developmental assessment is one of the most important parts of providing pediatric primary care. Besides providing a marker to evaluate the child, the assessment also affords an important learning tool for the parents. Pointing out milestones to be achieved in the near future and their impact on safety can help the family prepare appropriately (Table 14–2).

Discussion Source

Hill, N., & Sullivan, L. (1999). *Management Guidelines for Pediatric Nurse Practitioners.* Philadelphia: FA Davis, Pp. 1–31.

TABLE 14–2.
ANTICIPATED EARLY CHILDHOOD
DEVELOPMENTAL MILESTONES

Age	Able to Be Observed during Office Visit	Reported by Parent or Caregiver
Newborn	• Moves all extremities • Spontaneous stepping • Reacts to sound by blinking, turning • Responds to cries of other neonates • Well-developed sense of smell • Preference for higher-pitched voices Reflexes • Tonic neck • Palmar grasp • Babinski response • Rooting awake and sleep • Sucking	• Able to be calmed by feeding, cuddling • Reinforces presence of developmental tasks seen in examination room
1–2 months	• Lifts head • Holds head erect • Regards face • Follows objects through visual field • Moro reflex fading	• Spontaneous smile • Recognizes parents
3–5 months	• Grasps cube • Reaches for objects • Brings objects to mouth • Raspberry sound • Sits with support	• Laughs • Recognizes food by sight • Rolls back to side
6–8 months	• Sits briefly without support • Scoops small object with rake grip; some thumb use • Hand-to-hand transfers • Imitates "bye-bye"	• Rolls back to stomach • Recognizes "no"
9–11 months	• Stands alone • Imitates peek-a-boo and pat-a-cake • Picks up small object with thumb and index finger	• Cruises • Follows simple command, such as "Come here."

(continued)

TABLE 14–2. (continued)

Age	Able to Be Observed during Office Visit	Reported by Parent or Caregiver
12–15 months	• Walks solo • "Mama," "Dada" specific • Neat pincher grasp • Places cube in cup • Hands over objects on request • Builds tower of two bricks	• Says one to two words • Indicates wants by pointing • Scribbles spontaneously
15–20 months	• Points to several body parts • Throws a ball • Seats self in chair	• Uses a spoon with little spilling • Walks up and down steps with help • Understands two-step commands • Feeds self • Carries and hugs doll
24 months	• Speaks in phrases of two words or more • Kicks ball on request • Jumps with both feet • Uses pronouns • Developing handedness	• Runs • Copies vertical and horizontal line • Has 50-word vocabulary • Washes and dries hands • Parallel play
30 months	• Walks backward • Hops on one foot • Copies circle	• Gives first and last name • Uses plurals
36 months	• Holds crayons with fingers • About 75% of speech intelligible to people not in daily contact with child • Three-word sentences	• Walks down stairs alternating steps • Rides tricycle • Copies circles • Dresses with supervision
3–4 years	• Responds to command to place object in, on, or under a table • Knows gender • Draws circle when one is shown	• Takes off jacket and shoes • Washes and dries face • Cooperative play • Speech includes plurals, personal pronouns, verbs • Skips

(continued)

TABLE 14–2. (continued)

Age	Able to Be Observed during Office Visit	Reported by Parent or Caregiver
4–5 years	• Runs and turns while maintaining balance • Stands on one foot for at least 10 seconds • Counts to four • Draws a person without torso • Copies (+) by imitation • Verbalizes activities to do when cold, hungry, tired	• Buttons clothes • Dresses self (not including tying shoelaces) • Can play without adult input for about 30 minutes
5–6 years	• Catches ball • Knows age • Knows right from left hand • Draws person with six to eight parts, including torso • Identifies best friend • Likes teacher	• Able to complete simple chores • Understands concept of 10 items; likely counts higher by rote • Has sense of gender
6–7 years	• Copies triangle • Draws person with at least 12 parts • Prints name • Reads multiple single-syllable words	• Ties shoelaces • Counts to 30 or beyond • Able to differentiate morning from later in day • Generally plays well with peers • No significant behavioral problems in school • Can name intended career
7–8 years	• Copies a diamond • Reads simple sentences • Draws person with at least 16 parts	• Ties shoes • Knows day of the week
8–9 years	• Able to give response to question such as what to do if an object is accidentally broken	• Able to add, subtract, borrow, carry • Understands concept of working as a team

(continued)

Age	Able to Be Observed during Office Visit	Reported by Parent or Caregiver
TABLE 14–2. (continued)		
9–10 years	• Knows month, day, year • Gives months of the year in sequence	• Able to multiply and do complex subtraction • Has increased reading fluency
10–12 years	• Beginning of pubertal changes for many girls	• Able to perform simple division • Has complex reading skills • May have interest in opposite sex

QUESTIONS

26. When considering a person's risk for measles, mumps, and rubella (MMR), the NP considers the following:

    A. Children should have two doses before the sixth birthday.

    B. Considerable mortality and morbidity occur with all three diseases.

    C. Most cases in the United States occur in infants.

    D. The use of the vaccine is often associated with protracted arthralgia.

27. Which of the following is true about the MMR vaccine?

    A. It contains live virus.

    B. Its use is contraindicated with a history of egg allergy.

    C. Revaccination of an immune person is associated with risk of allergic reaction.

    D. One dose is recommended for young adults who have not been previously immunized.

ANSWERS

26. **A**

27. **A**

DISCUSSION

The MMR vaccine is a live, attenuated vaccine. The recommended schedule for early childhood immunization is two doses of MMR vaccine given between 12 and 15 months and 4 and 6 years (Fig. 14–1). Two immunizations 1 month apart are recommended for older children who were not immunized earlier in life. As with other immunizations, giving additional doses to those with an unclear immunization history is safe.

Rubella, also known as German measles, typically causes a relatively mild, 3- to 5-day illness with little risk of complication to the person infected. However, when rubella is contracted during pregnancy, the effects to the fetus can be devastating. Immunizing the entire population against rubella protects unborn children from the risk of congenital rubella syndrome. Measles can cause severe illness with serious sequelae, including encephalitis and pneumonia; sequelae of mumps include orchitis.

In the past, a history of egg allergy was considered a contraindication to receiving MMR vaccine. However, its use now appears safe, but a 90-minute observation is recommended. The MMR vaccine is safe to use during lactation, but its use in pregnant women is discouraged because of the possible risk of their developing congenital rubella syndrome from the live virus contained in the vaccine. However, this is likely a more theoretical than actual risk. MMR vaccine is well tolerated with rare reports of mild, transient adverse reaction such as rash and sore throat. Systemic reaction to MMR is rare.

Discussion Sources

Centers for Disease Control Recommended Childhood Immunization Schedule—United States. Available at http:wonder.cdc.gov/wonder/prevguid/m0053300/entire/htm.
U.S. Preventative Services Task Force (1996). *Guide to clinical preventive services* (2nd ed.). Baltimore: Williams & Wilkins.

QUESTIONS

28. When advising parents about influenza immunization, the NP considers the following about the vaccine:

    A. It may be given to at-risk infants older than age 6 months.
    B. Its use is limited to children older than age 2 years.
    C. It contains live virus.
    D. It's use is not recommended for household members of high-risk patients.

Recommended Childhood Immunization Schedule
United States, January - December 2000

Vaccines [1] are listed under routinely recommended ages. [Bars] *indicate range of recommended ages for immunization. Any dose not given at the recommended age should be given as a "catch-up" immunization at any subsequent visit when indicated and feasible.* (Ovals) *indicate vaccines to be given if previously recommended doses were missed or given earlier than the recommended minimum age.*

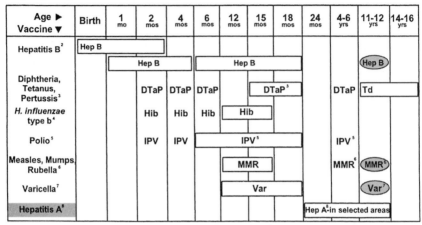

Age ▶ / Vaccine ▼	Birth	1 mo	2 mos	4 mos	6 mos	12 mos	15 mos	18 mos	24 mos	4-6 yrs	11-12 yrs	14-16 yrs
Hepatitis B [2]	Hep B											
		Hep B				Hep B					(Hep B)	
Diphtheria, Tetanus, Pertussis [3]			DTaP	DTaP	DTaP		DTaP [3]			DTaP	Td	
H. influenzae type b [4]			Hib	Hib	Hib	Hib						
Polio [5]			IPV	IPV		IPV [5]				IPV [5]		
Measles, Mumps, Rubella [6]						MMR				MMR [6]	(MMR [6])	
Varicella [7]						Var					(Var [7])	
Hepatitis A [8]										Hep A - in selected areas		

Approved by the Advisory Committee on Immunization Practices (ACIP), the American Academy of Pediatrics (AAP), and the American Academy of Family Physicians (AAFP).

On October 22, 1999, the Advisory Committee on Immunization Practices (ACIP) recommended that Rotashield® (RRV-TV), the only U.S.-licensed rotavirus vaccine, no longer be used in the United States (MMWR, Volume 43, Number 43, Nov. 5, 1999). Parents should be reassured that their children who received rotavirus vaccine before July are not at increased risk for intussusception now.

[1]This schedule indicates the recommended ages for routine administration of currently licensed childhood vaccines as of 11/1/99. Additional vaccines may be licensed and recommended during the year. Licensed combination vaccines may be used whenever any components of the combination are indicated and its other components are not contraindicated. Providers should consult the manufacturers' package inserts for detailed recommendations.

[2]Infants born to HBsAg-negative mothers should receive the 1st dose of hepatitis B (Hep B) vaccine by age 2 months. The 2nd dose should be at least one month after the 1st dose. The 3rd dose should be administered at least 4 months after the 1st dose and at least 2 months after the 2nd dose, but not before 6 months of age for infants.
Infants born to HBsAg-positive mothers should receive hepatitis B vaccine and 0.5 mL hepatitis B immune globulin (HBIG) within 12 hours of birth at separate sites. The 2nd dose is recommended at 1-2 months of age and the 3rd dose at 6 months of age.
Infants born to mothers whose HBsAg status is unknown should receive hepatitis B vaccine within 12 hours of birth. Maternal blood should be drawn at the time of delivery to determine the mother's HBsAg status; if the HBsAg test is positive, the infant should receive HBIG as soon as possible (no later than 1 week of age).
All children and adolescents (through 18 years of age) who have not been immunized against hepatitis B may begin the series during any visit. Special efforts should be made to immunize children who were born in or whose parents were born in areas of the world with moderate or high endemicity of hepatitis B virus infection.

[3]The 4th dose of DTaP (diphtheria and tetanus toxoids and acellular pertussis vaccine) may be administered as early as 12 months of age, provided 6 months have elapsed since the 3rd dose and the child is unlikely to return at age 15-18 months. Td (tetanus and diphtheria toxoids) is recommended at 11-12 years of age if at least 5 years have elapsed since the last dose of DTP, DTaP or DT. Subsequent routine Td boosters are recommended every 10 years.

[4]Three Haemophilus influenzae type b (Hib) conjugate vaccines are licensed for infant use. If PRP-OMP (PedvaxHIB® or ComVax® [Merck]) is administered at 2 and 4 months of age, a dose at 6 months is not required. Because clinical studies in infants have demonstrated that using some combination products may induce a lower immune response to the Hib vaccine component, DTaP/Hib combination products should not be used for primary immunization in infants at 2, 4 or 6 months of age, unless FDA-approved for these ages.

[5]To eliminate the risk of vaccine-associated paralytic polio (VAPP), an all-IPV schedule is now recommended for routine childhood polio vaccination in the United States. All children should receive four doses of IPV at 2 months, 4 months, 6-18 months, and 4-6 years. OPV (if available) may be used only for the following special circumstances:
1. Mass vaccination campaigns to control outbreaks of paralytic polio.
2. Unvaccinated children who will be traveling in <4 weeks to areas where polio is endemic or epidemic.
3. Children of parents who do not accept the recommended number of vaccine injections. These children may receive OPV only for the third or fourth dose or both; in this situation, health-care providers should administer OPV only after discussing the risk for VAPP with parents or caregivers.
4. During the transition to an all-IPV schedule, recommendations for the use of remaining OPV supplies in physicians' offices and clinics have been issued by the American Academy of Pediatrics (see Pediatrics, December 1999).

[6]The 2nd dose of measles, mumps, and rubella (MMR) vaccine is recommended routinely at 4-6 years of age but may be administered during any visit, provided at least 4 weeks have elapsed since receipt of the 1st dose and that both doses are administered beginning at or after 12 months of age. Those who have not previously received the second dose should complete the schedule by the 11-12 year old visit.

[7]Varicella (Var) vaccine is recommended at any visit on or after the first birthday for susceptible children, i.e. those who lack a reliable history of chickenpox (as judged by a health care provider) and who have not been immunized. Susceptible persons 13 years of age or older should receive 2 doses, given at least 4 weeks apart.

[8]Hepatitis A (Hep A) is shaded to indicate its recommended use in selected states and/or regions; consult your local public health authority. (Also see MMWR Oct. 01, 1999;48(RR12); 1-37).

FIG. 14–1. Immunizations

29. A 7-year-old child with type 1 diabetes mellitus is about to receive influenza vaccine. His parents and he should be advised that:

   A. The vaccine is more than 90 percent effective in preventing influenza.

   B. The vaccine's use is contraindicated during antibiotic therapy.

   C. Localized immunization reactions are fairly common.

   D. A short, intense, flulike syndrome typically occurs after immunization.

ANSWERS

28. A

29. C

DISCUSSION

Influenza is a viral illness that typically causes many days of incapacitation and suffering as well as the risk of death. The vaccine is about 70–80% effective in preventing influenza A and B and reducing the severity of the disease.

Having a mild illness or taking an antibiotic are not contraindications to any immunization, including influenza. Annual influenza vaccine is recommended for children with chronic health problems such as asthma. The vaccine does not contain live virus and is not shed; therefore, there is no risk of shedding an infectious agent to household contacts. This vaccine may be given to infants as young as age 6 months. Influenza vaccine is recommended for household members of high-risk patients in order to avoid transmission of infection.

Discussion Sources

Centers for Disease Control Recommended Childhood Immunization Schedule—United States. Available at http:wonder.cdc.gov/wonder/prevguid/m0053300/entire/htm.
U.S. Preventative Services Task Force (1996). *Guide to clinical preventive services* (2nd ed.). Baltimore: Williams & Wilkins.

QUESTIONS

30. Which of the following is true about the hepatitis B virus (HBV) vaccine?

    A. It contains live HBV.

    B. Children should have anti-HBs titers drawn after 3 doses of vaccine.

    C. Hepatitis B immunization should be offered to all children by their twelfth birthdays.

    D. Serologic testing for hepatitis B surface antigen (HBsAg) should be checked before initiating HBV in children.

31. You are doing rounds in the nursery and examine the neonate of a mother who is HBsAg-positive. Your most appropriate action is to:

    A. administer hepatitis B immune globulin (HBIG)

    B. isolate the child

    C. administer hepatitis B immunization

    D. give hepatitis B immunization and HBIG

ANSWERS

30. C

31. D

DISCUSSION

A small, double-stranded DNA virus that contains the inner protein of hepatitis B core antigen and an outer surface of hepatitis surface antigen causes hepatitis B. The virus is transmitted through exchange of body fluids. Hepatitis B infection can be prevented by limiting exposure to blood and body fluids as well as through immunization. Recombinant hepatitis B vaccine does not contain live virus and is well tolerated. Children should be immunized in early childhood. The well-child visit at ages 11 to 12 years offers an opportunity to update hepatitis B and other immunizations before adolescence.

Infants who have been infected perinatally with HBV have an estimated 25 percent lifetime chance of developing hepatocellular carcinoma or cirrhosis. As a result, all pregnant women should have screening with

HBsAg done at the first prenatal visit regardless of HBV vaccine history. The HBV vaccine is not 100 percent effective, and a woman may have carried HbsAg since before pregnancy. During the first 24 hours of life, a neonate born to a mother with HBsAg should receive HBV as well as HBIG in order to minimize the risk of perinatal transmission and subsequent development of chronic hepatitis B.

About 90–95% of those who receive the vaccine develop HBsAb (anti-HBs) after 3 doses, implying protection from the virus. As a result, routine testing for the presence of HBsAb after immunization is not generally recommended.

Administration of HBIG after exposure with a repeat dose in 1 month is about 75 percent effective in protecting from hepatitis B after percutaneous, sexual, or mucosal exposure to HBV. With postexposure HBIG, HBV vaccine series should be started.

Discussion Sources

Centers for Disease Control Recommended Childhood Immunization Schedule—United States. Available at http:wonder.cdc.gov/wonder/prevguid/m0053300/entire/htm.
Margolis, H., & Moyer, L. (1998). Ask the experts; Hepatitis B. Available at *http://www.medscape.com/scp/IIM/1998v15.n06.*
U.S. Preventative Services Task Force (1996). *Guide to clinical preventive services* (2nd ed.). Baltimore: Williams & Wilkins.

QUESTIONS

32. Which of the following is correct about the varicella vaccine?

A. It contains killed varicella zoster virus (VZV).

B. A short febrile illness is common during the first days after vaccination.

C. Children should have a varicella titer drawn before receiving the vaccine.

D. Mild cases of chickenpox have been reported in immunized patients.

33. Expected outcomes with the use of varicella vaccine include a reduction in the rate of all of the following except:

A. shingles

B. Reye syndrome

C. aspirin allergy

D. invasive varicella

34. A parent asks about varicella zoster immune globulin and you reply that it is a:

   A. synthetic product that is well tolerated
   B. pooled blood product that has been known to transmit infectious disease
   C. blood product obtained from a single donor
   D. pooled blood product with an excellent safety profile

ANSWERS

32. D
33. C
34. D

DISCUSSION

The VZV causes the highly contagious, systemic disease commonly known as chickenpox. Varicella infection usually confers lifetime immunity. However, reinfection may be seen in immunocompromised patients. More often, reexposure causes an increase in antibody titers without causing disease.

The VZV virus can lie dormant in sensory nerve ganglion. Later reactivation causes shingles, a painful, vesicular-form rash in a dermatomal pattern. About 15 percent of those who have had chickenpox develop shingles at least once during their lifetime. Shingles rates are markedly reduced in people who have received varicella vaccine compared with those who have had chickenpox.

A patient-reported history of varicella is considered a valid measurement of immunity, with 97–99% having serologic evidence of immunity. Among older children and adults with an unclear or negative varicella history, the majority are also seropositive. Confirming varicella immunity through varicella titers, even in the presence of a positive varicella history, should be done in health care workers because of their risk of exposure and potential transmission of the disease.

The varicella vaccine contains attenuated virus. The vaccine is administered in a single dose after the first birthday. Older children (age 13 years and older) and adults with no history of varicella infection or previous immunization should receive two immunizations 4 to 8 weeks apart. In particular, health care workers, family contacts of immunocompromised patients, and day care workers should be targeted for varicella vaccine. In addition, adults who are in environments with high risk of varicella transmission (e.g., college dormitories, military barracks, long-term care facilities) should receive the vaccine. The vaccine is highly protective against severe, invasive varicella. However, mild forms of chickenpox may be reported after immunization.

Varicella immune globulin, as with all forms of immune globulin (IG), provides temporary, passive immunity to infection. IG is a pooled blood product with an excellent safety profile. Although the majority of cases are seen in children younger than age 18 years, the greatest varicella mortality is found in persons ages 30 to 49 years.

Discussion Sources

Centers for Disease Control Recommended Childhood Immunization Schedule—United States. Available at http:wonder.cdc.gov/wonder/prevguid/m0053300/entire/htm.
Isada, C., Kasten, B., Goldman, M., et al. (1997). *Infectious Disease Handbook* (2nd ed.). Columbus, OH: Lexicomp.
U.S. Preventative Services Task Force (1996). *Guide to clinical preventive services* (2nd ed.). Baltimore: Williams & Wilkins.

QUESTIONS

35. An 11-year-old child presents with no documented primary tetanus immunization series. Which of the following represents the immunization needed?

   A. 3 doses of DTaP 2 months apart
   B. tetanus immune globulin now and 2 doses of tetanus–diphtheria (Td) 1 month apart
   C. Td now, with repeat in 1 and 6 months
   D. Td as a single dose

36. Problems after tetanus immunization typically include:

   A. localized reaction at site of injection
   B. myalgia and malaise
   C. low-grade fever
   D. diffuse rash

ANSWERS

35. C
36. A

DISCUSSION

Tetanus infection is caused by *Clostridium tetani*, an anaerobic, gram-positive, spore-forming rod. This organism, which is found in soil, particularly if it contains manure, enters the body through a contaminated wound and causes a life-threatening systemic disease characterized by painful muscle weakness and spasm ("lockjaw"). Diphtheria, caused by *Corynebacterium diphtheriae*, a gram-negative bacillus, is typically transmitted person-to-person or through contaminated liquids such as milk. Diphtheria is characterized by severe respiratory tract infection, including the appearance of pseudomembranous pharyngitis.

Tetanus and diphtheria are uncommon infections because of widespread immunization. A primary series of three Td vaccine injections sets the stage for long-term immunity. A booster Td dose every 10 years is recommended, but protection is likely for up to 20 to 30 years after a primary series. Using Td rather than tetanus toxoid for the primary series and booster doses in adults assists in keeping diphtheria immunity as well. At the time of wound-producing injury, tetanus immune globulin affords temporary protection for individuals who have not received tetanus immunization.

Tetanus immunization is well tolerated and has few adverse reactions. A short-term, localized area of redness and warmth is quite common and does not predict future problems with tetanus immunization.

Discussion Sources

Isada, C., Kasten, B., Goldman, M., et al. (1997). *Infectious Disease Handbook* (2nd ed.). Columbus, OH: Lexicomp.
U.S. Preventative Services Task Force (1996). *Guide to clinical preventive services* (2nd ed.). Baltimore: Williams & Wilkins.

QUESTIONS

37. Which of the following is the primary source of hepatitis A infection?

    A. blood products
    B. shellfish
    C. contaminated water supplies
    D. intimate person-to-person contact

38. When answering questions about hepatitis A vaccine, you consider that it:

  A. contains live virus

  B. should be given to children living in select high-risk states

  C. frequently causes systemic post-immunization reaction

  D. is 100 percent protective after a single injection

39. Usual treatment options for a child with hepatitis A include:

  A. alpha-interferon

  B. ribavirin

  C. acyclovir

  D. supportive care

ANSWERS

37. C

38. B

39. D

DISCUSSION

Hepatitis A infection is caused by HAV (hepatitis A virus), a small RNA virus. Transmitted primarily by fecal-contaminated drinking water and food supplies, hepatitis A is typically a self-limiting infection with a very low mortality rate that responds well to supportive care. Although raw shellfish growing in contaminated water can be problematic, fecal-contaminated water supplies are the most common source of infection. In developing countries with limited pure water, the majority of the children contact this disease by age 5 years. In North America, adults ages 20 to 39 years account for nearly 50 percent of the reported cases; children are more often affected than adults.

  Children who live in Arizona, Arkansas, California, Idaho, Nevada, New Mexico, Oklahoma, Oregon, South Dakota, Utah, and Washington state should be immunized against HAV because these states have two to three times the national average rate of hepatitis. Two doses of vaccine are recommended to ensure a greater immune response. Hepatitis A vaccine, which does not contain live vaccine, is usually well tolerated without systemic reaction.

Discussion Sources

Friedman, L. (1999). Liver, biliary tract and pancreas. In Tierney, L., McPhee, S., & Papadakis, M. *Current Diagnosis and Treatment* (38th ed.). Norwalk, CT: Appleton & Lange, Pp. 638–677.
U.S. Preventative Services Task Force (1996). *Guide to clinical preventive services* (2nd ed.). Baltimore: Williams & Wilkins.

QUESTIONS

40. Which of the following is true about oral poliovirus vaccine (OPV)?

   A. It contains killed virus.

   B. It is the preferred method of immunization.

   C. Two doses should be administered by a child's fourth birthday

   D. After administration of OPV, poliovirus may be shed from the stool.

41. Which of the following is true about inactivated poliovirus vaccine (IPV)?

   A. It contains live virus.

   B. It is the preferred method of immunization for immunocompromised children.

   C. Two doses should be administered by a child's fourth birthday

   D. After administration of IPV, poliovirus may be shed from the stool.

ANSWERS

40. **D**
41. **B**

DISCUSSION

Polioviruses are highly contagious and capable of causing paralytic, life-threatening infection. Transmitted fecal-orally, rates of infection among household contacts may be as high as 96 percent. However, since 1994, North and South America have been declared free of indigenous poliomyelitis, largely because of the efficacy of the OPV. This live virus vaccine is given orally with a small amount of the poliovirus shed through the stool. This shedding presents household members with possible exposure to poliovirus. Virtually all cases of paralytic poliomyelitis currently found in the United States are vaccine-associated (vaccine-associated paralytic poliomyelitis [VAPP]). Using IPV instead of OPV, a recommendation in the presence of patient immunosuppression or immunosuppressed household contact could eliminate VAPP. Due to VPP risk, OPV vaccine is no longer used in the United States.

Discussion Source

Zimmerman, R., & Spann, S. (1999). Poliovirus vaccine options. *American Family Physician.* 59 (1) 113–118.

QUESTIONS

42. Which of the following is most likely to have lead poisoning?

    A. a developmentally disabled 5-year-old child who lives in a 15-year-old house in poor repair
    B. an infant who lives in a 5-year-old home with copper plumbing
    C. a toddler who lives in a 45-year-old home
    D. a preschooler who lives nears an electric generating plant

43. You are devising a program to screen preschoolers for lead (Pb) poisoning. The most sensitive component of this campaign is:

    A. environmental history
    B. physical examination
    C. hematocrit level
    D. hemoglobin level

44. Patients with plumbism present with which kind of anemia?

    A. macrocytic, hyperchromic
    B. normocytic, normochromic
    C. hemolytic
    D. microcytic, hypochromic

45. Which of the following is the recommended screening for a child with significant risk of lead poisoning?

    A. start at age 3 months; repeat every 3 months
    B. start at age 6 months; repeat every 6 months
    C. start at age 1 year; repeat every year
    D. start at age 2 years; repeat annually

46. Intervention for a child with a Pb between 10–20 µg/dL usually includes all of the following except:

    A. removal from the lead source
    B. iron supplementation
    C. chelation therapy
    D. encouraging a diet high in vitamin C

47. Intervention for a child with a Pb of equal to 40–50 µg/dL usually includes:

    A. chelation
    B. calcium supplementation
    C. exchange transfusion
    D. iron depletion

ANSWERS

42. C
43. A
44. D
45. B
46. C
47. A

DISCUSSION

Lead poisoning, or plumbism, remains a significant public health problem. This is a reportable disease found in more than 2 million children and adults in the United States. Caused by exposure to lead in the environment, ingested lead inactivates heme synthesis by inhibiting the insertion of iron (Fe) into the protoporphyrin ring. This leads to the development of a microcytic, hypochromic anemia; basophilic stippling is noted on red blood cell morphology. In addition, lead is significantly toxic to the solid organs, bones, and the nervous system.

The major source of lead poisoning in children is lead-based paint. This paint has not been available in the United States for more than 20 years. However, the majority of homes built before 1957 contain lead paint. A diet low in calcium, iron, zinc, magnesium, and copper as well as high in fat, typical of children living in poverty, enhances lead absorption.

For lead poisoning to occur, there must be an intersection between the environmental hazard and the child. In older homes, the point of greatest risk is the window because the windowsills and putty have high lead concentration. Because toddlers are the ideal height to reach windowsills and are often drawn to open windows, the age of greatest risk is 2 to 3 years. Summer is the season of greatest risk. Children can acquire lead through two sources: inhaled paint powder and ingested paint chips. Inhalation of paint dust is a potent lead source for infants and in children with Pb below 45 µg/dL, although toddlers and children with Pb of more than 45 µg/dL are typically poisoned by also eating paint chips.

Besides paint, other lead hazards may be encountered. Lead-glazed pottery used to store and serve acidic beverages, soft water delivered by lead-lined pipes, lead-soldered vessels used for cooking, and fumes from burning casings of batteries can contribute to lead burden. In addition, soil around the base of the home may contain lead paint, and soil around highways often contains lead residual from automotive fuel. Certain folk medicines from the Middle East and Mexico may contain lead.

Clinical manifestation of lead poisoning is usually not apparent until a child's Pb level is markedly elevated. Because most children have low-level, chronic lead exposure with few or no symptoms, periodic screening of all children is recommended (Box 14–3).

BOX 14–3
PERIODIC CHILDHOOD LEAD SCREENING RECOMMENDATIONS

Low-risk children without significant lead exposure:

- Screen annually at ages 1–4 years

High-risk children with significant lead exposure (including living or spending a signficant amount of time in a home built before 1957, living in an older home being remodeled, living in a home built before 1957 that is being remodeled, having a household member with lead poisoning or an occupation with significant lead exposure or living near industry that may contaminate the environment with lead):

- Screen at age 6 months, repeat every 6 months as long as appropriate

Reference: Hill, N., & Sullivan, L. (1999). *Management Guidelines for Pediatric Nurse Practitioners*. Philadelphia: FA Davis, P. 467.

Primary prevention of lead poisoning should be the goal, with the goal of reducing risk for all children. After lead risk is identified, removing the child or limiting exposure is vital. Most children with Pb levels of 10 to 35 µg/dL are typically treated with removal from the source, improved nutrition, and iron therapy. With Pb levels of 36 to 50 µg/dL, chelation with an agent such as succimer along with the above listed intervention is indicated. With Pb levels of more than 51 µg/dL, hospital admission with expert evaluation is likely the most prudent course to avoid serious problems (including encephalopathy) associated with markedly elevated Pb levels.

Discussion Source

Hill, N., & Sullivan, L. (1999). *Management Guidelines for Pediatric Nurse Practitioners.* Philadelphia: FA Davis, Pp. 466–469.

QUESTIONS

48. The most likely causative organism of bronchiolitis is:

A. *Haemophilus influenzae*
B. parainfluenza virus
C. respiratory syncytial virus (RSV)
D. Coxsackie virus

49. One of the most prominent clinical features of bronchiolitis is:

A. fever
B. vomiting
C. wheezing
D. conjunctival inflammation

50. In the majority of children with bronchiolitis, intervention includes:

A. aerosolized ribavirin therapy
B. supportive care
C. oral theophylline therapy
D. ibuprofen therapy

51. Long-term sequelae of bronchiolitis may include:

A. recurrent airway reactivity
B. dilated terminal airways
C. hypoxemia
D. bronchopulmonary dysplasia

ANSWERS

48. C
49. C
50. B
51. A

DISCUSSION

Bronchiolitis is a common illness in early childhood; its peak incidence is in children younger than age 2 years. The most likely causative organism is RSV; it is less often caused by parainfluenzae and influenza virus and adenovirus. In most children, bronchiolitis runs a course of 2 to 3 weeks of mild upper respiratory symptoms with expiratory wheezing; supportive therapy is sufficient. In infants younger than age 3 months and children with chronic health problems, hypoxemia and hypercapnea is more common, necessitating hospital admission, hydration, and oxygenation. The use of corticosteroids and bronchodilators remains controversial. Long-term sequelae of bronchiolitis often include recurrent airway reactivity.

Discussion Source

Larsen, G., Accurso, F., Deterding, R., et al. (1999). Respiratory tract and mediastinum. In Hay, W., Hayward, A., Levin, M., & Sondheimer, J. *Current Pediatric Diagnosis and Treatment* (14th ed.). Stamford, CT: Appleton & Lange, Pp. 418–462.

QUESTIONS

52. You examine a newborn with a capillary hemangioma on her thigh. You advise her parents that this lesion:

    A. will likely increase in size over the first year of life
    B. should be treated to avoid malignancy
    C. usually resolves within the first months of life
    D. may develop a superimposed lichenification

53. You examine a 2-month-old infant with a port wine lesion over her right cheek. You advise the parents that this lesion:

    A. needs to be surgically excised
    B. grows proportionally with the child
    C. becomes lighter over time
    D. may become malignant

54. A 10-day-old child presents with multiple raised lesions over the trunk and nape of the neck resembling flea bites. The infant is nursing well and has no fever or exposure to animals. This may represent:

    A. erythema neonatorum toxicum
    B. milia
    C. neonatal acne
    D. staphylococcus skin infection

55. An Asian couple comes in with their 4-week-old infant who has blue-black macules scattered over the buttocks. These most likely represent:

    A. mottling
    B. Mongolian spots
    C. ecchymosis
    D. hemangioma

56. The most important aspect of skin care for patients with eczema is:

    A. frequent bathing with antibacterial soap
    B. consistent use of medium- to high-potency topical steroids
    C. application of lubricants
    D. treatment of dermatophytes

57. One of the more common sites for eczema in infants is the:

    A. dorsum of the hand
    B. face
    C. neck
    D. flexor surfaces

ANSWERS

52. A
53. B
54. A
55. B
56. C
57. B

DISCUSSION

A number of dermatologic conditions are found in early infancy. Parents understandably have concerns about these lesions. A thorough knowledge of the more common conditions is an important part of the NP's role.

Capillary hemanogioma is a congenital vascular malformation. The lesion becomes evident shortly after birth and grows rapidly in the first year, then plateaus in size and eventually regresses. About 90 percent are gone by age 9, usually leaving blush vascularity over the area. If the lesion is large or involves a vital organ such as the eye, treatment may be indicated. This can include the use of steroids, lasers, or alpha-interferon injection.

A port wine stain is a flat hemangioma with a stable course. These lesions have a predilection for appearing on the face and usually present at birth. Port wine stains tend to deepen in color as time goes on and grow proportionally with the child. Although not malignant, the lesions are often disfiguring and can be minimized or eliminated through the use of laser therapy.

Milia are typically white pinpoint papular lesions caused by sebaceous hyperplasia. The usual distribution is over the nose, cheeks, and other areas with an abundance of sebaceous glands. The cause is likely the maternal androgenic effect on the sebaceous glands. Benign in nature, milia resolve without special therapy by 4 weeks to 6 months of life.

Erythema toxicum neonatorum is a benign rash of unknown etiology that occurs in about 50 percent of term infants. Usually beginning in the first to tenth days of life, the lesions look like flea bites and are widely distributed; the palms and soles are spared. The lesions usually fade by 5 to 7 days after eruption without specific treatment.

Mongolian spots occur in about 90 percent of children of African and Asian ancestry and less than 10 percent of those of European ancestry. The distribution is usually over the lower back and buttocks but can occur widely. Caused by an accumulation of melanocytes, these are benign lesions that typically fade by age 7 without special therapy.

Acne neonatorum consists of open and closed comedones and pustules over the forehead and cheeks, similar to the adolescent version of the condition. The etiology is likely the effect of maternal androgens on the infant's skin. It usually resolves in about 4 to 8 weeks, but may persist up to age 6 months to 1 year. Low-dose benzoyl peroxide may be used.

Eczema or atopic dermatitis is one manifestation of a type I hypersensitivity reaction. This type of reaction is caused when IgE antibodies occupy receptor sites on mast cells causing a degradation of the mast cell and subsequent release of histamine, vasodilatation, mucous gland stimulation, and tissue swelling. Two subgroups, atopy and anaphylaxis, fall within the heading of type I hypersensitivity.

Within the atopy subgroup is a number of common clinical conditions such as allergic rhinitis, atopic dermatitis, allergic gastroenteropathy, and allergy-based asthma. Atopic diseases have a strong familial component and tend to cause localized rather than systemic reactions. Individuals with atopic disease are often able to identify allergy-inducing agents. Treatment for atopic disease of eczema includes avoidance of offending agents and minimizing skin dryness by limiting soap and water exposure as well as consistent use of lubricants. The NP should explain to the patient that the skin tends to be sensitive and needs to be treated with some care. When flare-ups occur, the skin eruption is largely caused by histamine release. Antihistamines and corticosteroids should be used to control eczema flare-ups. With an acute flare-up of eczema or with contact dermatitis, an intermediate- to higher-potency topical steroid is likely needed to control acute symptoms. After this is achieved, the lowest-potency topical steroid that yields the desired effect should be used.

Discussion Sources

Hill, N., & Sullivan, L. (1999). *Management Guidelines for Pediatric Nurse Practitioners.* Philadelphia: FA Davis, Pp. 53–88.
Morelli, J., & Weston, W. (1999). Skin. In Hay, W., Hayward, A., Levin, M., & Sondheimer, J. *Current Pediatric Diagnosis and Treatment* (14th ed.). Stamford, CT: Appleton & Lange, Pp. 341–359.

QUESTIONS

58. Which of the following is the most prudent first-line treatment choice for a toddler with acute otitis media (AOM) who attends large-group day care?

    A. ceftibuten

    B. high-dose amoxicillin

    C. cefuroxime

    D. azithromycin

59. The majority of AOM is caused by:

    A. select gram-positive and -negative bacteria

    B. gram-negative bacteria and pathogenic viruses

    C. rhinovirus and *Staphylococcus aureus*

    D. predominately beta-lactamase–producing organisms

60. Which of the following represents the best choice of clinical agents for a child who is severely allergic to penicillin who has his first case of AOM?

A. ciprofloxacin
B. clarithromycin
C. amoxicillin
D. cefixime

61. Which of the following does not represent a risk factor for recurrent AOM in younger children?

A. pacifier use after age 10 months
B. history of first episode of AOM before age 3 months
C. exposure to second-hand smoke
D. penicillin allergy

62. Which of the following antimicrobial agents affords the most effective activity against S. *pneumoniae*?

A. ciprofloxacin
B. cefixime
C. trimethoprim-sulfamethoxazole (TMP-SMX)
D. cefuroxime

63. A 3-year-old boy with AOM continues to have otalgia and fever after 3 days of amoxicillin at 40 mg/kg/d. Which of the following is recommended?

A. watch and wait
B. azithromycin
C. ibuprofen
D. amoxicillin with clavulanate

64. Which of the following is most consistent with the diagnosis of AOM?

A. ear pulling in the infant
B. tympanic membrane (TM) retraction
C. TM immobility to insufflation
D. anterior cervical lymphadenopathy

ANSWERS

58. B
59. A
60. B
61. D
62. D
63. D
64. C

DISCUSSION

In children, AOM is the most frequent diagnosis for office visits in children younger than age 15 years.

Streptococcus pneumoniae, Haemophilus influenzae, Moraxella catarrhalis, and a variety of viruses contribute to the infectious and inflammatory process of the middle ear. Nearly two-thirds of all children have at least one episode by their second birthday; one-third have more than three episodes.

Bottle feeding is a risk factor for AOM, with rates significantly lower among infants who were breast-fed for the first 6 to 12 months of life; boys and children of Native American ancestry are also at increased risk. Eustachian tube dysfunction usually precedes the development of AOM, allowing negative pressure to be generated in the middle ear and aspiration of pharyngeal pathogens. As a result, avoiding conditions that can cause Eustachian tube dysfunction can lead to a reduction in the occurrence of AOM (Box 14–4).

When out-of-home child care is needed, parents of younger children should be encouraged to choose small-group care with fewer than six

---

BOX 14–4
CAUSES OF EUSTACHIAN TUBE DYSFUNCTION

- Allergic rhinitis
- Upper respiratory infection
- Craniofacial abnormalities
- Passive cigarette smoke exposure
- Feeding in a supine position
- Pacifier use beyond age 10 months

children. Vaccines for influenza and pneumococcal vaccine have been advocated by some sources.

Streptococcus pneumoniae causes 40–50% of AOM; it is the least likely of the three major causative bacteria to resolve without antimicrobial intervention while causing the most significant symptoms. This organism has recently exhibited resistance to a number of antibiotic agents, including amoxicillin, cephalosporins, and macrolide. The mechanism of resistance is an alteration of intracellular protein-binding sites, which can typically be overcome by using higher doses of amoxicillin and select cephalosporins.

Hemophilus influenzae and *Moraxella catarrhalis* are gram-negative organisms capable of producing beta-lactamase. Although these two organisms have relatively high rates of spontaneous resolution (50 percent and 90 percent, respectively), without antimicrobial intervention, *H. influenzae* is the organism most commonly isolated from mucoid and serious middle ear effusion. Beta-lactamase production by organisms probably contributes less to AOM treatment failure than to prescribing an inadequate dosing of amoxicillin needed to eradicate drug-resistant *S. pneumoniae* (DRSP). Respiratory syncytial virus is commonly isolated from the middle ear fluid in children with AOM. Other common viral agents include human rhinovirus and coronavirus. AOM caused by these viral agents usually resolves in 7 to 10 days with supportive care alone.

Appropriate assessment is critical to arriving at the diagnosis of AOM. Ear pulling in preverbal children may be noted but is not considered diagnostic for the condition. The TM may be retracted or bulging and is typically reddened with loss of translucency and mobility on insufflation. With recovery, TM mobility returns in about 1 to 2 weeks, but middle ear effusion typically persists for 4 to 6 weeks.

Recurrent otitis media is defined as three episodes with documented resolution between illnesses within a 6-month period despite appropriate therapy or four or more episodes in the preceding 12 months. Approximately 15–25% of children age 2 years and younger have recurrent otitis media; having the first episode of AOM within the first 3 months of life is a potent risk factor for recurrent otitis media.

About 10 percent of children treated for AOM are unresponsive to the initial agent. AOM treatment failure is more common during the winter season and in children who have a history of recurrent otitis media. Children with AOM treatment failure present with persistent fever, otalgia, and irritability after 48 hours of antimicrobial therapy. Because the child's condition is unlikely to change after this short interval, persistence of TM redness, bulging, and immobility without other symptoms do not indicate treatment failure.

Repeated antibiotic use increases risk for colonization and disease caused by *S. pneumoniae,* the pathogen most likely to cause severe AOM symptoms and lead to complications such as recurrent otitis media. Considering this, clinicians can minimize DRSP development by judiciously prescribing antimicrobial agents. This includes prescribing an adequate dose of an antibiotic with strong activity against *S. pneumoniae* when antimicrobial therapy is needed for treating patients with AOM. In addition, it is equally important not to prescribe antibiotics when they are not required, such as in patients with viral upper respiratory infections or other self-limiting conditions.

Haemophilus influenzae is the most common pathogen cultured from middle ear exudate in children with chronic otitis media with effusion (Table 14–3). Two major factors probably contribute to this. First, although infection with a pathogen in those with AOM is often noted to spontaneously resolve without antimicrobial therapy, *H. influenzae* also has a propensity to adhere to virally infected or damaged tissue. As a result, continued pathogen colonization can be seen. In addition, clinicians often fail to prescribe an adequate dose of an antimicrobial agent with beta-lactamase inhibition or stability to reach therapeutic level in the middle ear (Tables 14–4 and 14–5).

Recent use of antimicrobial agents, age younger than 2 years, and attending day care increases a child's risk of infection with DRSP. As a result, a child who has had exposure to an antibiotic within the previous month should be given higher-dose amoxicillin or amoxicillin-clavulanate; cefuroxime axetil may be used as an alternative. With treatment failure on day 3 of therapy, daily intramuscular (IM) ceftriaxone for 3 days may be used. This supplies action against *S. pneumoniae* and beta-lactamase–producing organisms but carries with it the expense and inconvenience of repeated office visits as well as the discomfort of injections. Clindamycin may be used if DRSP is thought to be the offending pathogen, realizing that the agent has inadequate activity against *H. influenzae* or *M. catarrhalis.* In a child with AOM treatment failure on days 10 to 18 who has not recently taken antibiotics, the role of both DRSP and beta-lactamase–producing organisms must be considered. As a result,

TABLE 14–3. **DEFINITIONS OF OTITIS MEDIA TERMS**	
Acute otitis media	The presence of fluid in the middle ear in association with local or systemic illness including otalgia, otorrhea, fever
Otitis media with effusion	The presence of fluid in the middle ear in the absence of signs or symptoms of acute infection

TABLE 14–4.
SELECT ANTIBIOTICS USED IN THE TREATMENT OF
ACUTE OTITIS MEDIA

Antibiotic	Recommended Dosage	Comments
Usual dose amoxicillin	40 mg/kg/d divided into BID or TID doses	• First-line AOM therapy • Effective against non-resistant *S. pneumoniae* organisms • Ineffective against beta-lactamase–producing organisms
Higher-dose amoxicillin	80–90 mg/kg/d divided into BID or TID doses	• Effective against moderately resistant *S. pneumoniae* organisms
Amoxicillin with clavulanate (Augmentin)	Amoxicillin component 40–90 mg/kg/d with clavulanate 6.4 mg/kg/d divided into BID or TID doses	• Effective against susceptible beta-lactamase–producing organisms • In higher dose, effective against moderately resistant *S. pneumoniae* organisms
Ceftriaxone	50 mg/kg/d IM as one time or three daily doses	• Effective against moderately resistant *S. pneumoniae* organisms • Effective against susceptible beta-lactamase–producing organisms
Cefuroxime axetil	30 mg/kg/d divided into BID doses	• Effective against select beta-lactamase–producing organisms
Clindamycin	8–12 mg/kg/d divided into TID doses	• Effective against moderately resistant *S. pneumoniae* organisms • Ineffective against *H. influenzae* and *M. catarrhalis* organisms

TABLE 14–5.
RECOMMENDATIONS FOR TREATMENT
OF ACUTE OTITIS MEDIA

Condition	Dosage
Without antibiotic therapy in past month	• Usual-dose amoxicillin at 40 mg/kg/d • High-dose amoxicillin at 80–90 mg/kg/d
Treatment failure day 3	• High-dose amoxicillin-clavulanate • Cefuroxime • IM ceftriaxone in three daily doses
Treatment failure days 10–28	• Same as day 3 therapy
Antibiotic therapy within past month	• High-dose amoxicillin • High-dose amoxicillin-clavulanate • Cefuroxime
Treatment failure day 3	• IM ceftriaxone • Clindamycin • Tympanocentesis
Treatment failure days 10–28	• High-dose amoxicillin-clavulanate • Cefuroxime • Tympanocentesis

Reference: Dowell, S., Butler, J. Giebink, S., et al., and the Drug-Resistant *Streptococcus pneumoniae* Therapeutic Working Group (1999). Acute otitis media: Management and surveillance in an era of pneumococcal resistance: A report from the Drug-resistance *Streptococcus pneumoniae* Therapeutic Working Group. *Pediatric Infectious Disease Journal* 18:1–9.

therapeutic options include high-dose amoxicillin-clavulanate, cefuroxime axetil or IM ceftriaxone. If the patient has recently taken antibiotics, tympanocentesis should be considered to establish the offending organism.

The macrolides, in particular azithromycin and clarithromycin, are stable in the presence of beta-lactamase and provide reasonable gram-negative coverage. However, DRSP does not respond well to macrolides, limiting the usefulness of these products.

Trimethoprim-sulfamethoxazole has commonly been used as a first-line agent in treating patients with AOM. Although the agent is beta-lactamase stable with reasonable gram-negative activity, TMP-SMX *S. pneumoniae* resistance is more common than resistance to penicillin and is reported in approximately 25 percent of isolates.

The second- and third-generation cephalosporins are a heterogeneous group of antibiotics with varying beta-lactamase stability and antipneumococcal activity. In particular, cefaclor, cefixime, and cefabutin are active against *H. influenzae* and *M. catarrhalis* infection but are less active against *S. pneumoniae* infection, especially DRSP. Cefprozil and cefpodoxime also have similar limitations. Cefuroxime axetil and IM ceftriaxone have better activity against DRSP and beta-lactamase activity.

Appropriate follow-up visits are important in the care of children with AOM. Infants younger than age 3 months should be routinely seen 1 to 2 days after initiation of therapy because of increased risk of treatment failure. In children older than age 3 months, otalgia, fever, and other symptoms that persist beyond 3 days of therapy may indicate treatment failure. Repeat evaluation is in order. If the child appears to be recovering, a follow-up examination at 4 to 8 weeks to evaluate for otitis media with effusion (OME) and to reinforce AOM risk reduction is necessary. Eighty percent of children with OME clear the middle ear by 8 weeks. If OME persists beyond 8 weeks, the presence of communication problems and other symptoms dictate the need for further evaluation and treatment. Routine retreatment with antibiotics is not indicated for children with OME.

Discussion Sources

Berman, S., & Schmidt, B. (1996). Ear, nose and throat. In Hay, W., Groothuis, J., Hayward, A., & Levin, M. *Current Pediatric Diagnosis and Treatment* (12th ed.). Stamford, CT: Appleton & Lange, Pp. 454–492.

Dowell, S., Butler, J. Giebink, S., et al., and the Drug-resistant *Streptococcus pneumoniae* Therapeutic Working Group (1999). Acute otitis media: Management and surveillance in an era of pneumococcal resistance: A report from the Drug-resistance *Streptococcus pneumoniae* Therapeutic Working Group. *Pediatric Infectious Disease Journal* 18:1–9.

Dowell, S., Marcy, S., Phillips, W., et al. (1998). Otitis media: Principles of judicious use of antimicrobial agents. *Pediatrics* 101 (1) 166–178.

Pitkaranta, A., Virolainen, A., Jero, J., Arruda, E., Hayden, F. (1998). Detection of rhinovirus, respiratory syncytial virus, and coronavirus infections in acute otitis media by reverse transcriptase polymerase chain reaction. *Pediatrics* 102 (2) 291–302.

Poole, M. (1998). Declining antibiotic effectiveness in otitis media: A convergence of data. *Ear, Nose and Throat Journal* 77(6): 444, 447, 448.

US Department of Health and Human Services (1994). *Quick Reference Guide for Clinicians: Managing Otitis Media with Effusion in Young Children.* (AHCPR Publication No. 94–0623). Silver Spring, MD: US Department of Health and Human Services.

QUESTIONS

65. A 6-year-old girl presents with urinary tract infection (UTI). The most likely causative organism is:

   A. *Klebsiella pneumoniae*
   B. *Proteus mirabilis*
   C. *Escherichia coli*
   D. *Staphylococcus saprophyticus*

66. In caring for the patient in Question 65, your next best action is to prescribe:

   A. TMP-SMX
   B. amoxicillin
   C. ciprofloxacin
   D. metronidazole

67. Which of the following is a reasonable choice of an antibiotic for the treatment of a 7-year-old girl with a UTI and sulfa allergy?

   A. azithromycin
   B. ciprofloxacin
   C. TMP-SMX
   D. cefixime

68. The most likely diagnosis in the presence of a urinalysis revealing positive nitrite and leukocyte esterase is:

   A. purulent vulvitis
   B. gram-negative UTI
   C. cystitis caused by *S. saprophyticus*
   D. urethral syndrome

69. The notation of alkaline urine in a child with UTI may point to infection caused by:

   A. *Klebsiella* spp.
   B. *P. mirabilis*
   C. *E. coli*
   D. *S. saprophyticus*

70. Which of the following is most accurate information when caring for a 3-month-old boy with a UTI?

    A. This is a common condition.
    B. Systemic manifestation of this illness is rare.
    C. A structural abnormality of the urinary tract should be suspected.
    D. Pyuria is rarely found.

71. A 2-year-old boy is completing a course of antibiotic therapy for UTI and is doing well. Which of the following is the best advice to give his parents on his follow-up care?

    A. Return to the office if he develops a rash.
    B. He should continue on antimicrobial prophylaxis while awaiting the results of urologic evaluation.
    C. UTIs are common in toddlers who are still in diapers.
    D. Although serious, a childhood UTI rarely causes future urologic problems.

ANSWERS

65. C
66. A
67. D
68. B
69. B
70. C
71. B

DISCUSSION

Urinary tract infection, defined as the presence of bacteria in the urine with symptoms, is found in approximately 5 percent girls and 1–2 percent of boys during childhood. Before the first birthday, UTI is more common in boys; however, during the rest of childhood, frequency in girls outnumbers boys. One of the most potent risk factors for UTI in infant males is having an intact foreskin. Sequelae to UTI in childhood, whether accompanied by renal reflux or not, include postinfectious nephropathy and renal scarring. Hypertension and renal insufficiency may be sequelae of renal scarring.

The diagnosis of UTI in a younger child requires a high index of suspicion, as findings are often nonfocal and resemble many other common childhood episodic illnesses such as viral syndrome. However, if fever (> 102.2° F) without focal cause persists beyond 2 days, a urinalysis should be considered. A suprapubic tap or catheterized specimen should be obtained in infants, but a catheterized specimen is the preferred method of collection in toddlers. A midstream catch is acceptable in older children.

As with adults, UTIs in children can involve mucosal tissue (cystitis) or soft tissue (pyelonephritis). Most community-acquired infections are caused by enteric gram-negative rods from the *Enterobacteriaceae* group such as *E. coli* and *P. mirabilis*, as well as the less commonly encountered *K. pneumoniae*. These organisms are capable of reducing dietary nitrates to nitrites. This, coupled with the inflammatory changes seen in UTI, leads to the typical urinalysis dipstick's revealing the presence of leukocyte esterase, nitrites, and small amounts of protein. In children with UTIs caused by *P. mirabilis*, the urine is typically alkaline.

Acute, uncomplicated cystitis typically presents in an otherwise healthy older girl who complains of dysuria and frequency but does not have fever and constitutional symptoms. The physical examination may reveal suprapubic tenderness but also may not. The infection is limited to the bladder. Cystitis is usually easily eradicated with 3 to 7 days of antibiotic therapy with TMP-SMX. Alternatives include cephalexin and amoxicillin, but the clinician should realize there is a risk of treatment failure with *E. coli*. The fluoroquinolones are not currently labeled for use in children younger than age 18 years. Third-generation cephalosporins such as cefixime as well as amoxicillin with clavulanate offer reasonable alternatives if TMP-SMX use is not possible.

After the diagnosis of UTI, preadolescence girls and all boys with UTI should be considered for urologic evaluation. This evaluation should be initiated after the infection is clinically resolved and should be focused on ruling out structural abnormalities of the urinary tract, including urethral reflux and obstructive abnormalities. Voiding cystourethrography and renal ultrasound are reasonable first-line studies. In children younger than age 5 years, UTI antimicrobial prophylaxis should be continued while awaiting evaluation for reflux.

Discussion Sources

Hill, N., & Sullivan, L. (1999). *Management Guidelines for Pediatric Nurse Practitioners.* Philadelphia: FA Davis, Pp. 243–236.

Lum, G. (1999). Kidney and urinary tract. In Hay, W., Groothuis, J., Hayward, A., & Levin, M. *Current Pediatric Diagnosis and Treatment* (12th ed.). Stamford, CT: Appleton & Lange, Pp. 599–621.

QUESTIONS

72. You examine a 10-year-old boy with strep pharyngitis. His mother asks if he can get a "shot of penicillin." You consider the following when counseling her about the use of IM penicillin:

    A. There is nearly a 100 percent cure rate in strep pharyngitis when IM penicillin is used.
    B. Treatment failure rates with IM penicillin approach 20 percent.
    C. The risk of severe allergic reaction with IM products is similar to that of oral preparations.
    D. Injectable penicillin has a superior spectrum of antimicrobial coverage compared with the oral version of the drug.

73. You examine a 15-year-old child presenting with a 1-day history of sore throat, low-grade fever, maculopapular rash, and cervical and occipital lymphadenopathy. The most likely diagnosis is:

    A. scarlet fever
    B. roseola
    C. rubella
    D. rubeola

74. A 4-year-old child presents with fever, exudative pharyngitis, anterior cervical lymphadenopathy, and a fine, raised, pink rash. The most likely diagnosis is:

    A. scarlet fever
    B. roseola
    C. rubella
    D. rubeola

75. An 18-year-old woman has a chief complaint of a "sore throat and swollen glands" for the past 3 days. Her physical examination reveals exudative pharyngitis, minimally tender anterior and posterior cervical lymphadenopathy, and maculopapular rash. Abdominal examination reveals right and left upper quadrant abdominal tenderness. The most likely diagnosis is:

    A. group A beta-hemolytic strep pharyngitis
    B. infectious mononucleosis
    C. rubella
    D. scarlet fever

76. Which of the following is most likely to be found in the laboratory data of a person who has infectious mononucleosis?

    A. neutrophilia
    B. lymphocytosis with atypical lymphocytes
    C. positive antinuclear antibody
    D. macrocytic anemia

77. You examine 15-year-old boy who has infectious mononucleosis with marked tonsillar hypertrophy, exudative pharyngitis, difficulty swallowing, and a patent airway. You prescribe the following:

    A. amoxicillin
    B. prednisone
    C. ibuprofen
    D. acyclovir

78. A 2-year-old infant presents with a pustular, ulcerating lesion on the hands and feet as well as oral ulcers. The child is cranky, well hydrated, and afebrile. The most likely diagnosis is:

    A. hand-foot-and-mouth disease
    B. aphthous stomatitis
    C. herpetic gingivostomatitis
    D. Vincent's angina

79. A 6-year-old child presents with a 1-day history of fiery red, maculopapular facial rash concentrated on the cheeks. He has had mild headache and myalgia for the past week. The most likely diagnosis is:

    A. erythema infectiosum
    B. roseola
    C. rubella
    D. scarlet fever

ANSWERS

72. **B**
73. **C**
74. **A**
75. **B**
76. **B**
77. **B**
78. **A**
79. **A**

DISCUSSION

Developing an accurate diagnosis of an acute febrile illness with associated rash or skin lesion can be a daunting task. Knowledge of the infectious agent, its incubation period, mode of transmission, and common clinical presentation can be helpful (Table 14–6).

Discussion Source

Levin, M. Infections: Viral and rickettsial. (1999). In Hay, W., Groothuis, J., Hayward, A., & Levin, M. *Current Pediatric Diagnosis and Treatment* (12th ed.). Stamford, CT: Appleton & Lange, Pp. 960–994.

QUESTIONS

80. At which of the following ages in an infant's life is parental anticipatory guidance about teething most helpful?

    A. 2 months
    B. 4 months
    C. 6 months
    D. 8 months

81. At which of the following ages in a young child's life is parental anticipatory guidance about temper tantrums most helpful?

    A. 10 months
    B. 12 months
    C. 14 months
    D. 16 months

TABLE 14–6.
DIFFERENTIAL DIAGNOSIS OF COMMON RASH-PRODUCING FEBRILE ILLNESSES IN CHILDREN

Clinical Condition with Causative Agent	Presentation	Comments
Roseola infantum or exanthem subitum Agent: Human herpesvirus 6 (HHV-6)	Discrete rosy-pink macular or maculopapular rash lasting hours to 3 days that follows a 3- to 7-day period of fever	About 90% seen in children < 2 years Fever is often quite high Febrile seizures in 10% of children affected Supportive treatment needed
Erythema infectiosum (fifth disease) Agent: Human parvovirus B 19	3–4 days of mild flulike illness followed by 7–10 days of red rash that begins on face with "slapped cheek" appearance and spreads to trunk and extremities Rash onset corresponds with disease immunity of patient Viremic and contagious before but not after onset of rash	Droplet transmission Leukopenia may be noted Risk of hydrops fetalis when contracted by women during pregnancy Supportive treatment needed
Infectious mononucleosis (IM) Agent: Epstein-Barr viruses (human herpesvirus 4)	Rash: Macopapular rash in ~20%, rare petechial rash Fever, "shaggy" purple-white exudative pharyngitis, malaise, marked diffuse lymphadenopathy, hepatic and splenic tenderness and occasional enlargement Diagnostic testing: Heterophil antibody test (Monospot). Leukopenia with lymphocytosis with atypical lymphocytes	Incubation period 20–50 days > 90% will develop a rash if given amoxicillin or ampicillin during IM Potential for respiratory distress when enlarged tonsils and lymphoid tissue impinges on the upper airway; steroids may be used to relieve airway obstruction Avoid contact sports for at least 1 month because of risk of splenic rupture; otherwise, treatment is supportive

(continued)

TABLE 14–6. (continued)

Clinical Condition with Causative Agent	Presentation	Comments
Acute HIV infection Agent: Human immunodeficiency virus (HIV)	Macopapular rash, fever, mild pharyngitis, ulcerating oral lesions, diarrhea, diffuse lymphadenopathy	Most likely to occur in response to infection with large viral load Consult with HIV specialist concerning initiation of antiretroviral therapy
Scarlet fever Agent: Strep pyogenes (group A beta hemolytic streptococci)	Scarletina form, sandpaper-like rash occasionally present Severe sore throat usually with exudate Fever, headache, tender, localized anterior cervical lymphadenopathy Occasional presentation with mild sore throat and rash	When strep pharyngitis presentation includes rash, usually called scarlet fever Rate of long-term complication or seriousness of illness same as when rash is absent Rash may peel Hoarseness, cough, nasal discharge rarely associated with condition and suggest viral pharyngitis Treatment with oral penicillin; IM penicillin offers only advantage of enhanced compliance but not greater eradication rate than that of oral therapy
Rubella Agent: Rubella virus	Mild symptoms: fever, sore throat, malaise, nasal discharge Diffuse maculopapular rash lasting about 3 days Posterior cervical and postauricular lymphadenopathy 5–10 days before onset of rash Arthralgia in about 25% (most common in women)	Incubation period about 14–21 days with disease transmissible for ~1 week before onset of rash to ~2 weeks after rash appears Generally a mild, self-limiting illness Greatest risk is effect of virus on the unborn child, especially with first trimester exposure (~80% rate congenital rubella syndrome) Prevent with immunization

(continued)

TABLE 14–6. (continued)

Clinical Condition with Causative Agent	Presentation	Comments
Measles Agent: Rubeola virus	Usually acute presentation with fever, nasal discharge, cough, generalized lymphadenopathy, conjunctivitis (copious clear discharge), photophobia, Koplik spots (appear ~2 days before onset of rash as nearly pinpoint white lesions on mucous membranes, conjunctival folds) Pharyngitis is usually mild without exudate Macopapular rash onset 3–4 days after onset of symptoms, may coalesce to generalized erythema	Incubation period about 10–14 days with disease transmissible for ~1 week before onset of rash to ~2–3 weeks after rash appears CNS and respiratory tract complications common Prevent with immunization Supportive treatment as well as intervention for complications needed
Hand-foot-and-mouth disease Agent: Coxsackie virus A16	Prodrome of fever, malaise, sore mouth anorexia 1–2 days later, lesions Also can cause conjunctivitis, pharyngitis Duration of disease: 2–7 days Supportive treatment needed	Transmission via oral-fecal route or droplet Highly contagious with incubation periods of 2–6 weeks Supportive treatment needed

Reference: Hill, N., & Sullivan, L. (1999). *Management Guidelines for Pediatric Nurse Practitioners*. Philadelphia: FA Davis,. Pp. 468–470.

82. At which of the following ages in a young child's life is parental anticipatory guidance about using "time out" as a discipline method most helpful?

    A. 18 months
    B. 24 months
    C. 30 months
    D. 36 months

83. At which of the following ages in a young child's life is parental anticipatory guidance about electrical outlet safety most helpful?

    A. 4 months
    B. 6 months
    C. 8 months
    D. 10 months

84. At which of the following ages in a young child's life is parental anticipatory guidance about toilet readiness training most helpful?

    A. 12 months
    B. 15 months
    C. 18 months
    D. 24 months

85. At which of the following ages in a young child's life is parental anticipatory guidance about infant sleep position most helpful?

    A. birth
    B. 2 weeks
    C. 2 months
    D. 4 months

ANSWERS

80. C
81. B
82. B
83. C
84. C
85. A

DISCUSSION

Providing health advice to the growing family is a critical part of an NP's role. During anticipatory guidance counseling, an NP should review the normal developmental landmarks the child is expected to reach in the near future coupled with advice about how parents can cope with, adapt to, and avoid problems with these changes. This guidance is tailored to meet the needs of the family but typically follows a developmental framework.

Discussion Source

Brayden, R., & Headley, R. (1999). Ambulatory pediatrics. In Hay, W., Groothuis, J., Hayward, A., & Levin, M. *Current Pediatric Diagnosis and Treatment* (12th ed.). Stamford, CT: Appleton & Lange, Pp. 201–218.

QUESTIONS

86. Which of the following advice should you give to a breastfeeding mother whose infant has gastroenteritis?

    A. Discontinue breastfeeding.
    B. Give the infant oral rehydration solution.
    C. Continue breastfeeding.
    D. Supplement with flat ginger ale.

87. Which of the following is the advice you should give to the parents of a toddler with gastroenteritis?

    A. Try sips of cola.
    B. Give the child sips of an oral rehydration solution.
    C. Give the child sips of Gatorade.
    D. Try sips of water.

88. The onset of symptoms in food poisoning caused by *Staphylococcus* spp. is typically how many hours after the ingestion of the offending substance?

    A. 0.5 to 1
    B. 1 to 4
    C. 4 to 8
    D. 8 to 12

89. The onset of symptoms in food poisoning caused by *Salmonella* spp. is typically how many hours after the ingestion of the offending substance?

    A. 2 to 8
    B. 8 to 12
    C. 12 to more than 24
    D. 24 to 36

90. In order to obtain the most accurate hydration status in a child with acute gastroenteritis, an NP should ask about:

    A. the time of last urination
    B. thirst
    C. quantity of liquids taken
    D. number of episodes of vomiting and diarrhea

91. What percent of body weight is typically lost in a child with moderate dehydration?

    A. 2 to 3
    B. 3 to 5
    C. 6 to 10
    D. 11 to 15

92. Clinical features of shigellosis include all of the following except:

    A. bloody diarrhea
    B. high fever
    C. malaise
    D. vomiting

ANSWERS

86. C
87. B
88. B
89. C
90. A
91. C
92. D

DISCUSSION

Acute gastroenteritis is a common episodic disease of childhood. Usually viral in nature, the child presents with vomiting and diarrhea of short duration that typically are free of blood and pus. In addition the child usually does not have a fever. Usually there is a history of contacts with children who have similar symptoms. The duration of illness is usually short (less than 4 days with no sequelae). One of the most important parts of the assessment of a child with acute gastroenteritis is determining hydration status. Asking about last urination provides a helpful way of evaluating this. If the child has voided within the previous few hours, the degree of dehydration is minimal. A number of other clinical parameters are helpful in assessing for dehydration (Table 14–7). Although mild

TABLE 14–7.
CLINICAL PRESENTATION OF PATIENTS WITH DEHYDRATION

Clinical Presentation	Mild Dehydration	Moderate Dehydration	Severe Dehydration
Decrease in body weight, %	3–5	6–10	11–15
Skin turgor	Normal	Slightly to moderately decreased	Markedly decreased with tenting possible
Capillary refill	2–3 seconds	3–5 seconds	> 5 seconds
Tears	Normal to slightly decreased	Slightly decreased	Markedly decreased to absent
Pulse	Normal	Normal	Tachycardia
Blood pressure	Normal	Normal	Low
Mucous membranes	Dry	Dry	Parched
Urine output	Mildly decreased	Decreased	Anuria

Reference: Ford, D. (1999). Fluid, electrolyte and acid-base therapy. In Hay, W., Hayward, A., Levin, M., & Sondheimer, J. *Current Pediatric Diagnosis and Treatment* (14th ed.) Stamford, CT: Appleton & Lange.

dehydration can usually be managed with frequent small-volume feedings of oral rehydration solutions such as Pedialyte, a child with moderate to severe dehydration likely needs parenteral fluids. Sports drinks such as Gatorade and soda are not appropriate for rehydration solution. The use of antidiarrheal agents is usually discouraged because of the risk of increasing the severity of illness if a toxin-producing bacteria is the causative agent.

Warning signs during acute gastroenteritis include fever coupled with bloody or pus-filled stools. If these are present, consider a bacterial source of infection such as shigellosis. Stool culture should be obtained and appropriate antimicrobial therapy initiated.

Improperly handled food is a common source of gastrointestinal infection. Knowledge of the timing of the onset of symptoms is helpful when attempting to discern the offending organism. Most food poisoning episodes are short and self-limiting, resolving over a few hours to days without special intervention.

Discussion Sources

Ford, D. (1999). Fluid, electrolyte and acid-base therapy. In Hay, W., Groothuis, J., Hayward, A., & Levin, M. *Current Pediatric Diagnosis and Treatment* (12th ed.). Stamford, CT: Appleton & Lange, Pp. 1108–1117.

Hill, N., & Sullivan, L. (1999). *Management Guidelines for Pediatric Nurse Practitioners.* Philadelphia: FA Davis, Pp. 215–218.

QUESTIONS

93. The most common reason for precocious puberty in girls is:

    A. ovarian tumor

    B. adrenal tumor

    C. exogenous estrogen

    D. early onset of normal puberty

94. The most common reason for precocious puberty in boys is:

    A. testicular tumor

    B. a number of relatively uncommon health problems

    C. exogenous testosterone

    D. early onset of normal puberty

ANSWERS

93. D
94. B

DISCUSSION

Precocious puberty in girls has long been defined as the onset of secondary sexual characteristics before the eighth birthday. More recent study reveals that there may be a group of girls who have the onset of slowly developing secondary sexual characteristics between ages 6 and 8 years as a benign variant. As a result, the most common reason for precocious puberty in girls is early onset of normal puberty. However, a subset of girls, particularly those with pubertal changes noted before the sixth birthday, often have significant health problems such as ovarian or adrenal tumors. Expert evaluation and referral are indicated. Evaluation typically includes obtaining bone age, levels of follicle-stimulating hormone and luteinizing hormone, and abdominal ultrasound. Treatment depends on the cause. In the absence of an adrenal or ovarian tumor, counseling about the nature of the process of early puberty should be discussed with the child and family. Because girls typically achieve nearly all of their adult height 1 year after the first menstrual period, a girl achieving menarche at a premature age may have short stature. If the child and family wish to attempt to halt the onset of puberty, a gonadotropin-releasing hormone analog may be given by injection to counteract the effects of endogenous hormones. The long-term effect of this therapy on fertility is not known.

Premature thelarche is a relatively common, benign process in which breast enlargement is noted in female toddlers. Present unilaterally or bilaterally, there are no other signs of puberty, including accelerated linear growth. Reassurance and ongoing monitoring is the typical course of treatment. In premature adrenarche, a parent usually reports that the child between ages 5 and 6 years has body odor, pubic hair, and, rarely, axillary hair. There are no other signs of puberty, including accelerated linear growth. Reassurance and ongoing monitoring is the typical course of treatment.

Precocious puberty in boys is defined as the onset of secondary sexual characteristics before the ninth birthday. Overall, this condition is less common in boys than girls and is less likely to be a benign normal variation. Gonadal and adrenal tumors as well as a number of genetically based diseases are the most likely causes. Prompt referral to expert care is indicated.

Discussion Source

Gotlin, R., Kappy, M., Slover, R. & Zeiter, P. (1999). Endocrine disorders. In Hay, W., Groothuis, J., Hayward, A., & Levin, M. *Current Pediatric Diagnosis and Treatment* (12th ed.). Stamford, CT: Appleton & Lange, Pp. 812–850.

QUESTIONS

95. An innocent murmur has which of the following characteristics?

    A. occurs late in systole
    B. has a localized area of auscultation
    C. is softer when the patient moves from supine to standing position
    D. frequently obliterates the S₂ heart sound

96. The murmur of atrial septal defect is usually:

    A. found in children with symptoms of cardiac disease
    B. first found on a 2- to 6-month well-child examination
    C. found with mitral valve prolapse
    D. presystolic in timing

97. A Still's murmur:

    A. is seen in the presence of cardiac pathology
    B. has a humming, vibratory quality
    C. is a reason for denying sports participation clearance
    D. has the ability to become louder then the patient is standing

ANSWERS

95. C
96. B
97. B

DISCUSSION

The ability to appropriately assess children with a heart murmur is an important part of the role of an NP. Knowledge of the most common murmurs, their clinical presentation, and their impact on a child's health are critical to appropriate assessment. It is also necessary to be able to determine the need for specialty referral (Table 14–8).

TABLE 14–8.
DIFFERENTIAL DIAGNOSIS OF COMMON HEART MURMURS IN CHILDREN

When evaluating a child with cardiac murmur:
- Ask about the major symptoms of heart disease: chest pain, congestive heart failure symptoms, palpitations, syncope, activity intolerance, and poor growth and development
- The bell of the stethoscope is most helpful for auscultating lower-pitched sounds, and the diaphragm is better for those with higher pitch.
- Systolic murmurs are graded on a 1 to 6 scale, from barely audible to audible with stethoscope off the chest. Diastolic murmurs are usually graded on the same scale but abbreviated to grades 1 to 4 because these murmurs will not be loud enough to reach grades 5 and 6.
- A critical part of the evaluation of a child with a heart murmur is the decision to offer antimicrobial prophylaxis. No prophylaxis is needed with benign murmurs. Please refer to the American Heart Associations Guidelines for the latest in advice.

Murmur	Important Cardiac Examination Findings	Additional Findings	Comments
Newborn	Gr 1–2/6 early systolic, vibratory, heard best at LLSB with little radiation. Pulses intact, otherwise well neonate	Subsides or disappears when pressure applied to abdomen	Heard in first few days of life; disappears in 2–3 weeks. Benign condition
Still's (vibratory innocent murmur)	Gr 1–3/6 early systolic ejection, musical or vibratory, short, often buzzing, heard best midway between apex and LLSB	Softens or disappears when sitting, standing, or with Valsalva maneuver. Louder when supine or with fever or tachycardia	Usual onset age 2–6 years; may persist through adolescence. Benign condition

(continued)

TABLE 14–8. (continued)

Murmur	Important Cardiac Examination Findings	Additional Findings	Comments
Hemic	Gr 1–2/6 systolic ejection, high-pitched, heard best in pulmonic and aortic areas	Heard only in the presence of increased cardiac output, such as fever, anemia, stress	Disappears when underlying condition resolves Usually seen without cardiac disease Most often heard in children and younger adults with thin chest walls
Venous hum	Gr 1–2/6 continuous musical hum heard best at the URSB and ULSB and the lower neck	Disappears in supine position, when jugular vein is compressed Common after age 3 years	Believed to be produced by turbulence in the subclavian and jugular veins Benign condition
Pulmonary outflow ejection murmur	Gr 1–2/6 soft, short, systolic ejection murmur, heard best at LLSB, usually localized	Softens or disappears when sitting, standing, or with Valsalva maneuver Louder when supine	Heard throughout childhood Benign condition but has qualities similar to murmurs caused by pathologic condition such as ASD, COA, PS

(continued)

TABLE 14–8. (continued)

Murmur	Important Cardiac Examination Findings	Additional Findings	Comments
Patent ductus arteriosus	Gr 2–4/6 continuous murmur heard best at ULSB and left infraclavicular area	In premature newborns, seen with active precordium. In older children, with full pulses	Normal ductus closure occurs by day 4 of life Often isolated finding but may be seen with COA, VSD Accounts for +/−12% of all congenital heart disease Twice as common in females In preterm infants < 1500 g, rate as high as 20-60%
Atrial septal defect	Gr 1-3/6 systolic ejection murmur heard best at the ULSB with widely spilt fixed S_2	Accompanying mid-diastolic murmur heard at the fourth ICS LSB common caused by increased flow across tricuspid valve	Two times as common in females Child may be entirely well or present with CHF Often missed in the first few months of life or even entire childhood Watch for children with easy fatigability Cyanosis rare

(continued)

TABLE 14–8. (continued)

Murmur	Important Cardiac Examination Findings	Additional Findings	Comments
Ventricular septal defect	Gr 2–5/6 regurgitant systolic murmur heard best at LLSB Occasionally holosystolic, usually localized	Thrill may be present as well as a loud P_2 with large left-to-right shunt	Usually without cyanosis Children with small- to moderate-sized left-to-right shunt without pulmonary hypertension likely to have minimal symptoms Larger shunts may result in CHF with onset in infancy
Aortic stenosis	Gr 2–5/6 systolic ejection murmur heard best in ULSB or a second RICS, possibly with paradoxically split S_2	Ejection click at apex, third LICS, second RICS Radiation or thrill to the carotid arteries	More common in males than females In children, usually caused by unicuspid (if noted in infancy) or bicuspid (if noted in childhood) valve Mild exercise intolerance common
Coarctation of the aorta (COA)	Gr 1–5/6 systolic ejection murmur heard best at the ULSB and left interscapular area (on back)	Weak or absent femoral pulses, hypertension in arms	Often seen with AS, MR Presence of dorsalis pedis pulse in child essentially rules out this condition

(continued)

TABLE 14–8. (continued)

Murmur	Important Cardiac Examination Findings	Additional Findings	Comments
Mitral valve prolapse	Gr 1–3/6 midsystolic click followed by a late systolic murmur heard best at the apex	Murmur heard earlier in systole and often louder with standing or squatting	Often with pectus excavatum, straight back (> 85%)
Pulmonic valve stenosis	Gr 2–5/6 heard best at ULSB, ejection click at second LICS	Radiates to the back S2 may be widely split	No symptoms with mild to moderate disease Usually a fusion of valvular cusps

References: Park, M. (1996). *Pediatric Cardiology for Practitioners.* St. Louis: Mosby-Yearbook.
Wolfe, R., Bouchek, M., Schaeffer, M., & Wiggins, J. (1995). Cardiovascular disease. In Hay. W. Groothuis, J., Hayward, A., & Levin, M. *Current Pediatric Diagnosis and Treatment* (12th ed.), Pp. 544–607.

Discussion Sources

Park, M. (1996). *Pediatric Cardiology for Practitioners.* St. Louis: Mosby-Yearbook.
Wolfe, R., Bouchek, M., Schaeffer, M., & Wiggins, J. (1995). Cardiovascular disease. In Hay, W., Groothuis, J., Hayward, A., & Levin, M. *Current Pediatric Diagnosis and Treatment* (12th ed.). Stamford, CT: Appleton & Lange, Pp. 544–607.

Index

Pages followed by t indicate tables; pages bold type indicate boxes; pages italics indicate figures